Hiatt · Phillips · Morgenstern (Eds.) Surgical Diseases of the Spleen

Springer
Berlin
Heidelberg
New York
Barcelona
Budapest
Hong Kong
London
Milan
Paris
Santa Clara
Singapore
Tokyo

J. R. Hiatt E. H. Phillips L. Morgenstern (Eds.)

Surgical Diseases of the Spleen

Contributors

A. Allins W. Arnaout R. W. Busuttil R. A. Duensing
R. Friedman F. J. Giles J. R. Hiatt F. Hulka
M. S. Komaiko L. R. Kong J. E. Korman S. W. Lim
L. Morgenstern R. J. Mullins R. S. Neiman
E. H. Phillips S. I. Schwartz J. E. Skandalakis
R. E. Stiehm D. D. Trunkey M. Wakim W. A. Wilcox
R. A. Williams

With 113 Figures, many in Color, and 24 Tables

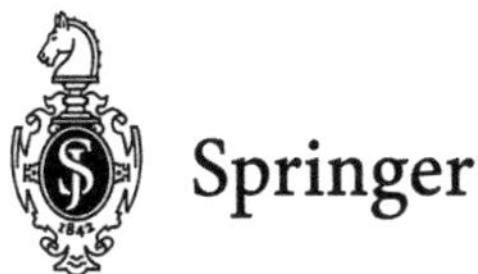

Springer

Jonathan R. Hiatt, M.D.
Director, Surgical Residency Program
and Trauma Services
Cedars-Sinai Medical Center
8700 Beverly Boulevard
Los Angeles, CA 90048-1865, USA

Edward H. Phillips, M.D.
Director, Endoscopic Surgery
Cedars-Sinai Medical Center
8700 Beverly Boulevard
Los Angeles, CA 90048-1865, USA

Leon Morgenstern, M.D.
Emeritus Director of Surgery
Cedars-Sinai Medical Center
444 South San Vincente Boulevard
Los Angeles, CA 90048, USA

ISBN-13: 978-3-642-64461-0   e-ISBN-13: 978-3-642-60574-1
DOI:10.1007/ 978-3-642-60574-1

Library of Congress Cataloging-in-Publication Data
Surgical diseases of the spleen/J.R. Hiatt, E.H. Phillips, L. Morgenstern (eds.) p.cm. Includes bibliographical references and index. 1. Splenectomy. 2. Spleen – Diseases. I. Hiatt, J.R. (Jonathan R.), 1951. II. Phillips, Edward H., 1947. III. Morgenstern, Leon. [DNLM: 1. Splenic Diseases – surgery. 2. Splenectomy – methods. 3. Spleen – pathology. WH 600 S9613 1997] RD547.5.S87 1997 617.5′51059–dc20 DNLM/DLC for Library of Congress

© Springer-Verlag Berlin Heidelberg 1997

Softcover reprint of the hardcover 1st edition 1997

Production: PRO EDIT GmbH, D-69126 Heidelberg
Illustrations: T.C. Hengst, Thousand Oaks, CA, USA
Typesetting: K+V Fotosatz GmbH, D-64743 Beerfelden

SPIN 10515104 24/3135-5 4 3 2 1 0 – Printed on acid-free paper

To Jo Carol, Joseph and Jeremy

JONATHAN R. HIATT

*With gratitude – To my father, the consumate physician
who taught by example*
*To my teachers, colleagues, and most of all, patients,
who truly educated me*
To my wife and children for their loving support and daily surprises

EDWARD H. PHILLIPS

To Laurie and David

LEON MORGENSTERN

*The editors express deep gratitude to Peggy Acoca
for expert clerical assistance*

Preface

Among all of the organs in the surgeon's workaday world, the spleen has been something of an orphan for the better part of this century. Hidden deep within a recess of the left upper quadrant – more rarely subject to diseases than other solid viscera and by far the most fragile of the organs – the spleen eluded prominence and singularly defied progress in surgical innovation and research. Its emergence from orphanage into the realm of modern surgical practice represents the subject and the rationale for this book. The century closes with a vastly different view of the spleen than the one with which it began.

What was it that brought the spleen out of its figurative hiding place into the more prominent position it holds today? First, it was the discovery of the causal association of specific hematologic disorders with the spleen, such as proposed by Micheli in 1911 for autoimmune hemolytic anemia and Kaznelson in 1916 for idiopathic thrombocytopenic purpura. Splenectomy for these disorders was shown to be highly effective, if not curative. Also, the parallel development of hematology and pathology gave rise to an ever-expanding and increasingly sophisticated list of disorders related to splenic anomalies, dysfunction, infections, and tumors. "Leukocythemia," at the turn of the century the generic neoplastic disorder, evolved into a complex classification of lymphomas and leukemias. The list continues to grow and change. For all of these disorders, as Crosby has commented, "Splenectomy goes in and out of fashion." The staging of Hodgkin's disease, for example, which in some centers was a leading indication for splenectomy in the 1970s and 1980s, has fallen out of favor; so has splenectomy as a primary approach for hairy cell leukemia and thrombotic thrombocytopenic purpura. Splenectomy for Gaucher's disease has yielded to treatment with enzyme replacement therapy, although the latter is usually unaffordable by the majority of patients with the disease.

A dramatic change in surgical attitudes toward splenectomy for trauma and some benign splenic disorders began in the early 1960s: with partial splenectomies performed by Campos Christo for trauma and Morgenstern for a hematologic disorder, the myth of the "surgical inviolability" of the spleen was successfully challenged and discredited. It was not, however, until the 1980s that the conservative approach to splenic injuries (with conservation of functioning splenic tissue as a primary goal) achieved prominence in trauma centers worldwide. Validating the shift toward splenic salvage for trauma, rather than wholesale extirpation of the organ, was a growing body of evidence that the spleen had important immunologic functions. Peculiarly, this validation was recognized widely only after the techniques of splenic conservation were perfected. Evidence continues to accumulate that the spleen has hitherto undiscovered immunologic functions, and new techniques of splenic conservation continue to evolve, including the use of absorbable mesh, more effective methods of hemostasis, and nonoperative management, which is the ultimate technique for conservation.

As the century draws to a close, the most dramatic development in splenic surgery is the successful application of laparoscopic techniques to splenectomy, both total and partial. Laparoscopic splenectomy is rapidly becoming the procedure of choice for idiopathic thrombocytopenic purpura in adults and older children. The laparoscopic approach is less well suited to the splenomegaly of neoplastic or hematologic diseases, but the barriers there are also falling quickly, as techniques, instrumentation, and surgical skills continue to improve.

It would be a blatant omission to neglect the important role that various imaging modalities have assumed in the diagnosis and, occasionally, the treatment of splenic diseases. The supersedance of the physical examination by imaging studies is often alluded to jokingly, but the truth is that the spleen is very photogenic. Radionuclide studies, ultrasonography, computed tomography, and magnetic resonance imaging have all made diagnosis more precise, treatment more timely, and followup more meaningful. The new and constantly improving imaging techniques have been a great boon to splenic surgery.

There is little doubt that some diseases for which splenectomy is currently indicated will be treated by alternative methods, as has happened with hairy cell leukemia and Gaucher's disease. The converse phenomenon – new diseases which create new indications for splenectomy – is also real: Witness the broad new spectrum of splenic disorders, inflammatory and neoplastic, secondary to the human immunodeficiency virus. Also, the spleen may serve as a home for genetically altered hepatocytes or other cell lines, and the ultimate role for the organ in transplant surgery has yet to be explored.

This volume undertakes to present what we believe is the latest and best information on the surgery of the spleen. In medical history, the spleen is a treasure trove of fact, fable, and fantasy. It took its early place in medicine as the source of black bile, one of the four cardinal humors. The relation of black bile to the emotion of melancholy even found its way into the literature of the nineteenth century in the works of the poets Baudelaire and Verlaine. To the spleen were also assigned the sometimes contradictory attributes of anger, laughter, scorn, and, in Elizabethan times, even a reproductive function. At present, the major functions of this mysterious organ are hematologic and immunologic. What the future holds in store for the spleen in terms of functions as yet undiscovered and techniques as yet untried can only be imagined and reserved for future editions of the present volume.

LEON MORGENSTERN
JONATHAN R. HIATT
EDWARD H. PHILLIPS

Los Angeles, California, 1996

Contents

Section I: Basic Concepts

A History of Splenectomy 3
L. Morgenstern

Anatomy and Embryology of the Spleen 15
L. Morgenstern and J.E. Skandalakis

Pathology of the Spleen 25
R.S. Neiman

The Spleen in Infection and Immunity 53
R.E. Stiehm and Mary Wakim

Spleen Imaging 61
M.S. Komaiko

Section II: Splenic Diseases

Benign Neoplasms of the Spleen 91
L. Morgenstern

Malignant Splenic Lesions 105
F.J. Giles and S.W. Lim

Splenectomy for Hematologic Disorders 131
S.I. Schwartz

Infections of the Spleen 143
R.A. Williams and R.A. Duensing

Metabolic Disorders and the Spleen 161
W.A. Wilcox

Portal Hypertension and Disorders of the Splenic Circulation ... 175
R.W. Busuttil and W. Arnaout

Section III: Splenic Surgery

Open Splenectomy 197
J. R. HIATT, A. ALLINS, and L. R. KONG

Laparoscopic Splenectomy 211
E. H. PHILLIPS, J. E. KORMAN, and R. FRIEDMAN

Splenic Trauma 233
D. D. TRUNKEY, FRIEDA HULKA, and R. J. MULLINS

Partial Splenectomy 263
L. MORGENSTERN

Subject Index 281

List of Contributors

ALLINS, A.
Department of Surgery, Cedars-Sinai Medical Center,
8700 Beverly Boulevard, Los Angeles, CA 90048, USA

ARNAOUT, W.
Liver and Pancreas Transplantation, Cedars-Sinai Medical Center,
8635 West Third Street, Suite #590-W, Los Angeles, CA 90048, USA

BUSUTTIL, R. W.
Liver and Pancreas Transplantation, Cedars-Sinai Medical Center,
8635 West Third Street, Suite #590-W, Los Angeles, CA 90048, USA

DUENSING, R. A.
Department of Surgery, UCI Medical Center,
Building 53, Route 81, 101 The City Drive, Orange, CA 92668, USA

FRIEDMAN, R.
Department of Surgery, Cedars-Sinai Medical Center,
8700 Beverly Boulevard, Los Angeles, CA 90048, USA

GILES, F. J.
Hematology/Oncology, Department of Medicine, Cedars-Sinai Medical
Center, 8700 Beverly Boulevard, B-209, Los Angeles, CA 90048, USA

HIATT, J. R.
Cedars-Sinai Medical Center, Department of Surgery, Room 8215,
8700 Beverly Boulevard, Los Angeles, CA 90048-1865, USA

HULKA, FRIEDA
Department of Surgery, Oregon Health Sciences University,
3181 W. San Jackson Park Road, Portland, OR 97201-3098, USA

KOMAIKO, M. S.
Department of Imaging/Radiology, Cedars-Sinai Medical Center,
8700 Beverly Boulevard, Room 5416, Los Angeles, CA 90048, USA

KONG, L. R.
Department of Surgery, Cedars-Sinai Medical Center,
8700 Beverly Boulevard, Los Angeles, CA 90048, USA

KORMAN, J. E.
Department of Surgery, Cedars-Sinai Medical Center,
8700 Beverly Boulevard, Los Angeles, CA 90048, USA

LIM, S. W.
Hematology/Oncology, Department of Medicine, Cedars-Sinai Medical
Center, 8700 Beverly Boulevard, B-209, Los Angeles, CA 90048, USA

MORGENSTERN, L.
Emeritus Director of Surgery, Cedars-Sinai Medical Center, 444 South
San Vincente Boulevard, MGB-602, Los Angeles, CA 90048, USA

MULLINS, R. J.
Professor of Surgery, Oregon Health Sciences University,
3181 W. San Jackson Park Road, Portland, OR 97201-3098, USA

NEIMAN, R. S.
Director, Division of Hematopathology, Professor of Pathology
and Laboratory Medicine, Indiana University School of Medicine,
Riley Hospital for Children 0969, 702 Barnhill Drive, Indianapolis,
IN 46202-5200, USA

PHILLIPS, E. H.
Director, Endoscopic Surgery, Cedars-Sinai Medical Center,
8700 Beverly Boulevard, Suite 8215, Los Angeles, CA 90048-1865, USA

SCHWARTZ, S. I.
Professor and Chair, Department of Surgery, Strong Memorial Hospital
of the University of Rochester, 601 Elmwood Avenue, Rochester,
NY 14642, USA

SKANDALAKIS, J. E.
Centers for Surgical Anatomy & Technique, Emory University School
of Medicine, 1462 Clifton Road NE, Suite 303, Atlanta, GA 30322, USA

STIEHM, R. E.
Professor of Pediatrics, UCLA School of Medicine, 10833 Le Conte
Avenue, Room 22-387 MDCC, Los Angeles, CA 90095, USA

TRUNKEY, D. D.
Professor and Chairman, Department of Surgery, Oregon Health
Sciences University, 3181 SW Sam Jackson Park Road, Portland,
OR 97201-3098, USA

WAKIM, MARY
Department of Pediatrics, UCLA School of Medicine, 10833 Le Conte
Avenue, Room 22-387 MDCC, Los Angeles, CA 90095, USA

WILCOX, W. A.
Director, Skeletal Dysplasia, Cedars-Sinai Medical Center,
8700 Beverly Boulevard, SSB-364, Los Angeles, CA 90048, USA

WILLIAMS, R. A.
Vice Chairman, Department of Surgery, UCI Medical Center, Building 53,
Route 81, Room 207C, 101 The City Drive, Orange, CA 92668, USA

Section I: Basic Concepts

A History of Splenectomy

L. MORGENSTERN

> "... the 10 organs that minister to the soul are: the gullet for the passage of food, the windpipe for voice, the liver for anger, the gall for jealousy, the lungs to absorb liquids, the stomach to grind food, the spleen for laughter, the kidneys to advise, the heart to give understanding, and the tongue to decide."
>
> *The Midrash*

Historically, more functions have been attributed to the spleen than to any other parenchymatous organ. Ancient writings described the spleen as an organ which inhibited the running capacity of horses and men. Talmudic reference is made to the spleen as the seat of laughter. In ancient Greece it was known as the organ which produced black bile, the cardinal humor of melancholy. To this, Galen added the concept of the spleen as a filter. In Shakespeare and other authors, literary allusions abound with the spleen as the seat of conflicting emotions such as joy, anger, spite, whim, malice, impetuosity, among others.

But no organ shares its rich and colorful history of partial or total extirpation. The history of splenectomy has been recorded many times [1–9]. This chapter will summarize the salient features of this history, adding the revolutionary concepts which have taken hold the last half of this century.

Age of Fable

One of the earliest references to splenectomy is found in the monumental *Natural History* of C. Pliny (23–79 A.D.) in this oft-quoted passage [10]:

This member [the spleen] hath a propriete by itself sometimes, to hinder a man's running: whereupon professed runners in the race that be troubled with the splene have a device to burn and waste it with a hot yron. And no marveile: For why? They say that the splene may be taken out of the body by way of incision, and yet the creature live nevertheless: But if it be man or woman that is cut for the splene, he or she looseth their laughter by the means. For sure it is intemperate laughers have always great spleens.

Propagation of this myth can also be found in the apocryphal references in ancient literature to removal of the spleen in marathon runners and in horses to increase their speed. In the First Book of Kings (I Kings 1:5), Adonijah attempted to usurp the throne of King David, preparing chariots and horsemen and fifty men to run before him. The Talmudic interpretation (Tracate Sanhedrin 2.6) of this passage included the remarkable fact that "they all had their spleens removed." The Talmudic scholar Rashi (1040–1105) commented that this was due to a feeling of heaviness imparted by the spleen, the removal of which helped increase running speed.

The giraffe, noted for its speed in running, was erroneously believed to be spleenless. The myth persisted into the middle ages and beyond. The German author Murer wrote: "Ich han mir lon dass milz Schnyden/Dass ich mag laufen wegt und veer." ("I have let them cut my spleen that I may run faster and further").

The allusion to speed (among numerous other functions) can also be found in Shakespeare: "I am scalded with my violent motion/And spleen of speed to see your majesty." (*King John*, 5.7.49)

But strangest of all is the persistence of the myth into the twentieth century. At Johns Hopkins University in 1922, Macht and Finesilver [11] subjected the ancient myth to the experimental method. They tested trained splenectomized and nonsplenectomized mice for running speeds over a cotton rope. The winners? The mice that had been splenectomized!

The Sixteenth Century

Paracelsus (1490–1541) was among the first to reject the humoral theory of disease. He wrote that the spleen was a superfluous organ [rather than the important repository of black bile] "which could create fever, hardening and putrefaction" and therefore should be excised when diseased. In 1549, 8 years following Paracelsus' death, his pupil Fioravanti prevailed upon an "old man Andriano Zaccarello" (Fig. 1) who was skilled with the knife, to operate upon a patient, a Greek woman of 24, who suffered from "very great enlargement of the spleen." The dauntless Zaccarello reportedly cut the good lady's spleen out using nothing but a razor. Within 24 days, the woman was well enough to attend mass. So wondrous a feat was her cure that the excised spleen was exhibited in the town square for the townspeople to see. Was this "first" splenectomy fact or fable? Only Fioravanti's bare account is left for the reader to judge for himself.

Vesalius (1514–1564) is said to have performed splenectomies in animals, with no adverse effects. He was among the first of many physician-anatomists to show that the spleen was not an organ vital to life.

The first of a large group of partial splenectomies for spleens purportedly prolapsed through abdominal wounds was by Viard, who performed this operation on two occasions in 1581. It was the progenitor of a remarkable se-

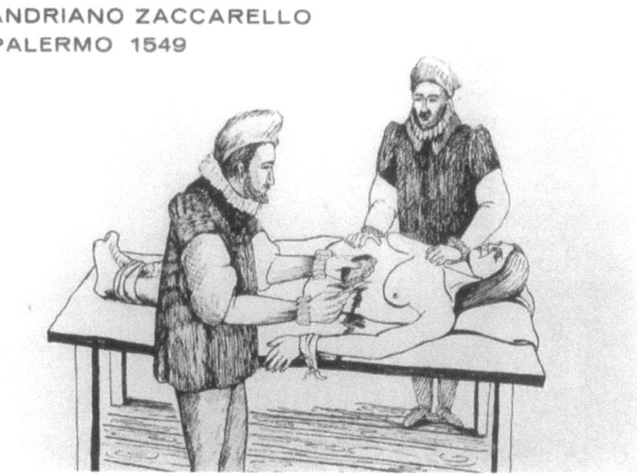

Fig. 1. The first recorded elective splenectomy was performed by Andriano Zaccarello, under less than optimal conditions. Although the patient reportedly survived, the authenticity of this improbable operation is questionable

ries of partial splenectomy for traumatic splenic prolapse, as will be described below.

The Seventeenth Century

Splenectomies in dogs by a number of investigators continued to provide evidence that the spleen was a dispensable organ. Among those early experimental surgeons were Timothy Clark (1663) of England and Zambeccari of Italy (1680). The latter's feat was described during the next century by Giovanni Morgagni, who also described splenectomies in dogs with no threat to their well being.

The nature of abdominal wounds in the centuries preceding our own was obviously quite different. We are more accustomed to injuries due to blunt trauma at high speeds, high velocity missiles and only rarely traumatic lacerations large enough to allow the relatively fixed spleen to prolapse. This was apparently not so in past centuries. In 1676 Timothy Clark, in a remarkably brief case report [12], described the removal of a spleen from a butcher who attempted suicide by plunging his knife into the left upper quadrant. "The man recovered rapidly." In 1684, Daniel Cruger of Germany described an abdominal wound in "a man named Scultetus," gravely wounded on his left side, causing the prolapse of a large portion of the spleen. The prolapsed portion of the spleen was excised by a surgeon from Colberg, Nicolaus Matthias. He was "restored ... to health within the space of 3 weeks"... He lived happily thereafter.

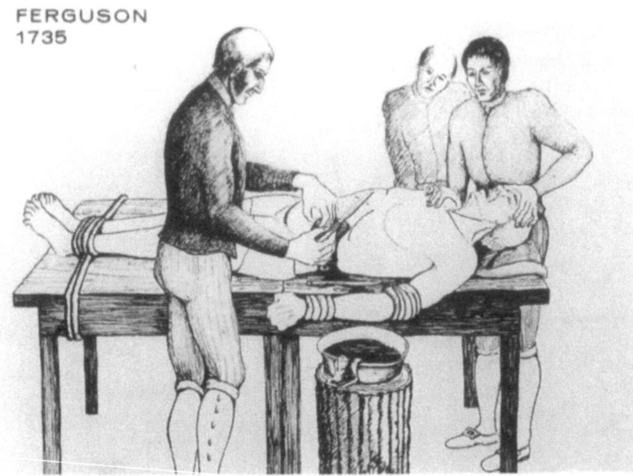

Fig. 2. Ferguson's report appeared in 1738, although his excision of a partially extruded spleen was performed several years earlier. Recovery was remarkably uneventful

The Eighteenth Century

In 1738, John Ferguson of Scotland (Fig. 2) reported the case of Thomas Conway, who received a wound with a Skane or great knife which went into the left hypochondrium. Twenty-four hours after the injury Ferguson found the "spleen out of the wound" and its exposed part "cold, black and mortified ..." Ferguson proceeded to place "a ligature of strong waxed thread above the unsound Part and cut off three ounces and a half of the spleen ... After bathing all of the Parts with warm wine", the spleen was returned to the abdominal cavity, "leaving the Ends of the threads out of the Wound." Conway recovered with "no inconvenience from want of the Part of the spleen which he lost."

There were other partial splenectomies. In 1743, Mr. Wilson, a surgeon in a regiment of British Dragoons, amputated a portion of spleen in a soldier with a penetrating wound in the left upper quadrant. The patient recovered "with no stronger inclination for women than before." In 1797 Dorsch removed over half the spleen in a 35-year-old man who suffered a knife wound between the ribs. The patient survived 23 years. By the close of the eighteenth century partial splenectomies, all occasioned by prolapse of a portion of spleen through a left upper quadrant wound, outnumbered total splenectomies by a wide margin.

The Nineteenth Century

The first authenticated case of splenectomy for disease was performed by Quittenbaum of Rostock, Germany (Fig. 3), in 1826. It was the first of a se-

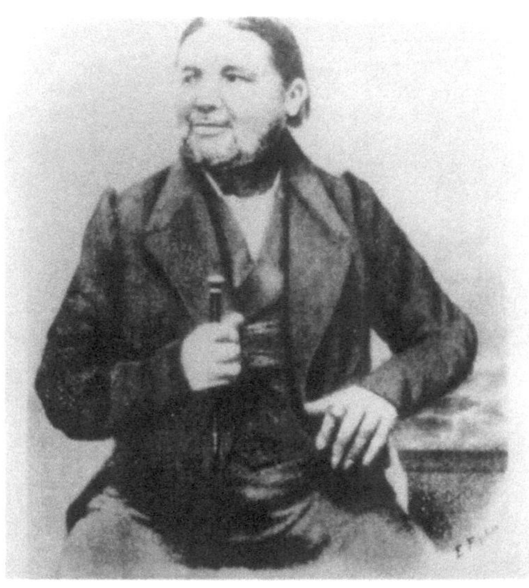

Fig. 3. Carl Freiderich Quittenbaum (1793–1852) is given credit for the first elective splenectomy for splenic disease. The unfortunate patient died within 6 h after operation

ries of valiant tries but disappointing failures. Quittenbaum removed the spleen of a woman with cirrhosis and ascites "more from the patient's urgent entreaty rather than the surgeon's judgement." The woman lived only 6 h. Thirty years later (1855), Kuchler of Darmstadt removed a massively enlarged spleen from a 36-year-old patient with a history of malarial fever. The excised spleen weighed 1500 g. The patient died 4 h postoperatively of hemorrhage from a branch of the splenic artery. This led one of Kuchler's contemporaries (and probable rival), Gustav Simon, to declare in 1857 that extirpation of the spleen was "a bad operation ... in fact an outright error." Controversy raged between the two men before surgical associations and medical faculties for several years, with no resolution of the controversy nor any love lost between the two protagonists. History has sided with Kuchler.

The next well-recorded splenectomies were performed in England by Sir Thomas Spencer Wells (Fig. 4). In 1865, he removed the spleen of a 34-year-old woman, under chloroform anesthesia, for a spleen so enlarged that its lower pole could be palpated vaginally. The operation lasted only 35 min and the excised spleen weighed over 6 lbs. Things seemed to be going well for the first 6 days, but in the early hours of the seventh day her condition took a rapid turn for the worse and she expired. Death was probably due to sepsis. One year later, in 1866, Thomas Bryant of the Guy's Hospital in London excised the enlarged spleen of a 20-year-old male suffering from "leucocythemia," the generic term then for leukemia. An interesting side note, as recorded in the case report, is that the operation was performed in a "private room in the hospital." Death occurred within less than 3 h due to hemorrhage from an unidentified vessel. At the same hospital a year later, in 1867, Thomas Bryant operated on a young woman with massively enlarged spleen extending "underneath ... Poupart's ligament." Difficulties in hemostasis

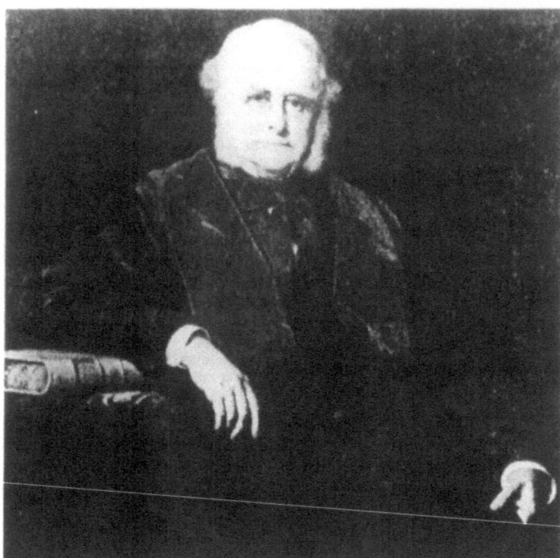

Fig. 4. Sir Thomas Spencer Wells (1818–1897) attempted his first splenectomy in 1865, but the patient succumbed on the seventh day. His second and third cases also ended fatally. Finally, his fourth attempt in 1877, probable congenital hemolytic anemia, was successful

were apparent during the operation, despite successful ligature of the splenic pedicle. Death ensued within 15 min after closure of the abdomen from uncontrollable hemorrhage.

In the same year, 1867, Jules Péan of France (Fig. 5), operating upon a 20-year-old woman for an abdominal tumor presumed to be ovarian in origin, ascertained instead that a large cyst containing 3 l of fluid was arising from the spleen. Initially, he attempted to remove the cyst piecemeal, but a torn branch of the splenic vein forced him to proceed with a total splenectomy. The operation took a little over 2 h, with little further blood loss. The successful outcome was pointedly stressed in the title of an article published within months of the operation: "(...ablation of a splenic cyst and complete extirpation of hypertrophial spleen); recovery!" Thus, the honor of the first successful splenectomy for splenic pathology fell to France and her master surgeon Jules Péan.

In 1877, Spencer Wells, undaunted by his previous failures, attempted a fourth splenectomy, this time with success. The patient was a 22-year-old woman with recurrent attacks of jaundice and splenomegaly. Although the spleen ruptured during removal and "a good deal of blood was lost," the patient recovered and lived many years thereafter. The condition was probably congenital hemolytic icterus, although this condition was not described until years later. In the report of this case Wells also summarized the world experience with splenectomy up to that time; using compilations of at least three other authors in his sources.

By 1877 splenectomy had been performed just over 50 times, for conditions such as "leucemia," malaria, cysts, wandering spleen and "simple hypertrophy." All but one of the splenectomies for "leucemia" ended fatally. Of the successes, seven had been for wandering spleen and six for splenic cysts of varying etiologies. The overall mortality rate for splenectomy exceeded

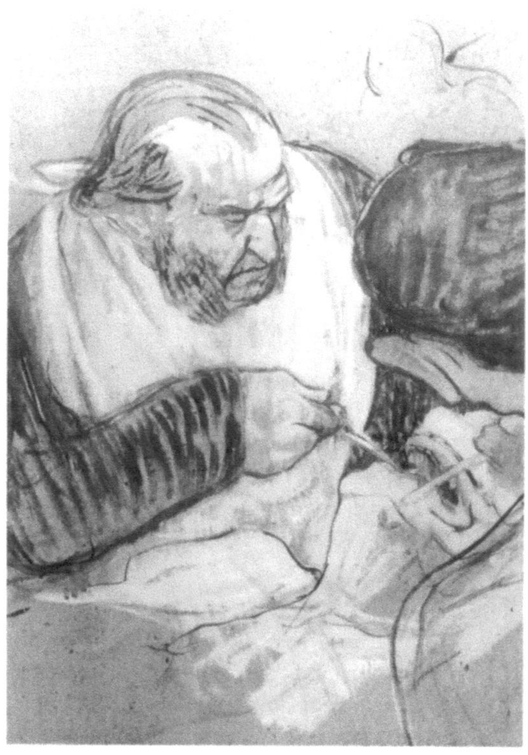

Fig. 5. Jules Péan (1830–1898) must receive credit for the first successful splenectomy for splenic disease (a splenic cyst) in 1867. He mentioned the segmental distribution of the splenic vasculature and attempted partial splenectomy, but abandoned the attempt because of hemorrhage

70%, predominantly in splenectomies performed for hematological disease. Such were the gloomy early statistics for an operation that was later to become commonplace and rarely fatal.

Curiously, reports of partial splenectomy for spleens protruding through abdominal wounds continued to appear throughout the nineteenth century, much as they did in preceding centuries. This remarkable tendency of the spleen to prolapse into the wound, allowing for partial resection, was a phenomenon destined to disappear later. The wounds included stab wounds, shotgun wounds, penetrating wounds by ox-horns, iron pins, wheel-spokes and sundry other missiles. They make for fascinating surgical lore in the colorful language of the early case reports.

Of splenectomies performed for trauma, the credit for the first recorded case is given to a British naval surgeon, E. O'Brien, Esq. (Fig. 6), who, in 1816, while stationed in San Francisco, excised a protruding spleen (out again!) from a Mexican tailor who had been stabbed by his female victim during an attempted rape. The pedicle of the spleen was ligated and splenectomy performed. Despite a concomitant kidney injury, the patient recovered.

In 1892 a splenectomy for trauma more akin to what is seen today was performed by O. Reigner of Breslau, Germany. The patient, a 14-year-old la-

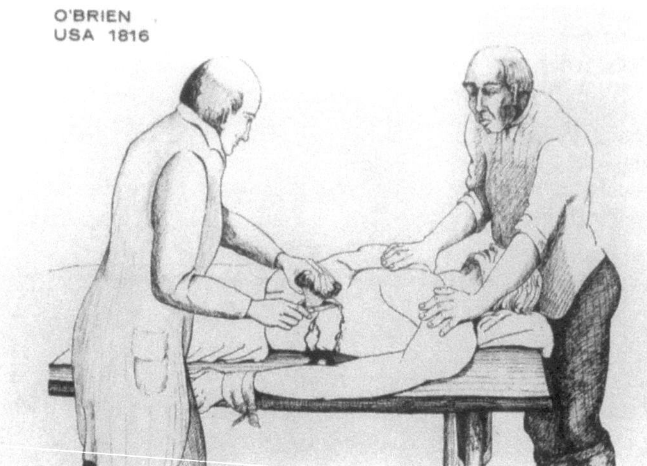

Fig. 6. E. O'Brien reported the first successful splenectomy for trauma in America in 1816. As was common in these early reports, the spleen had prolapsed through a larger left upper quadrant wound

borer, fell from a scaffold and struck his abdomen en route. After observing the patient's rising pulse, diminishing urinary output and progressive abdominal distention overnight, Dr. Reigner operated and found the spleen completely transected. Despite a complicated course unrelated to the removal of the spleen, the patient recovered.

That not all injuries of the spleen mandated splenectomy was presciently noted by Theodor Billroth in 1881, after observing an injured spleen in a man who had died of a head injury incurred 5 days previously: "From the appearance of the rent, and the small quantity of blood effused, we concluded that the injury might have healed completely."

By the closing decades of the nineteenth century, little progress was made in the techniques of splenectomy or its outcome, despite the competence of master surgeons deservedly famous in other arenas of abdominal surgery. They included such names as Czerny, Langenbuch, Trendelenburg, Billroth, Rydigier, Roswell Park and others, all of whom performed splenectomies with dismal outcomes, usually death. By 1900, one author, Bessel-Hagen [13] was able to compile 360 cases of splenectomy for various diagnoses, with operative mortality just under 40%.

Thereafter, the number of splenectomies in Europe and the North American continent grew rapidly in number as more specific indications for splenectomy became recognized. In 1895 J. Bland Sutton had described two successful splenectomies for what was probably congenital hereditary spherocytosis. He had also reported a splenectomy for wandering spleen. Both conditions were specific indications for splenectomy. In 1911 Micheli first reported a successful splenectomy for autoimmune hemolytic anemia. Another landmark event in the evolution of the hematological indications for splenectomy occurred in 1916, when a Czech medical student, Paul Kaznelson, suggested to his professor that the spleen was the site of platelet destruction in the case of a 36-year-old woman with idiopathic thrombocytopenic purpura. Splenectomy resulted in dramatic improvement. Subsequent cases confirmed this causal relationship, planting this disease firmly among the prime indications for splenectomy.

The typical experience with splenectomy by 1920 in a major surgical center (The Mayo Clinic) is related by Moynihan [2] describing the "modern position of the operation of splenectomy" up to that time. Of a total of 243 splenectomies there were 26 hospital deaths, a mortality rate of just under 11%. Some of the diagnoses appear unfamiliar today, such as "splenic anemia," for which splenectomy carried a high mortality rate. Fifty-three splenectomies were done for "pernicious anemia," 32 for "hemolytic icterus" and 26 for "myelogenous leukemia." This latter group probably included cases of lymphatic leukemia, judging from the relatively low mortality rate (3.8%). There were ten splenectomies for "septic splenomegalia," with two hospital deaths. The remaining indications for splenectomy were varied, including hepatic cirrhosis (presumably with congestive splenomegaly), Gaucher's disease, tuberculosis, wandering spleen and others.

As the century progressed, indications for splenectomy were increasingly molded by the developments in hematology and neoplastic diseases. Splenectomy for certain diseases went "in and out of fashion," as noted by the hematologist William Crosby [14]. Splenectomy for Banti's Disease ("splenic anemia" or congestive splenomegaly) was fashionable for a brief interval and then fell into disrepute. Splenectomy for the leukemias was only rarely indicated, except for the relatively rare hairy cell leukemia. Splenectomy for the massive splenomegaly of myeloid metaplasia was a hotly debated issue, resolved in favor of splenectomy in selected cases. The list of hemolytic syndromes, lipid storage diseases, and autoimmune disorders grew longer and longer with each passing year. Advances in chemotherapy for malignancies altered the indications for splenectomy in non-Hodgkin's as well as in Hodgkin's lymphoma. In the 1970s staging splenectomies for Hodgkin's disease were one of the most common elective splenic procedures performed. Changing concepts in the staging and treatment of this disease, however, led to a marked decrease in this procedure in the ensuing decades.

Trauma as an indication for splenectomy became increasingly common as the century progressed. Splenectomies for trauma included not only those performed for blunt or penetrating injury, but also for injuries incurred "accidentally" during other surgical procedures. Such splenectomies were euphemistically called "incidental" splenectomies and in many hospitals constituted between 20%–40% of all splenectomies performed. Although successful splenorrhaphies had been performed and reported earlier in the century in both American [15] and European [16, 17] hospitals, by the 1940s splenectomy had become the standard practice for even the most trivial injury. A notable exception was the recognition by pediatric surgeons that splenic injuries could be treated nonoperatively in children [18, 19].

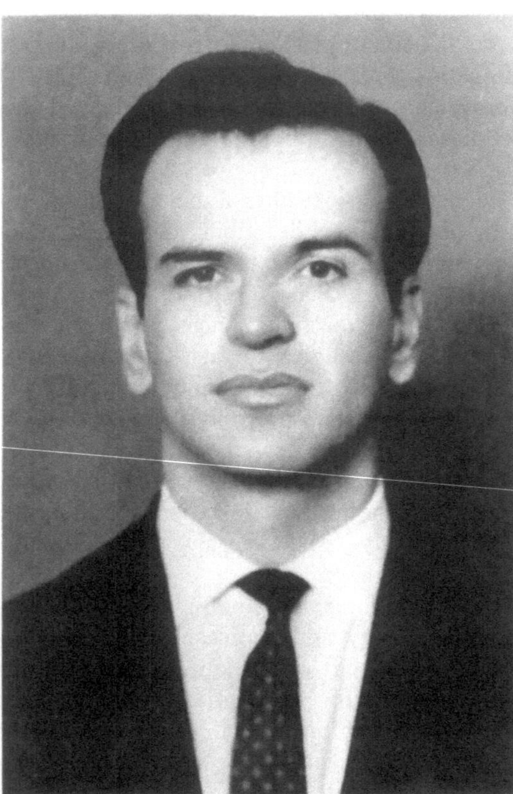

Fig. 7. Marcel Campos Christo of Brazil (1920–) was the first to perform planned partial splenectomies for trauma. His first report, in 1962, of eight cases marked the beginning of a new era in splenic surgery

The epoch of splenic "inviolability" ended in 1962 when Marcelo Campos Christo of Brazil (Fig. 7) reported eight cases of segmental resection of the spleen for injuries due to both penetrating and blunt trauma [20]. This daring departure from the then current surgical practice was based on his own and previous author's studies on the segmental nature of the splenic vasculature. Seven of the eight patients recovered without incident; the eighth, victim of a gunshot wound, succumbed 1 month postoperatively of complications unrelated to the splenic surgery. Campos Christo's work received little notice until considerably later in the 1960s, when splenic salvage began to receive increasing attention. Morgenstern [21] reported on successful subtotal splenectomies for hematologic disease. Reports of splenic salvage following trauma, utilizing topical hemostasis, splenorrhaphy or partial resection appeared in increasing numbers from surgical centers worldwide [22–25].

Concurrent with the development of surgical techniques for splenic salvage was a growing body of literature on the immunological functions of the spleen and its importance in the prevention of overwhelming postsplenectomy sepsis [26, 27]. Validation of splenic salvage procedures by a larger body of clinical and experimental evidence stressing the spleen's immunologic importance spurred the trend toward splenic salvage even further.

The number of total splenectomies performed for trauma, both iatrogenic or otherwise, declined dramatically thereafter. Nonoperative management of splenic injury, initially popular only in pediatric practice, was extended to include adults, in carefully selected cases. The technique of partial splenectomy was increasingly employed in conditions other than trauma, to include Hodgkin's disease, Gaucher's disease, schistosomiasis, and splenic cysts. The latter lesion is the only indication which has been of proven value in follow-up observations.

As the century draws to a close, the latest development in the history of splenectomy is the application of laparoscopic techniques to selected splenic conditions. The first laparoscopic splenectomies were performed in the early 1990s by Phillips and Carroll [28], Cuschieri et al. [29], Thibault et al. [30] and Delaitre et al. [31]. What at first seemed an almost impossible technical feat, considering the complicated and fragile vasculature of the spleen, eventually yielded to the ingenuity and expertise of the laparoscopic surgeons. It has been a fitting and dramatic development at the close of the twentieth century for a procedure which has had such a colorful history. Currently, the principal indications for the laparoscopic approach have been idiopathic thrombocytopenic purpura (ITP), splenic cysts, congenital spherocytic anemia and autoimmune hemolytic anemia. It has also been reported in cases of trauma and staging for Hodgkin's disease. The approach is too recent to evaluate in the latter conditions. For ITP it seems to be an ideal procedure for surgeons with the appropriate level of training and skill. Laparoscopic splenectomy is treated in greater detail in the chapter by Phillips in this volume.

Omitted from this account are the numerous technical advances which have influenced the history of splenectomy and splenic salvage. For diagnosis, these include the advances in imaging devices such as ultrasound, scintiscans and computed tomographic scans. Notable developments in operative technique include a host of topical hemostatic agents, the hemoclip, surgical staplers, synthetic meshes and a vast armamentarium of laparoscopic instruments and devices. All have had a bearing on the techniques of splenic surgery.

This history of splenic surgery and splenectomy has been painted in detail in some areas and in broad strokes in others. The spleen has always been a "mysterious" organ of seemingly occult function as well as a forbidding organ of extreme vulnerability for the surgeon. But on both fronts it has yielded considerable ground. The ensuing chapters bear eloquent proof of this statement.

References

1. Morgenstern L (1974) The surgical inviolability of the spleen: historical evolution of a concept. In: Proceedings of the XXIIIth international congress of the history of medicine, vol 1. Wellcome Institute of the History of Medicine, London, pp 62–68
2. Moynihan B (1920) The surgery of the spleen. Br J Surg 8:307
3. Meade RH (1968) Surgery of the spleen. In: An introduction to the history of general surgery, chap 19. Saunders, Philadelphia, pp 256–260

4. Ellis H (1988) Clio chirurgica: the spleen. Silvergirl, Austin, pp 7–80
5. Pugh HL (1946) Splenectomy, with special reference to its historical background (Collective Review). Int Abstr Surg 83(3):209–224
6. Sherman R (1980) Perspectives in management of trauma to the spleen: 1979 Presidential address, American Association for the Surgery of Trauma. J Trauma 20(1):1–13
7. Crosby WH (1983) An historical sketch of splenic function and splenectomy. Lymphology 16:52–55
8. Pool EH, Stillman RG (1923) History of splenectomy. In: Surgery of the spleen, chap XIII. Appleton, New York, pp 297–309
9. Coon WW (1991) The spleen and splenectomy (The Surgeon's Library). Surg Gynecol Obstet 173:407–414
10. Krumbhaar EB (1915) The history of extirpation of the spleen. N Y Med J 101:232–234
11. Macht DI, Finesilver EM (1922) The effect of splenectomy on integration of muscular movements in the rat. Am J Physiol 62:525–530
12. Clark DT (1673–1674) De lienis resectione in cane (et homine) vivo (Observatio 164–165). Misc Curiosa Acad Nat Curios S1(4–5):198–199
13. Bessel-Hagen F (1900) Ein Beitrag zur Milzchirurgie. Verh Dtsch Ges Chir 29:714–757
14. Crosby WH (1985) Splenectomy: in and out of fashion (editorial). Arch Intern Med 145(2):226–227
15. Mayo WJ (1910) Principles underlying surgery of the spleen. JAMA 54:14–18
16. Zikoff V (1895) O prishivanii selezyonki (on suturing the spleen). Vrach 16:995–1000
17. James RL (1892) A case of gunshot wound of the spleen, suturing of the diaphragm; recovery. No Am Pract 4:232–233
18. Douglas GJ, Simpson JS (1971) The conservative management of splenic trauma. J Pediatr Surg 6:565–570
19. Touloukian RJ (1985) Splenic preservation in children. World J Surg 9:214–221
20. Campos Christo M (1962) Segmental resections of the spleen: report on the first eight cases operated on. O Hospital 62:187–203
21. Morgenstern L, Kahn FH, Weinstein IM (1966) Subtotal splenectomy in myelofibrosis. Surgery 60(2):336–339
22. Morgenstern L (1977) The avoidable complications of splenectomy. Surg Gynecol Obstet 145:525–528
23. Buntain WL, Lynn HB (1979) Splenorrhaphy: changing concepts for the traumatized spleen. Surgery 86(5):748–760
24. Morgenstern L, Shapiro SJ (1979) Techniques of splenic conservation. Arch Surg 114:449–454
25. Morgenstern L (1985) Conservative surgery of the spleen. In: Cuschieri A, Hennessy TPJ (eds) Current operative surgery: general surgery. Bailliere Tindall, London, pp 74–92
26. Balfanz JR, Nesbit ME Jr, Jarvis C, Krivit W (1976) Overwhelming sepsis following splenectomy for trauma. J Pediatr 88(3):458–460
27 Singer DB (1973) Postsplenectomy sepsis. Perspect Pediatr Pathol 1:285–311
28. Carroll B, Phillips E (1991) Laparoscopic splenectomy. Surg Endosc 6:183–185
29. Cuschieri A, Shimi S, Banting S, Vander Valpen G (1992) Technical aspects of laparoscopic splenectomy: hilar segmental devascularization and instrumentation. J R Coll Surg Edinb 37(6):414–416
30. Thibault C, Mamazza J, Létourneau R, Poulin E (1992) Laparoscopic splenectomy: operative technique and preliminary report. Surg Laparosc Endosc 2(3):248–253
31. Delaitre B, Maignien B (1992) Laparoscopic splenectomy – technical aspects. Surg Endosc 6:305–308

Anatomy and Embryology of the Spleen

L. Morgenstern, in collaboration with J.E. Skandalakis

> "The neighbouring organ [the spleen] is situated on the left-hand side, and is constructed with a view of the keeping the liver bright and pure – like a napkin, always prepared and at hand to clean the mirror."
> *Plato*, Fourth Century B.C.

The aim of this chapter is to emphasize key elements in surgical anatomy and embryology of importance and relevance to surgical practice. The anatomy and embryology of the spleen are well described in standard texts on those subjects [1]. Detailed anatomical and embryological descriptions have been purposely omitted from this chapter, which concentrates on the surgical relevance of spleen-related structures and their development. A number of the subjects considered here are treated in greater detail in the chapters which follow.

Anatomy

The spleen is the largest reticuloendothelial organ in the body. Although its characteristic shape is well known, its appearance is variable, as manifested by clefts in the parenchyma of various depths and in various locations. The normal human spleen weighs approximately 150 to 250 g and is about the size of a clenched fist. Its juxtaposition in the left upper quadrant to the ninth, tenth, and 11th ribs renders it extremely vulnerable to injury when these ribs are fractured. The spleen must double in size, at least, before its anterior border will project beyond the left costal margin. There are two surfaces: the parietal surface is related to the diaphragm, while the visceral surface is related to the left colon, left kidney, pancreatic tail, and stomach.

The splenic capsule in humans is relatively thin and is composed of a layer of mesothelial cells under which are several cell layers of fibroelastic tissue. The capsule is susceptible to tears or avulsion by either direct trauma or injudicious traction on adjacent structures. From the splenic capsule arise the trabeculae, which traverse the parenchyma. The capsule and trabeculae contain blood vessels, lymphatics, and nerves. In other mammals, smooth muscle is present in the capsule and trabeculae; humans have few, if any, smooth muscle cells in these structures.

Splenic Artery

The splenic artery is one of the three main branches of the celiac axis. It differs from its sister branches, the left gastric and hepatic arteries, by its length and marked tortuosity.[1] From its origin at the celiac axis, it winds sinuously toward the spleen on the superior surface of the pancreas, from which it is generally free but in which it may sometimes be imbedded (see Fig. 6 in the chap. by Phillips, this volume). In its course, it is in close juxtaposition to the splenic vein, especially at the bottom of its U-shaped bends, where injury to the vein (or pancreas) may occur when the artery is being isolated or ligated; the artery is best controlled at the apex of these bends.

As the splenic artery traverses the pancreatic area through the lesser sac, it gives off a variable number of branches into the pancreatic parenchyma [3, 4]. The first major branch to the spleen, the superior polar artery, generally occurs within 2–3 cm of the splenic hilum and heads superiorly to supply the upper pole. The remaining branches of the splenic artery, as have been described by many authors, vary in size and in number from three to five, or occasionally more, supplying the blood to the splenic parenchyma in a segmental fashion (Fig. 1). Ligation or occlusion of these branches results in segmental devascularization, a maneuver which is utilized in subtotal or segmental splenectomy (see the chap. by Morgenstern, "Partial splenectomy", this volume).

The spleen also derives a portion of its blood supply from branches of the left gastroepiploic artery, which traverse the gastrosplenic omentum or ligament. These arteries also vary in size and length. The shortest are generally found in the area of the upper pole of the spleen and are the most difficult

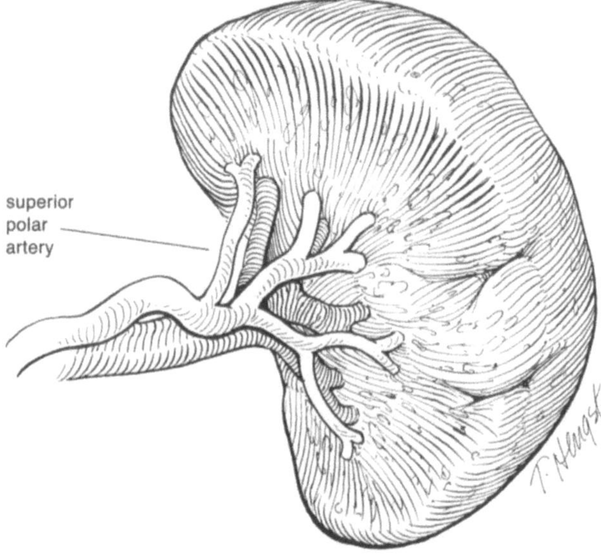

Fig. 1. Arterial branches in the splenic hilum include the superior polar artery and a variable number of segmental arteries

---

[1] A bruit has been described in one report, attributed to the tortuosity of the artery [2].

and treacherous to isolate for ligation, presenting a risk of injury to both spleen and stomach. Those in the lower portion of the gastrosplenic omentum are easily visualized and amenable to ligation without difficulty.

If the spleen has not been mobilized, ligation of the splenic arteries is permissible and the spleen remains viable if the collateral circulation is intact (polar arteries, short gastric arteries, and left gastroepiploic arteries). If the color of the spleen is changed, however, and there is evidence of ischemia, a splenectomy should be performed. In general, the splenic artery should be only be ligated if absolutely necessary (i.e., during splenectomy).

With splenic enlargement, large arterial branches which do not follow the pattern described above may result from parasitization of neighboring structures such as the omentum, mesentery, or peritoneum. This is especially true in the lower pole with massive splenomegaly, where large arterial branches may be encountered arising from the omentum or the intestinal mesentery.

Splenic Vein

The splenic vein follows a course from the spleen to the portal vein, without the characteristic tortuosity of the splenic artery. The vein lies in close juxtaposition to the artery, especially in its distal two thirds, and is most closely apposed to the artery at the bottom of the U-shaped arterial bends. Splenic veins are characteristically fragile and are more troublesome to the surgeon than their arterial counterparts. The arborization of the venous system follows the arterial distribution closely, including the branches into the pancreatic parenchyma. Avulsion of these small veins can be of particular annoyance to the surgeon near the tail of the pancreas or when avulsed flush with the pancreatic parenchyma when freeing the splenic artery. These branches become engorged in patients with portal hypertension and may be the cause of major hemorrhage if not controlled with great care during isolation of the splenic vein for a distal splenorenal shunt. At the hilum of the spleen, larger branches are subject to tearing and avulsion, requiring gentleness and care in mobilization of, and traction on, the spleen.

With massive splenomegaly, the splenic vein and its tributaries are large and thinwalled. The main splenic vein in spleens weighing between 1500 and 2000 g may approach the size of a normal inferior vena cava. Similarly, the short gastric veins are markedly enlarged and engorged. The most superior of the short gastric veins are most susceptible to avulsion and traction injury, either on the splenic or gastric side. Since these veins may be extremely short, adequate exposure for their control is of utmost importance.

Splenic Parenchyma

The normal color of the sectioned spleen parenchyma is dark red or reddish purple. Very dark spleens suggest hemolysis, as seen in the hemolytic anemias and other hemolytic syndromes.

The cut surface of the spleen is finely granular. In the normal spleen, the white pulp – or Malpighian corpuscles – appear as whitish nodules, varying in size from a fraction of a millimter to 1 mm. The major portion of the splenic substance is composed of the red pulp. In disorders or neoplasms of the white pulp, such as lymphomas or leukemias, the white pulp stands out as easily identifiable nodules, varying in size from millimeter-sized nodules to that of coalesced nodules several centimeters in size.

On the sectioned splenic parenchyma, the smaller branches of the splenic artery may be identified by their thicker walls and diminished tendency to retract within the parenchyma. This renders them fairly easy to identify, grasp, and ligate with clips in the course of partial splenectomy (see the chap. by Morgenstern, "Partial Splenectomy", this volume). The sectioned veins, in contrast, are flush with or retracted within the parenchyma, either as thin, simple or V-shaped slits. They are best handled by suture ligation or, when small enough, by electrocautery, argon beam coagulation, or topical hemostatic agents.

The younger the spleen, the greater the tendency for effective autohemostasis; the older the spleen, the greater the tendency of the parenchyma to bleed, even after trivial injury. This difference explains the increased likelihood of successful nonoperative management of splenic injury in children and young adults.

The Pancreatic "Connection"

The tail of the pancreas is in close apposition to the hilum of the spleen, in some cases being intimately adherent to it. The pancreas shares small branches from the splenic artery and vein which may give rise to troublesome bleeding. The edge of the pancreatic tail, no matter how closely apposed to the hilum, must be clearly identified and separated from the vascular structures of the hilum before these are clamped, divided, and ligated.

The danger of inadvertent pancreatic injury is especially present with neoplastic splenomegaly, which may distort the normal anatomical relationship of pancreatic tail to spleen. Accidental injury to the pancreatic tail may be responsible for pancreatic fistula, pancreatitis, or pancreatic pseudocyst in the wake of a difficult splenectomy. These are potentially disastrous complications, particularly in patients with hematologic disorders and immune suppression.

Ligaments of the Spleen
(see Figs. 2, 3, 4 in the chap. by Hiatt, this volume)

Much has been written of the splenic ligaments, their location and importance. Suffice it to say, for surgical purposes, that there are a few "ligaments" or peritoneal attachments which are constant and others which are variable.

Fig. 2. Polysplenia in a patient with *situs inversus*

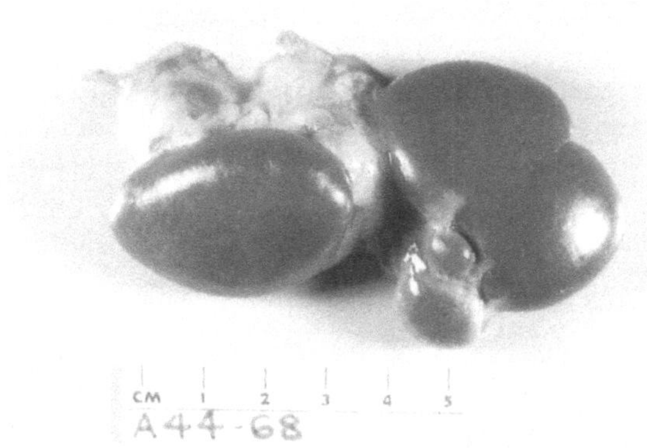

Fig. 3a,b. Laparoscopic view of large accessory spleen in splenic hilum of a patient with immune thrombocytopenic purpura. **a** Prior to dissection. **b** Dissection and removal of accessory spleen

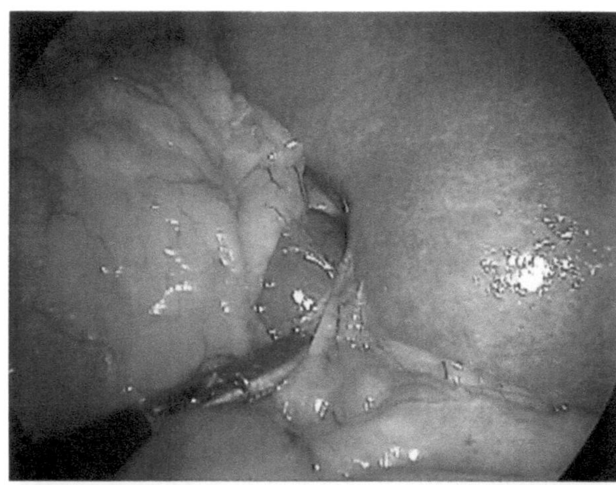

a

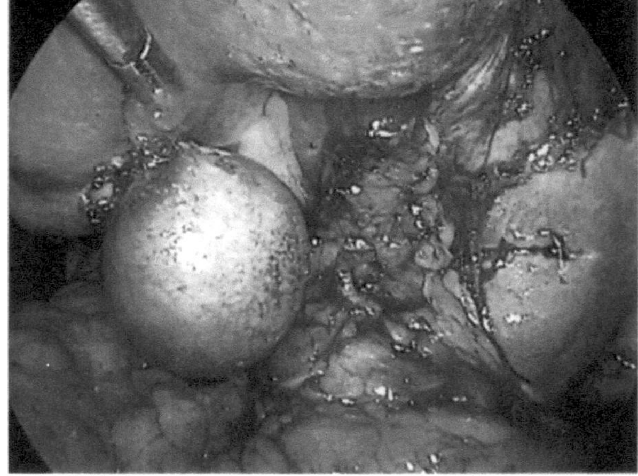

b

The "Constant" Ligaments

The Splenogastric Ligament. Splenogastric ligament is synonymous with the gastrosplenic omentum, and through it course the short gastric vessels. Its extent is variable, but usually it extends from the upper pole of the spleen to its lower third, sometimes leaving a portion of the lower third unattached to the gastrosplenic omentum. Occasionally, the entire medial surface of the spleen will be attached to the stomach in a broad band of vascular peritoneal reflection.

The Splenocolic Ligament. The peritoneal fold from the splenic flexure of the colon to the lower pole of the spleen is short and not as vascular as the gastrosplenic ligament, nor is its attachment as broad. Mobilization of the splenic flexure of the colon, preparatory to resection or anastomosis, requires section of this structure. Undue traction is a cause of traumatic avulsion of the lower pole.

The Splenorenal Ligament. The splenorenal ligament is actually the posterior peritoneum which has parted above the underlying kidney to encompass the hilar vessels and the tail of the pancreas. It is the fold of peritoneum immediately posterior and parallel to the spleen which is incised surgically as one of the most important steps in mobilization of the spleen. It is generally less vascular than either the splenogastric or splenocolic ligament in normal spleens, but may contain sizable vessels in cases of splenomegaly.

The Splenophrenic Ligament. In inflammatory and neoplastic disorders of the spleen, the attachment to the diaphragm may be extensive and dense. With normal spleens, very little sharp dissection is necessary to free the occasional peritoneal folds extending from the superior pole to the diaphragm. In abnormal spleens, with dense adhesions to the diaphragm, incision or perforation of the diaphragm is a constant danger and not an uncommon surgical complication.

The Spleno-omental Ligament. A constant fold of peritoneum attaches to the lower pole of the spleen from the omentum, close to the splenic flexure of the colon. This is separate from the splenocolic ligament and is the peritoneal fold which is most commonly responsible for iatrogenic injury to the lower pole of the spleen during operations in the left upper quadrant. It has been labeled the "criminal fold" by Morgenstern and usually contains one or more small vessels, which in normal spleens may be controlled by electrocautery. With larger spleens, or in patients with coagulation disorders, these vessels require individual ligation. Minor injuries due to excessive traction on the spleno-omental fold, avulsing the capsule of the spleen or underlying splenic parenchyma, were in the past responsible for many unnecessary splenectomies involving normal spleens. Newer techniques of hemostasis have fortunately made splenectomy for such injuries a relative rarity.

Splenopancreatic Ligament. The peritoneum between the tail of the pancreas and the splenic hilum, approaching and encompassing the hilar vessels, has sometimes been called the splenopancreatic ligament. It is hardly identifiable as a discrete structure, compared with the aforementioned ligaments.

Other Ligaments Involving the Spleen

Occasionally, other peritoneal folds involving contiguous organs, such as folds between the diaphragm and colon, are added to those ligaments which regularly involve the spleen. The phrenico-colic ligament acts as a slinglike suspensory mechanism, supporting the lower pole of the spleen. Also, there are a variable number of inconstant folds of peritoneum which may attach to or near the spleen. These must be divided in splenectomy but hardly merit a unique anatomical designation.

Lymphatic Drainage

The splenic lymphatics have their origin in the splenic capsule and the trabeculae. The splenic lymph node chain includes suprapancreatic nodes, infrapancreatic nodes, and afferent and efferent lymph vessels. The largest group of "splenic lymph nodes," the splenopancreatic nodes, is located along the splenic artery. A small number, however, can be found near the short gastric vessels. The stomach and pancreas also drain into the splenic nodes.

Embryology

The splenic primordium, taking origin from the primitive mesoderm, becomes evident during the fifth week of gestation. It begins as an outgrowth from the dorsal mesogastrium, acquires its distinctive vasculature and cellular composition in the ensuing weeks, and soon begins its leftward drift and axial rotation to eventually settle in the left upper quadrant of the abdomen. From this bare outline of early development can be derived those anomalies of the spleen which are of clinical importance to the surgeon.

Anomalies and Congenital Splenic Conditions

Asplenia [5] is probably the rarest of splenic anomalies and invariably occurs in association with serious cardiovascular malformations which are incompatible with life beyond infancy. Other associated anomalies involve the lungs, liver, and intestinal tract.

Congenital hyposplenia has been reported but is also very uncommon. Such patients bear the hematologic stigmata of asplenic patients and are subject to overwhelming post-splenectomy sepsis (see chaps. by Stiehm and Trunkey, this volume).

Polysplenia [6] refers to multiple splenic nodules or masses in place of the normal solitary splenic structure (Fig. 2). It may be a throwback to the primitive evolutionary stages of splenic development when the spleen was multinodular, as in the primitive sharks. Polysplenia in humans rarely exceeds ten splenic masses and more frequently consists of only several splenic units. It also is associated with serious cardiovascular anomalies which are usually lethal in early infancy. In one of the editors' cases, it was associated with *situs inversus.*

Splenogonadal fusion occurs with maldevelopment and maldescent of splenic tissue along with the left gonadal elements, both in males and females; the majority of cases occur in males. In males, splenic tissue is found attached to the left testicle; in females, the attachment is to the ovary. These are incidental findings during operations such as herniorrhaphy, orchiopexy, or exploratory laparotomy. Splenogonadal fusion may be associated with malformation of the extremities, a condition known as peromelia.

Accessory spleens are the most common of all splenic anomalies. The great majority of them are encountered in the vicinity of the splenic hilum; the second most common location is along the pancreatic border, in the splenogastric omentum, or near the splenic flexure. They have been described in other locations as well, including the omentum and presacral area. In a recent case of one of the editors (E.H.P.), an accessory spleen was found near the gallbladder on the right side. They have also been found imbedded within the tail of the pancreas, thus not detectable during laparotomy or laparoscopy.

The number of accessory spleens can vary from one to as many as five or more. They are present in up to 20% of patients, with an apparent increase in frequency having been reported in patients with hematologic disease. Accessory spleens differ in size as well as location. The largest accessory spleen in the editors' experience has been one measuring 3.5 cm in length and weighing 45 g. Ordinarily, accessory spleens do not exceed 1.0–2.0 cm in diameter and are attached to a small mesosplenium carrying their vascular supply.

The surgical indications for removal of accessory spleens vary with the conditons. In nonhematologic and nonneoplastic conditions (trauma, for example), they should not be removed. Although it is doubtful that even multiple accessory spleens can achieve the necessary aggregate splenic mass for immunologic competence, there is no reason to remove good splenic tissue if it can be preserved. On the other hand, in conditions such as idiopathic thrombocytopenic purpura and hemolytic syndromes, it is imperative to remove all splenic tissue, including the accessories. Leaving the latter carries a risk of recurrence of the disease for which splenectomy is being performed. The same holds true for neoplastic disorders which may be of multicentric origin. However, in some of the storage disorders, benign causes of hypersplenism (such as congestive splenomegaly), hamartomatosis, and other benign conditions, accessory spleens should be preserved.

While it has been argued that it is more difficult to detect and remove accessory spleens via the laparoscopic route than by open splenectomy, this is not true (Fig. 3). The excellent view afforded by modern laparoscopes and the the excellent maneuverability of the instruments in the hands of skilled laparoscopists permit as good an opportunity, if not a better one, to discover accessory spleens (see the chap. by Phillips, this volume). Those that are beyond visualization or palpation, as occur with intrapancreatic accessories, are missed by either method.

Accessory spleens can be demonstrated by radionuclide imaging studies. Such studies may therefore be useful preoperatively when removal of all splenic tissue is mandatory. They are also useful in cases of recurrent disease, such as with idiopathic thrombocytopenic purpura, to locate accessory spleens which are functional but were missed during the original operation.

Wandering or ectopic spleen, as the name implies, is a spleen which has lost its domicile in the left upper quadrant and has migrated elsewhere [7]. The condition results from the extensive laxity or absence of the "ligamentous" or peritoneal attachments of the spleen, allowing the organ to drop from its secure position to almost anywhere in the abdomen or even the pelvis. The migration is aided and abetted by the gradual lengthening of the splenic pedicle as time and traction exert their influence. Thus, the spleen may fall to the left lower quadrant or "float" in the right lower quadrant, palpable as a mass which is usually not suspected to be the spleen. On long pedicles and highly mobile, wandering spleens are extremely subject to torsion and infarction and may eventuate in an acute abdominal emergency.

Some of the earliest recorded splenectomies in the nineteenth century were for wandering spleens. The fourth successful splenectomy in the United States was performed for this indication in 1874. However, splenectomy for a wandering spleen is only the treatment of choice when the spleen is infarcted. Since this condition is more commonly detected in children than in adults, splenic salvage is indicated for spleens which are viable. Splenopexy in the left upper quadrant is a preferable alternative. If in the surgeon's opinion the spleen itself will not accept sutures of sufficient strength to hold it, the spleen may be capped with polyglycolic acid mesh and then sutured to the parietal peritoneum.

There are two remaining congenital conditions or disorders of the spleen which deserve mention. *Hamartomas* are focal collections or nodules of splenic tissue which lack the normal anatomical organization of splenic elements. They may be solitary or multiple. On occasion, they may be diffuse throughout the spleen, causing splenomegaly and hypersplenism. They are more frequently found in association with splenomegaly due to hematologic disease, which may raise some doubts as to their mode of origin. *Nonparasitic splenic cysts*, the great majority of which are epithelial cysts with mesothelial or mesothelial-derived linings, are considered to be of congenital origin. They are discussed more fully in the chapter by Morgenstern "Benign Neoplasms of the Spleen" (this volume).

References

1. Skandalakis JE, Colborn GL, Pemberton LB et al (1990) The surgical anatomy of the spleen. Probl Gen Surg 7:1
2. Smythe CM, Gibson DB (1963) Upper-quadrant bruit due to tortuous splenic artery. New Engl J Med 269:1308–1309
3. Michels NA (1942) The variational anatomy of the spleen and splenic artery. Am J Anat 70:21–72
4. Liu DL, Xia S, Su W, Ye Q Gao Y, Qian J (1996) Anatomy of vasculature of 850 spleen specimens and its application in partial splenectomy. Surgery 119:27–33
5. Majewski JA, Upshur JK (1978) Asplenia syndrome: a study of congenital anomalies in 16 cases. JAMA 240:1508–1510
6. Skandalakis JE, Gray SW (eds) (1994) Embryology for surgeons. Williams and Wilkins, Baltimore
7. Allen KB, Andrews G (1989) Pediatric wandering spleen – the case for splenopexy: review of 35 reported cases in the literature. J Pediatr Surg 24:432–435

Pathology of the Spleen

R. S. Neiman

"Enlargement of the spleen ... is caused by the flux of some humors which rush down, thick and tenacious. Such faulty humors may cause the spleen to become abnormally larger."
Galen, Second Century A.D.

Introduction

Our understanding of pathologic processes of the spleen have been hampered by a number of factors. The first is our limited experience in studying specimens of that organ. Many of the disorders involving the spleen are part of a disseminated lymphoreticular or hematopoietic process that can be more advantageously and more efficiently studied by biopsy of another involved organ such as a lymph node or the bone marrow. Diagnostic splenectomy is usually performed only if there is no evidence of disease in those organs. In addition, many pathologic processes in the spleen are self-limited. As a result, the organ is removed for study only in those cases in which the disease persists for abnormally prolonged periods of time. In addition, one does not usually biopsy the spleen, so that studies of the morphologic changes as disease processes evolve cannot be performed as in the bone marrow or liver. In the case of therapeutic splenectomy, the procedure is usually performed only after other modalities of therapy, such as corticosteroids, cytotoxic drugs or radiotherapy, which alter splenic morphology, have been administered. The potentially richest source of spleens for pathologic study, the autopsy, is of limited value because of the rapid postmortem change that affects the spleen and by the fact that in the majority of cases prior therapeutic intervention has altered the basic pathology of the organ.

The understanding of splenic pathology is further hampered by the underlying nature of that organ. The majority of splenectomy specimens are enlarged and bloody and seldom get the prompt and careful fixation needed to preserve the pathologic changes. It is no wonder that Galen's "organ of great mystery" remains mysterious!

There is much that one can do to minimize these problems, but cooperation between the surgeon and pathologist is necessary. Surgeons must recognize that, even in cases of therapeutic splenectomy or in cases of splenectomy after splenic rupture, there may be unsuspected underlying pathology which can be recognized if the specimen is submitted to the pathology laboratory in the fresh state as quickly as possible. Failure to deliver the specimen to the pathology laboratory can result in significant alteration in an organ which autolyses quite rapidly, obscuring meaningful pathologic changes. Pathologists must recognize that even in cases of therapeutic splenectomy and splenectomy secondary to rupture it is important to document possible underlying pathology and that this cannot be as successfully achieved if prompt attention to processing of splenic tissue is not undertaken. The prompt delivery of the splenectomy specimen to the pathology laboratory in the fresh state also provides an opportunity to perform additional ancillary studies that may prove invaluable in the diagnosis. These include touch imprints of the spleen, which are particularly useful in diagnosing such diseases as immune thrombocytopenic purpura (ITP), autoimmune hemolytic anemia and myeloproliferative disorders, as well as newer technologies such as flow cytometric, molecular biologic and cytogenetic studies that are becoming standard diagnostic techniques in the workup of many splenic disorders.

Surgeons must recognize that rapid, 1-day pathology sign out of splenectomy specimens is seldom of practical value. Because of the slow degree of penetration of fixative into splenic tissue, rapid processing of the organ frequently results in poor sections with little cellular detail and subsequent difficulty in the recognition of pathologic changes. Overnight fixation of tissue blocks is therefore highly desirable. It is better to wait an additional day for a more reliable diagnosis.

The role of frozen sections in splenic diagnosis is somewhat controversial. Touch imprints are frequently more reliable than an extremely difficult technical process of obtaining a frozen section in an enlarged bloody organ. Therefore, frozen sections of spleens should be discouraged where possible. However, if diagnostic splenectomy reveals the presence of tumor masses or focal lesions in the spleen, frozen section may be a valuable procedure.

The type of fixative used in processing sections of spleen is of less importance than the care taken in fixation. Most pathologists use hematoxylin and eosin (H&E) stains to evaluate splenic sections. However, periodic acid-Schiff (PAS) stains better highlight the cordal-sinusoidal relationships and provide differential staining of such cells as plasma cells, megakaryocytes, and granulocytes.

Normal Spleen Weight

The normal weight of the spleen may vary significantly [1, 2]. Factors responsible for this variation include whether the organ is obtained at autopsy or surgically and the subjects' age, gender or race. The normal surgically removed spleen may weigh as much as 250 g. With the progressive atrophy that accompanies senescence [3], the organ may weigh as little as 50 g. In general, weights tend to be lower in females and in races other than Caucasians [1].

Accessory Spleens

Accessory spleens, or splenunculi, are incidental findings that are noted frequently at autopsy [4]. They may single or multiple and occur most frequently in the hilum, in the gastrosplenic ligament or the tail of the pancreas [5]. They appear to be morphologically identical to the normal spleen. However, whether they provide significant normal function is questionable and probably relates to their size. They may be of clinical importance if overlooked in patients who undergo splenectomy because of hypersplenism. There are reported cases of recurrence of the symptoms of ITP because of splenunculi which were not removed at the time of splenectomy [6].

Splenosis

Splenosis refers to the regrowth of splenic tissue following splenectomy, or more commonly after traumatic rupture [7]. Splenosis has been attributed to autotransplantation of splenic tissue [7, 8]. Although these implants usually occur in the peritoneal cavity, they have been reported in other more distant sites such as pleura, pericardium, and in skin scars.

Splenic Function

Pathologic processes in the spleen can best be understood in the light of splenic function (Table 1). Four functions have been historically ascribed to the spleen. They are: (1) filtration, (2) immunologic, (3) reservoir (storage), and (4) hematopoietic. The first two functions are the dominant ones in humans. The filtration function refers to the removal from the circulating blood of abnormal or senescent red blood cells, the removal of red cell inclusions, and the removal of particulate antigens, such as microorganisms or antigen-antibody complexes. The immunologic function is essentially the same as that of other lymphoid organs in the body, except that the spleen monitors systemic blood-borne antigen as opposed to regional lymphatic and blood-borne antigen in the case of such organs as lymph nodes.

Although the reservoir function is not as great in humans as in other mammals, the organ still normally sequesters about one third of the total platelet mass and significant numbers of granulocytes. There is controversy

Table 1. Splenic functions

Major Functions
  I . Filtration
      A. Culling – erythrocyte (or other blood cell) destruction
          1. Physiologic (as red blood cells age)
          2. Pathologic
              a. Associated with blood cell abnormalities
              b. Associated with primary splenic changes
      B. Pitting (face lifting of erythrocytes)
          1. Removal of cytoplasmic inclusions
          2. Remodeling of cell membranes
      C. Erythroclasis – destruction of abnormal red blood cells with liberation into circulation of erythrocyte fragments
      D. Removal of other particulate material (bacteria, colloidal particles)
 II. Immunologic
      A. Trapping and processing of antigen
      B. Homing of lymphocytes
      C. Lymphocyte transformation and proliferation
      D. Antibody and lymphokine production
      E. Macrophage activation

Minor Functions
  I. Reservoir
      A. Storage or normal sequestration primarily of platelets, granulocytes, iron
 II. Hematopoietic
      A. Erythropoiesis, granulopoiesis, megakaryopoiesis (probably does not occur in humans)
      B. Lymphocyte and macrophage production

as to whether the human spleen has a hematopoietic function. Work done in our laboratory suggests that it does not [9–11]. The majority of pathologic processes in the spleen involve abnormalities of the filtration or immunologic functions and involve either the red pulp (filtration) or the white pulp (immunologic).

Hyposplenism

Hyposplenism refers to the defective or absent function of the spleen (Table 2). It may be congenital or acquired. The most common cause is splenectomy. In rare cases hyposplenism may occur in the presence of an intact or even an enlarged spleen. The characteristic finding associated with depressed splenic function is the presence of Howell-Jolly bodies in the blood (Table 3). However, depressed splenic function may also be documented by the presence of increased numbers of pits in the red cell membrane when blood is studied by phase contrast microscopy [12].

Table 2. Disorders associated with hyposplenism

I. Congenital
  A. Asplenia
  B. Hypoplasia
  C. Congenital immunodeficiency disorders

II. Acquired
  A. Splenectomy
  B. Acquired atrophy and/or infarction
    1. Sickle cell disease
    2. Vascular disorders (vasculitides, thromboembolic conditions)
    3. Essential thrombocythemia
    4. Malabsorption syndromes
    5. Autoimmune diseases
    6. Irradiation
    7. Cytotoxic chemotherapy
    8. Chronic alcoholism
    9. Hypopituitarism
  C. Functional asplenia with normal-sized or enlarged spleen
    1. Infiltration by leukemia, lymphoma, multiple myeloma
    2. Amyloidosis
    3. Sarcoidosis
    4. Vascular tumors
  D. Depressed immune function
    1. Physiologic in neonates and elderly
    2. Acquired immunodeficiency syndrome (AIDS)
    3. Irradiation
    4. Cytotoxic chemotherapy
    5. Immunosuppressive agents, including corocosteroids
    6. Endocrine disorders
      a. Hypothyroidism
      b. Hypopituitarism
      c. Diabetes mellitus
    7. Chronic alcoholism

Hypersplenism

Hypersplenism is the most frequent indication for splenectomy. It can be best defined as the presence of cytopenia of one or more peripheral blood cell lines in the presence of a normally compensating bone marrow and corrected or ameliorated following splenectomy. It is usually, but not invariably, associated with splenomegaly. Disorders causing hypersplenism can be divided into two functional groups (Table 4): (1) those in which the spleen is intrinsically normal and in which hypersplenism results from the increased destruction of abnormal blood cells and (2) those primary disorders of the spleen which result in the increased destruction of normal blood cells. Among the first category are such conditions as congenital disorders of red cells, autoimmune hemolytic anemias, and ITP. Conditions associated with the second category include infiltrative vascular and proliferative diseases of the spleen itself. There is evidence to suggest that splenomegaly for whatever

Table 3. Postsplenectomy blood picture

I.	Erythrocyte inclusions
	A. Howell-Jolly bodies
	B. Heinz bodies
	C. Pappenheimer bodies
II.	Poikilocytosis
	A. Target cells
	B. Acanthocytes
	C. Nucleated red blood cells (rarely)
III.	Thrombocytosis (usually transient)
IV.	Leukocytosis
	A. Lymphocytosis (may persist)
	B. Monocytosis (may persist)
	C. Eosinophilia

reason causes an increased splenic blood flow and a larger filtration fraction of blood cells than occurs in the normal spleen, particularly with respect to platelets [13]. This is particularly the case when disorders involving the red pulp are the cause of splenomegaly. However, functional hyposplenism may occur in patients whose spleens are of normal size.

Splenic Rupture

Rupture of the spleen may be divided into three types: traumatic, pathologic, and spontaneous. The three types overlap, because spleens involved by pathologic processes predispose the organ to rupture either spontaneously or secondary to trauma, particularly if they are greatly enlarged. Pathologic mechanisms by which spleens may become predisposed to rupture include infiltration and destruction of trabecular structures and capsule by reactive lymphoid cells [14], as in infectious mononucleosis, or by neoplastic cells, as in the leukemias. Rupture is also a complication of splenic infarction or may occur secondary to vascular embolization, vasculitis, septicemia, or blockage of splenic vessels by intrinsic splenic diseases. Rupture may also occur as a complication of nonhematopoietic tumors of the spleen, most notably metastatic neoplasms and malignant vascular tumors. Although traumatic rupture may occur in a normal spleen, in virtually all cases so-called spontaneous rupture occurs in a spleen with a (clinically undetected) pathologic process.

Pathologic conditions of the spleen can be divided basically into two categories: disorders of the red pulp and disorders of the white pulp. Although this is a useful subdivision, there are many overlaps. Disorders of the white pulp include both benign and malignant lymphoproliferative conditions. Disorders of the red pulp are associated with alterations in the cords and

Table 4. Disorders associated with hypersplenism

I. Disorders associated with sequestration of abnormal blood cells in an intrinsically normal spleen
    A. Congenital disorders of erythrocytes
        1. Hereditary spherocytosis
        2. Hereditary elliptocytosis
        3. Hemoglobinopathies, e.g., sickle cell disease, unstable hemoglobins
    B. Acquired disorders of erythrocytes
        1. Autoimmune hemolytic anemias
        2. Parasitic diseases, e.g., malaria, babesiosis
    C. Autoimmune thrombocytopenia
    D. Autoimmune neutropenia

II. Disorders of the spleen resulting in sequestration of normal blood cells
    A. Disorders of cordal macrophages
        1. Banti's syndrome
        2. Storage diseases
        3. Parasitic diseases, e.g., kala-azar
        4. Langerhans cell histiocytosis
        5. Infection-associated and familial hemophagocytic syndromes
        6. Malignant histiocytosis
    B. Infiltrative disorders
        1. Leukemias
        2. Lymphomas
        3. Plasma cell dyscrasias
        4. Myeloid metaplasia
        5. Chronic infections, e.g., tuberculosis, brucellosis
        6. Metastatic carcinoma
    C. Vascular abnormalities
        1. Vascular tumors
        2. Peliosis
    D. Splenic cysts
    E. Hamartomas

III. Miscellaneous Conditions
    A. Hyperthyroidism
    B. Hypogammaglobulinemia
    C. Progressive multifocal leukoencephalopathy

sinuses and are the most frequent ones associated with the clinical phenomenon of hypersplenism.

Gross examination of the spleen usually reveals one of three patterns. The first two represent diseases involving the white pulp. In one (Fig. 1), uniform expansion of the lymphoid tissue of the spleen occurs as a result of either a benign or malignant process. Examples include the so-called primary splenic lymphomas, low-grade malignant lymphomas of either B or T-cell type, and ITP. The second pattern, that of a single or few enlarged white pulp nodules (Fig. 2), is most frequently seen in Hodgkin's disease and in high-grade malignant lymphomas. All non-Hodgkin's lymphomas may involve the red pulp to a variable degree and some, particularly T-cell lymphomas, may involve the red pulp exclusively.

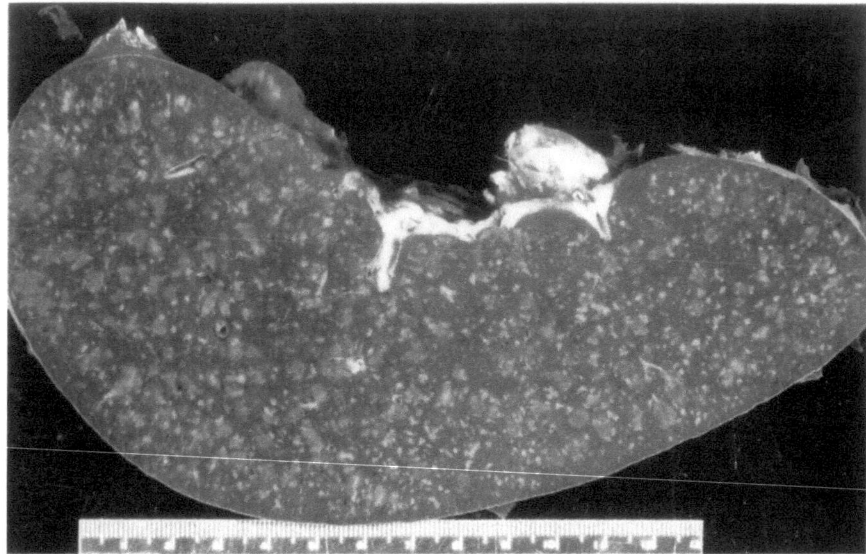

Fig. 1. Cross section of the spleen in a characteristic example of low-grade non-Hodgkin's lymphoma. Note the uniform involvement of all of the splenic white pulp causing a miliary pattern. This pattern is typical of low-grade non-Hodgkin's lymphomas and of systemic immune reactions involving the spleen

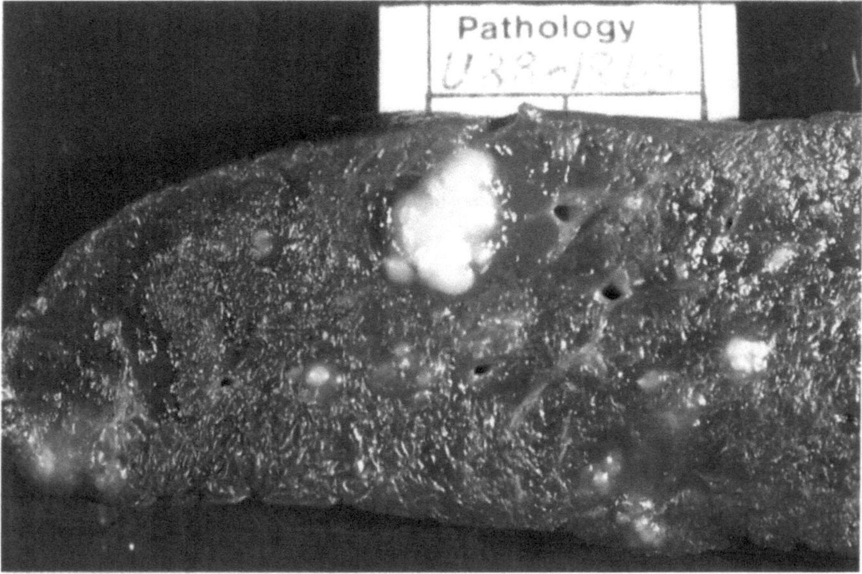

Fig. 2. Cross section of spleen in a case of malignant lymphoma, large cell type. In contrast to benign immunologic reactions and low-grade lymphomas, this pattern of involvement of the white pulp is characteristic of high-grade lymphomas and of Hodgkin's disease

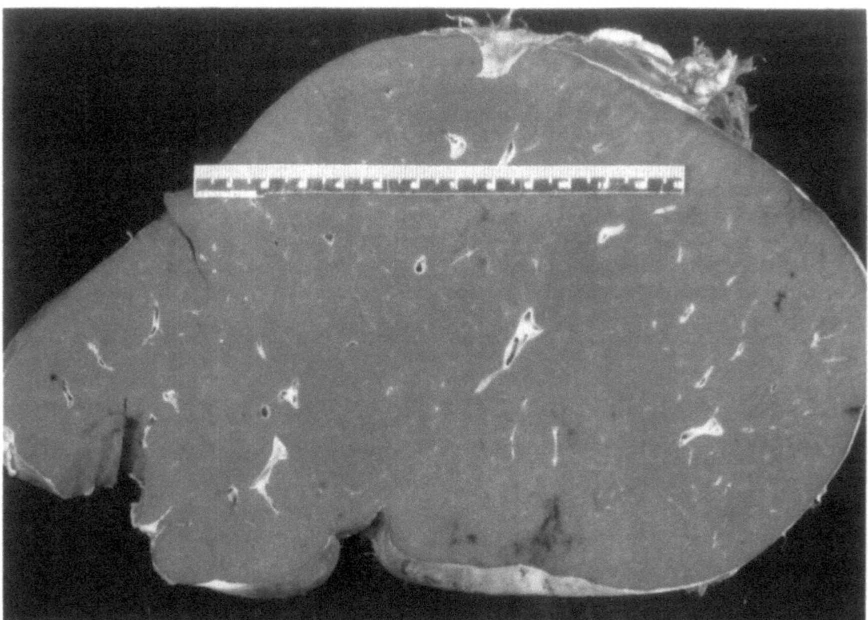

Fig. 3. Cross section of a greatly enlarged spleen in a patient with agnogenic myeloid meta-plasia removed because of hypersplenism. Note the relatively homogeneous character of the spleen with the loss of normal white pulp

The third pattern of involvement of the spleen is that of expansion of the red pulp, in which either reactive or infiltrative processes expand the cords and/or sinuses of the red pulp of the spleen with varying degrees of encroachment upon and atrophy of the white pulp (Fig. 3). Conditions corresponding to this pattern of involvement include leukemias, myeloproliferative disorders, and storage diseases.

Diseases of the White Pulp

We have divided splenic lymphoid tissue changes into seven types (Table 5). The functional and morphologic status of the splenic white pulp depends upon the age of the patient, his or her immunologic status, and the administration of therapeutic agents that alter immune functions such as cytotoxic agents or corticosteroids. With very few exceptions, diseases involving the white pulp represent proliferations of lymphoreticular tissue. They may be benign or malignant and usually are part of a systemic process.

The normal spleen in the pediatric age group contains white pulp that displays secondary germinal centers, a reflection of the heightened immunologic status of children and their almost constant exposure to antigens not pre-

Table 5. Types of splenic white pulp

I.   Inactive of hypoplastic – small lymphocytes
II. Early activated – small and large lymphocytes and immunoblasts
III. Evolving activated – germinal centers with marginal zones and perivascular plasma cells
IV. Granulomatous (histiocytic)
V.   Lymphomatous – monomorphous proliferation of small or large lymphocytes without germinal centers
VI. Hodgkin's disease – pleomorphic proliferation of lymphoreticular cells with Reed-Sternberg cells or their variants
VII. Dysproteinemic – lymphocytes, plasmacytoid lymphocytes and plasma cells and their precursors

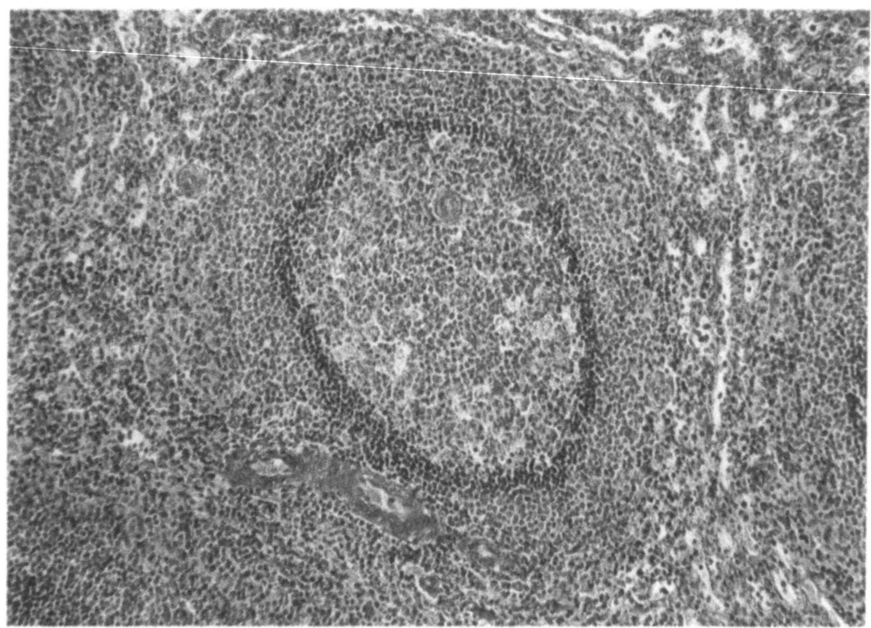

Fig. 4. Photomicrograph of splenic white pulp showing the characteristic features of the evolving activated immune response. There is a tripartite germinal center composed of a central area of follicular B lymphocytes, a dark outer mantle zone, and a lighter peripheral marginal zone. This pattern is characteristic in the pediatric age group and is also typical of the spleen in older patients who have immune reactions such as autoimmune disorders. PAS stain original magnification, ×100

viously encountered by their immune systems (Fig. 4). In adult life these germinal centers are usually smaller and less frequent and are usually only present in the acute phases of systemic immunologic reactions such infections or autoimmune disorders. Atrophy of the white pulp (Fig. 5) is usually associated with immunosuppression, cytotoxic drugs, or radiotherapy. However, it may be seen less frequently in the pediatric age group in congenital

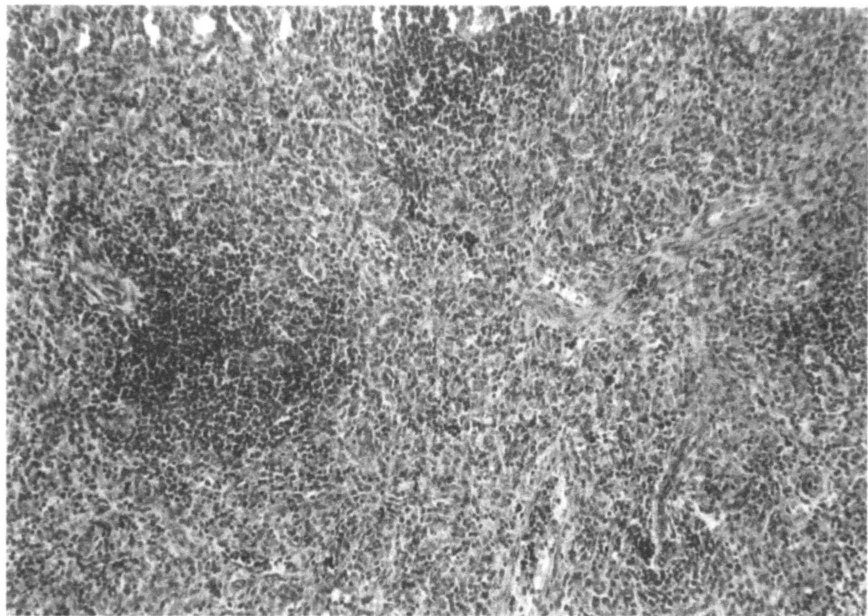

Fig. 5. Photomicrograph of cross section of spleen in a stillborn infant. The splenic white pulp displays no evidence of secondary germinal center formation. This picture is also characteristic of spleens in elderly patients. H&E stain original magnification, ×50

immunodeficiency. With increasing age the white pulp atrophies, in parallel with the decreased immunologic potential of older patients; and is a major factor in the shrinkage of that organ in senescence [3]. Activated germinal centers in spleens in the geriatric age are almost always abnormal but may represent a physiologic and self-limited response to antigen.

Activated Immune Response

The evolution of the immune response in human spleens has not been well studied, but has been assumed to be similar to that in experimental animals, which have been more closely observed. We have divided the morphologic features of the immune reaction arbitrarily into two categories: the early activated and evolving activated phases [15] (Table 6). The early activated phase is exemplified by the changes seen in infectious mononucleosis. In that disorder, immunologic activation occurs in the splenic white pulp as a manifestation of blood-borne antigen which is trapped in that organ. In this group of diseases lymphocytes in all stages of transformation are seen in the white pulp and along the trabeculae of the spleen, as well as surrounding penicilliary arterioles (Fig. 6). Secondary germinal centers are usually not present, but the white pulp may still be expanded. Spleens are generally enlarged but

Table 6. Types of splenic white pulp: activated

I. Early activated – small and large lymphocytes and immunoblasts
   A. Infectious mononucleosis
   B. Herpes simplex
   C. Other viral diseases (Korean epidemic hemorrhagic fever)
   D. Graft rejection
   E. Anti-lymphocyte serum (? B-cell stimulation)
   F. Corticosteroid – treated evolving immune responses (ITP, AIHA)

II. Evolving activated – germinal centers and perivascular plasma cells
   A. The norm in children and young adults
   B. ITP
   C. AIHA
   D. Felty's syndrome (rheumatoid arthritis)
   E. Systemic lupus erythematosis
   F. Chronic uremia with hypersplenism (hemodialyzed)
   G. Viral hepatitis
   H. Many systemic infections and chronic inflammatory states

ITP, immune thrombocytopenic purpura; AIHA, antibody-induced hemolytic anemia.

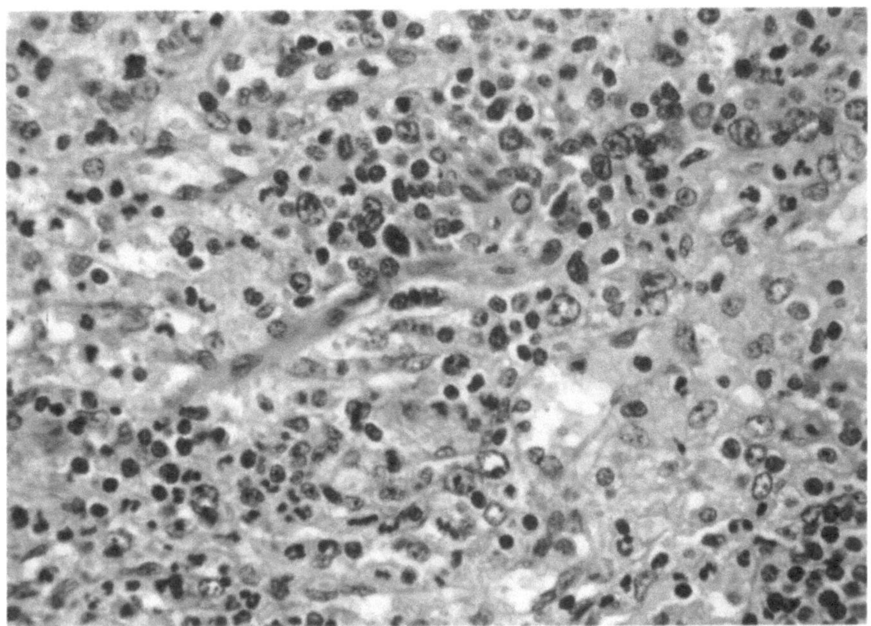

Fig. 6. Photomicrograph of a trabecular artery and vein adjacent to white pulp in a patient with infectious mononucleosis. There is a pleomorphic infiltrate of small lymphoid cells, plasma cells, and large transformed lymphocytes. Note that the lymphoid cells infiltrate the wall of the blood vessel. This cellular infiltration is thought to be the mechanism by which spleens are predisposed to rupture in infectious mononucleosis. PAS stain original magnification, ×400

usually not greatly so. The list of disorders causing early activation of the spleen is long and the reaction is not pathognomonic for one particular disease. Because this process represents part of a disseminated disorder and is frequently caused by a self-limited disease, diagnostic splenectomy is usually not performed in this stage of the immune reaction. However, because the lymphoid proliferation frequently infiltrates trabecular structures and the capsule of the spleen in this group of diseases, there is a tendency for so-called spontaneous rupture to occur and splenectomy is frequently required as an emergency procedure.

This is the most well recognized benign process of the white pulp of the spleen and is characteristic of a wide variety of systemic immune reactions. It is identical in its morphologic features and its etiology to the follicular hyperplasia of lymph nodes but differs from that condition in that it represents an immune reaction to systemic blood-borne antigen as opposed to the regional antigen causing follicular hyperplasia in lymph nodes. This process may be seen in a host of both self-limited and autoimmune processes and is perhaps most characteristically seen in untreated ITP. In this group of disorders, the white pulp demonstrates secondary germinal center formation with frequent tingible-body macrophages, with well-defined mantle and marginal zones surrounding the center (Fig. 4). Plasmacytosis in the red pulp and around penicilliary arteries is also noted. This morphologic picture is physiologic in children and young adults and represents the heightened immunologic status of young patients and is not necessarily evidence of any pathologic process. However, in patients over the age of approximately 30 years, it represents a reaction to antigen.

Granulomas of the Spleen

Three types of granulomas may involve the spleen (Table 7). The first are those associated with infectious diseases such as fungal and mycobacterial organisms. These granulomas may occur anywhere in the red or white pulp and appear morphologically indistinguishable from granulomas caused by similar organisms elsewhere in the body.

The second type of granuloma is presumed to be associated with altered immune function and resembles the granulomas of sarcoidosis (Fig. 7). These lesions have been reported in malignant lymphoma, Hodgkin's disease, chronic uremia, sarcoidosis, and IgA deficiency [16]. They always occur in close apposition to the afferent arterioles of the splenic white pulp and are not caused by infectious agents. It is thought that they represent an altered immune reaction in patients with an underlying disorder associated with T-cell abnormalities [16].

The third form of granuloma is the lipogranuloma, an incidental finding, usually associated with the white pulp and of little clinical significance. The etiology of lipogranulomata is not known, but they have no clinical significance.

Table 7. Granulomatous disorders of the spleen

I.   Infectious granulomas
      A. Bacterial
         1. Catalase-producing organisms (chronic granulomatous disease)
         2. Mycobacterial infection
            a. Tuberculosis
            b. Leprosy
            c. Atypical mycobacterial
         3. Tularemia
         4. *Yersinia*
         5. Tertiary syphilis
         6. Brucellosis
      B. Fungal
         1. Histoplasmosis
         2. Blastomycosis
         3. Coccidioidomycosis
         4. Sporotrichosis
      C. Protozoal
         1. Toxoplasmosis
         2. *Pneumocystis carinii*
         3. Leishmaniasis (kala-azar)
      D. Schistosomiasis

II.   Granulomas associated with altered immune function
      A. Sarcoidosis
      B. Hodgkin's disease
      C. Malignant lymphomas
      D. Chronic uremia
      E. Combined immunodeficiency
      F. Selective IgA deficiency

III. Lipogranulomas

Malignant Lymphomas

All histologic subtypes of malignant lymphoma may involve the spleen. In the vast majority of cases, splenic involvement is part of a disseminated process. However, there is a clinical entity that has been referred to as primary splenic lymphoma or malignant lymphoma presenting with massive splenomegaly, in which the spleen is the primary or only organ of involvement. It is probable that these cases were once included under the heading of nontropical splenomegaly syndrome [17], and many of theses cases were formerly misdiagnosed as hairy-cell leukemia [18]. This clinical presentation of malignant lymphoma is thought to include several variants of low-grade B-cell lymphoma of the mantle cell or marginal zone cell type [19]. Because some cases may present with circulating abnormal cells that superficially resemble hairy cells, they have also been termed splenic lymphoma with villous lymphocytes by clinical hematologists [20]. All low-grade lymphomas involve the spleen in a miliary pattern, representing the relatively uniform involvement of all splenic white pulp (Fig. 1). The pattern of splenic involvement in these

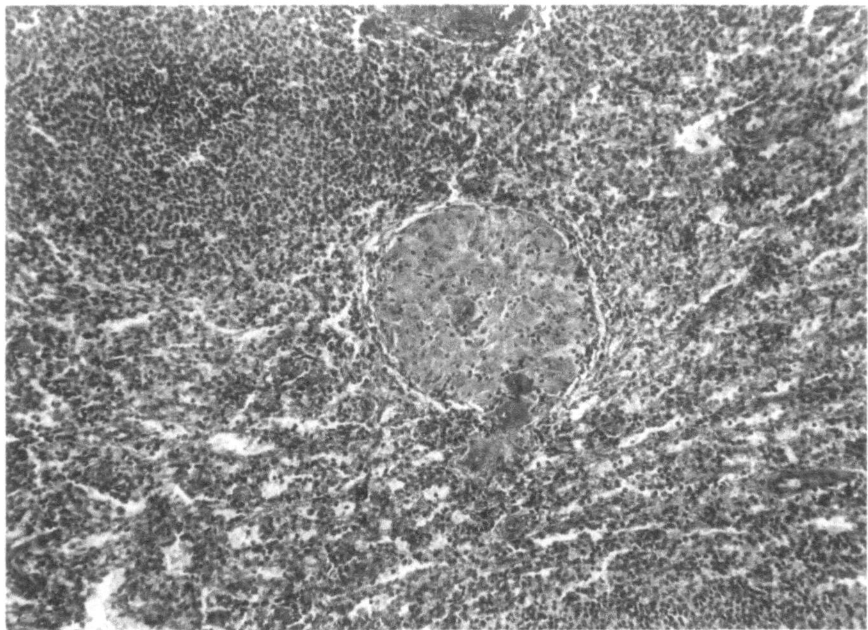

Fig. 7. Photomicrograph of a noncaseating sarcoid-like granuloma in a spleen obtained from a staging laparotomy in a patient with Hodgkin's disease. These granulomas are not infectious. PAS stain original magnification, ×100

cases is often very subtle and frequently requires immunologic or molecular techniques to confirm the diagnosis. Recently, marginal zone cell lymphomas involving the spleen have been described in patients with no splenomegaly [21]. The diagnosis is made incidently because of traumatic rupture or because of splenectomy for unrelated causes. Although so-called primary splenic lymphomas presenting with significant splenomegaly usually have evidence of disseminated disease upon careful staging, the primary lymphomas with no splenomegaly are usually confined to that organ.

Rarely, high-grade malignant lymphomas may involve the spleen exclusively [22, 23]. These present as isolated, single or few-tumor masses that are usually readily apparent by radiologic techniques. In the majority of cases, they represent large-cell or immunoblastic lymphoma.

Hodgkin's Disease

Staging laparotomy with splenectomy is less frequently performed in cases of Hodgkin's disease now than a decade or more ago because of the greater ability of noninvasive techniques to evaluate the spread of the disease and because of the development of new therapeutic modalities of combination chemotherapy. Since long-term survival using chemotherapy is now commonplace, it has replaced radiation therapy as the primary modality for treating Hodgkin's disease. As a result, there is less need to perform splenectomy as part of the workup for Hodgkin's disease.

The spleen is the most common extranodal site in Hodgkin's disease, being involved in approximately one third of cases. There is no correlation between splenic enlargement and the likelihood of involvement. All histologic subtypes of Hodgkin's disease have been reported to involve the spleen, but lymphocyte predominance is by far the rarest [24]. In all cases, splenic involvement by Hodgkin's disease may be detected by gross examination of serial slices of the removed spleen. However, splenic involvement may be very subtle and is easily missed if the organ is not meticulously examined (Fig. 8). Because of this fact, partial splenectomy in the staging of Hodgkin's disease is ill-advised.

Miscellaneous Lymphoproliferative Disorders

Under the heading of miscellaneous lymphoproliferative disorders are included a heterogeneous group of benign, malignant, and borderline

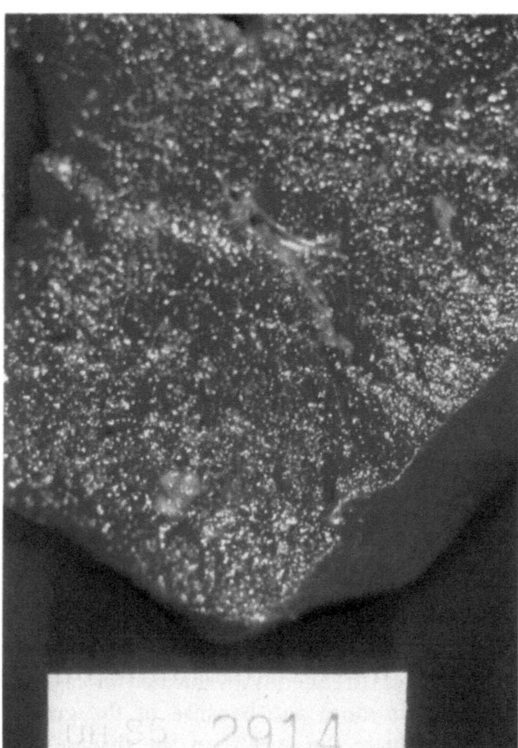

Fig. 8. Cross section of a spleen from a staging laparotomy for Hodgkin's disease. The white nodule near the bottom edge of the section was the only focus of Hodgkin's disease found in this case. Splenic involvement in Hodgkin's disease may be as subtle as this and requires careful examination by the pathologist

lymphoproliferative disorders. They include the heavy chain diseases, angioimmunoblastic lymphadenopathy, Castleman's disease, posttransplant lymphoproliferative disorders, lymphoproliferation in association with combined variable immunodeficiency, and the early stages of HIV infection. They may involve the spleen either in isolation or as part of a systemic process and may or may not produce splenomegaly. These disorders may involve either the red or the white pulp, or both. Because of the controversial nature of these conditions and the difficulty in characterizing them, fresh tissue is usually needed to perform immunologic, cytogenetic, and molecular genetic studies.

Disorders of the Red Pulp

Disorders of the red pulp include a wide variety of diseases, both benign and malignant, that have in common the expansion of the cords and/or sinuses (Table 8). They are most frequently associated with the clinical manifestations of hypersplenism. Hypersplenism may occur in association with any pathologic process in which the spleen becomes significantly enlarged because massive splenomegaly is associated with an increased percentage of total blood volume passing through the spleen [13, 25]. This increased infiltration fraction results in an increased percentage of total blood cells being sequestered (and destroyed) by the spleen. Although this may occur with any disorder causing significant splenomegaly, it is most characteristic in disorders which cause expansion of the red pulp, or, in the case of thrombocytopenia, with vascular tumors of the spleen. Hypersplenism may occur because of an intrinsic pathologic process within the spleen (example: hairy cell leukemia) or may occur because of an intrinsic abnormality in the circulating blood cells themselves (example: hereditary spherocytosis).

Nonneoplastic Disorders of Circulating Blood Cells

Among the nonneoplastic disorders of circulating blood cells are intrinsic diseases of red blood cells, white blood cells, and platelets in which the blood cell abnormality results in exaggerated sequestration and destruction of these cells by the spleen [26]. Foremost of these disorders is hereditary spherocytosis (Fig. 9). Other disorders with similar pathophysiology include hereditary elliptocytosis, the early splenomegalic phase of sickle cell disease, and autoimmune hemolytic anemias. Also included are autoimmune disorders involving granulocytes and platelets such as autoimmune neutropenia and ITP. The pathophysiology of splenic sequestration in essential thrombocythemia is similar. In all of these conditions, a hereditary or acquired abnormality of the circulating blood cell predisposes it to be preferentially se-

Table 8. The pathology of the red pulp

I. Expansion of cords of Billroth
   A. Because of pooling of abnormal blood cells in at least initially normal cords
      1. Hereditary spherocytosis
      2. Hereditary elliptocytosis
      3. Splenomegalic sickle cell disease
      4. Antibody-induced hemolytic anemia with significant spherocytosis
      5. Thrombocythemic states
   B. Widening of pulp cords because of proliferation of cordal macrophages
      1. Post blood transfusion
      2. Banti's syndrome
      3. Storage diseases
      4. Parasitic diseases, e.g. kala azar, malaria
      5. Langerhans cell histiocytosis
      6. Infection-associated and familial hemophagocytic syndromes
      7. Malignant histiocytosis
      8. Agnogenic myeloid metaplasia
   C. Widening of pulp cords because of infiltration by
      1. Inflammatory cells
      2. Malignant cells
         a. Hairy cell disease
         b. Chronic leukemias
         c. Acute leukemias
         d. Systemic mast cell disease
         e. Metastatic carcinoma (rare)
      3. Extramedullary hematopoiesis

II. Dilatation of the sinuses
   A. Because of congestion
      1. Passive congestion
      2. Hereditary (nonspherocytic) hemolytic anemias
      3. Homozygous hemoglobin C disease
      4. Some cases of antibody-induced hemolytic anemia
      5. Polycythemia vera
   B. Because of other factors
      1. Secondary (compensatory) extramedullary hematopoiesis
      2. Agnogenic myeloid metaplasia
      3. Metastatic carcinoma (occasionally)

III. Vascular tumors and miscellaneous conditions
     1. Hemangioma
     2. Hemangiosarcoma
     3. Inflammatory pseudotumor
     4. Peliosis

questered and destroyed in the spleen. The spleen itself is normal and maintains normal but heightened function.

In the case of hereditary spherocytosis, the abnormality is in the surface membrane of the red cell.

Spherocytes are less deformable than normal red cells, with the result that they lodge within the cords of the spleen and are unable to pass through the small pores between the sinus-lining cells. A similar mechanism applies with

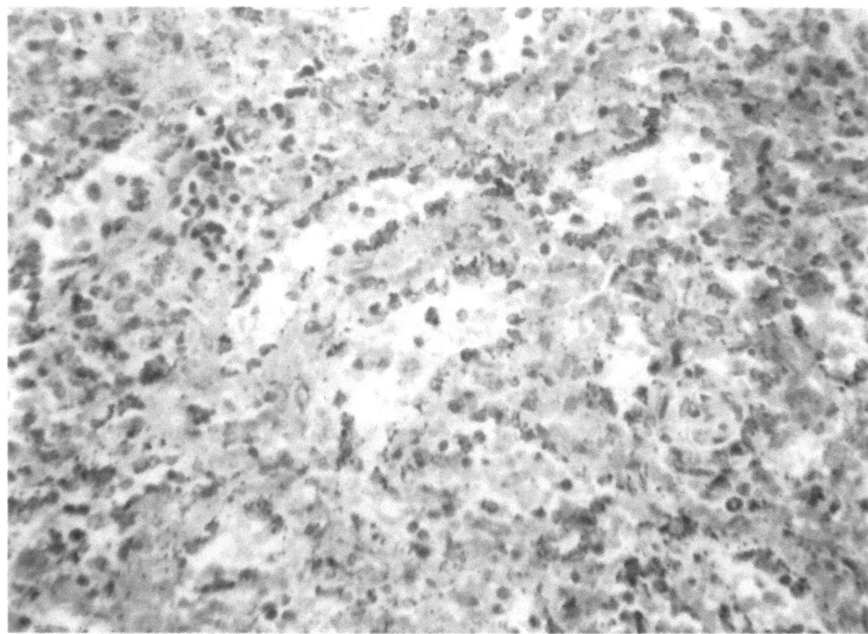

Fig. 9. Photomicrograph of splenic red pulp in hereditary spherocytosis. Note that the cords of Billroth are filled with spherocytic red cells and that the sinuses are relatively empty. The mechanical inability of red cells to deform in this condition is responsible for their retention and destruction in the spleen. H&E stain original magnification, ×100

elliptocytosis and sickle cell disease. In the case of red cells or white cells that are antibody-coated as in the autoimmune disorders, the antibody attached to the cell makes it recognizable by the spleen and it is removed from the circulation. In the case of essential thrombocythemia, the platelets are normally sequested in the spleen, but in that disorder the platelets are more sticky than normal platelets, with the result that they are filtered out in increased numbers (Fig. 10).

In the majority of these diseases, splenectomy is therapeutically beneficial because it removes the major source of accelerated cell destruction. However, it is not curative. In essential thrombocythemia, splenectomy is contraindicated because of the resultant increase in platelet count after splenectomy and the risk of thrombotic events.

Disorders of Cordal Macrophages

In this group of splenic disorders, the macrophages of the cords of Billroth proliferate either as a secondary reaction or because of a hereditary disorder. Splenic enlargement with resultant hypersplenism results from an increase of

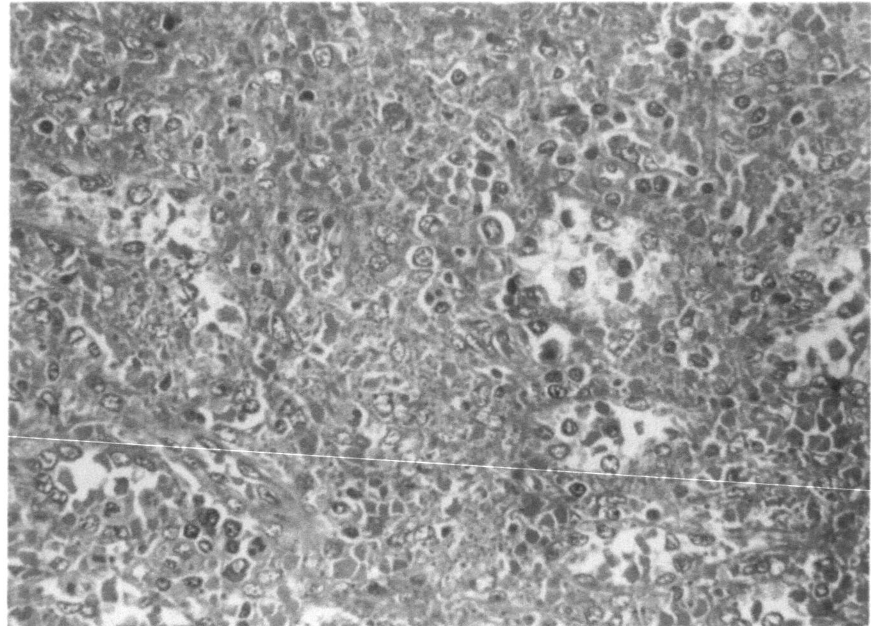

Fig. 10. Photomicrograph of splenic red pulp in a case of essential thrombocythemia. Note the masses of platelets retained in the cords. Epon embedded section, toluidine blue stain. Original magnification, ×400

the pool of splenic macrophages and expansion of the red pulp cords. Included in this group are storage diseases such as Gaucher's disease, Niemann-Pick disease, and ceroid histiocytosis [27] (Fig. 11). In addition, viral or infection-associated hemophagocytic syndrome also maybe placed in this category [28, 29].

Leukemias

All types of leukemias, whether acute or chronic, lymphoid or myeloid, may involve the spleen (Fig. 12). However, significant involvement is much less common in the acute leukemias than in the chronic leukemias. In all leukemic disorders, infiltration of both the cords and sinuses of the red pulp occurs. Splenectomy is usually not performed in leukemic disorders unless it is necessary for diagnosis or unless the patient becomes hypersplenic. The typical leukemic disorder associated with hypersplenism is hairy cell leukemia (Fig. 13). In this low-grade disorder of B lymphocytes, patients usually present with splenomegaly and pancytopenia. Splenectomy is frequently performed both for diagnostic purposes and to alleviate the blood cytopenias. Recently, advances in chemotherapy have rendered splenectomy in hairy cell

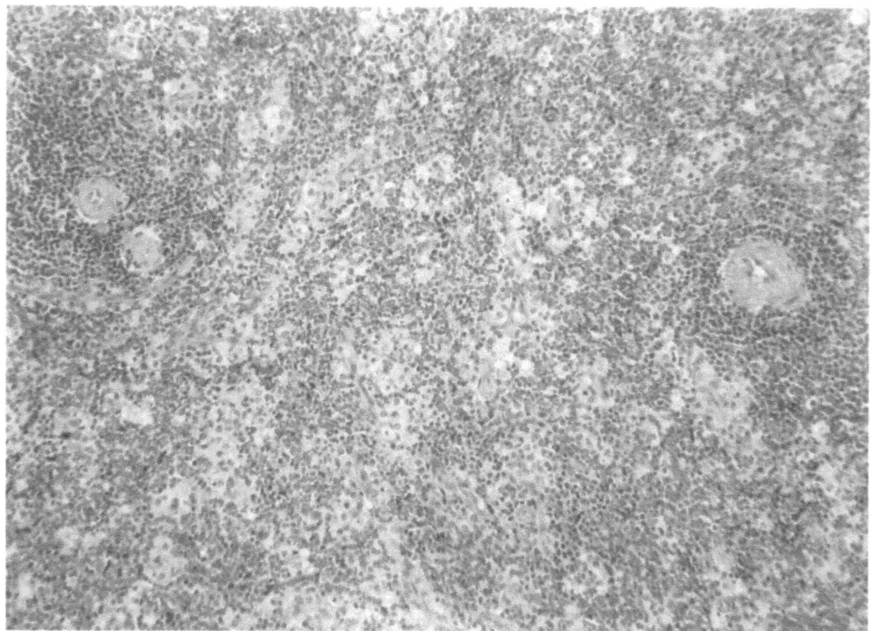

Fig. 11. Photomicrograph of spleen in ceroid histiocytosis. Note the numerous ceroid histiocytes in the red pulp. H&E stain, original magnification, ×100

leukemia less necessary. The advent of such therapeutic agents as interferon and 2-chlorodeoxyadenosine [30] have resulted in significant control of the disease without requiring splenectomy.

Early splenectomy in chronic myelogenous leukemia (CML) was once advocated as a method to prevent the development of extramedullary blast transformation [31, 32]. However, several studies of early splenectomy in this disorder have shown no survival advantage [33, 34]. As a result, early splenectomy in CML is no longer performed. However, the spleen is frequently removed in patients with CML before bone marrow transplantation.

Myeloproliferative Disorders

The myeloproliferative disorders include polycythemia vera (PV), agnogenic myeloid metaplasia (or myelofibrosis with myeloid metaplasia) (AMM), essential thrombocythemia (ET), and chronic myelogenous leukemia (CML). The reasons for splenomegaly differ in each of these disorders. In the uncomplicated erythrocytotic phase of PV, the spleen is enlarged because of engorgement of the organ as part of the increased blood volume that occurs in this disorder [35]. In AMM, splenomegaly is due to the increasing numbers

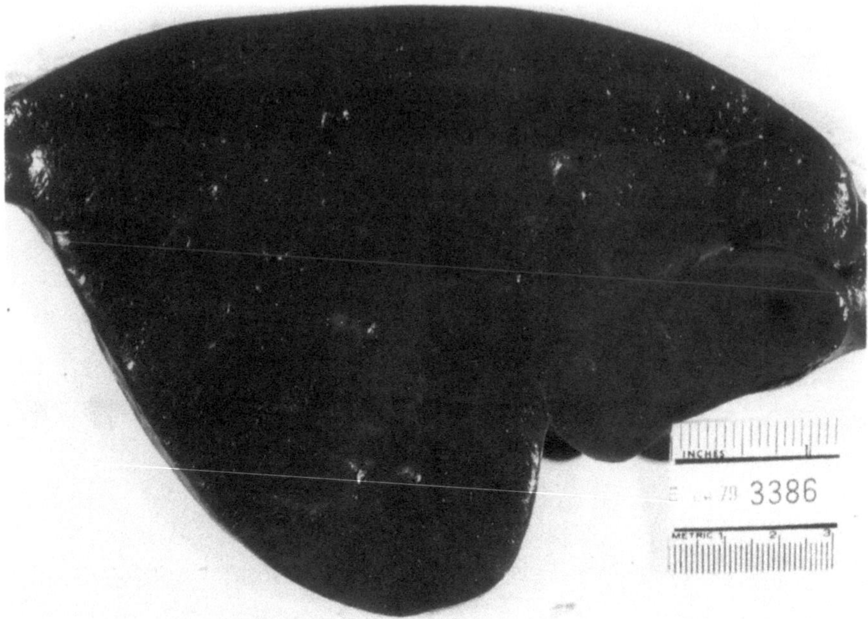

Fig. 12. Cross section of spleen in a case of hairy cell leukemia. Note the homogeneous appearance to the section and the loss of visible white pulp. This gross appearance is typical of all types of chronic leukemias

of hematopoietic precursor cells which gradually fill the spleen, causing progressive splenomegaly; as well as a secondary proliferation of cordal macrophages (Fig. 14). The pathology of CML has been discussed above. In ET, splenomegaly is due to sequestration of large numbers of platelets in the red pulp. As the disease progresses, the spleen becomes progressively atrophic because of infarction secondary to the platelet masses which obstruct vascular structures [36]. Splenectomy is contraindicated in both PV and ET and has been considered contraindicated in AMM because of the fear of postoperative infectious complications and because it was felt that the spleen was the only major source of hematopoietic cells in patients with a failing marrow [37]. It has been performed, however, in the later stages of AMM to alleviate progressive and massive enlargement of the spleen with resultant pain, hypersplenism, portal hypertension, and pressure symptoms [38, 39]. Splenic hematopoiesis in AMM appears to be quite ineffective and is usually greatly exceeded by splenic trapping and destruction of blood cells [40]. As a result in almost all cases, splenectomy results in increased blood cell counts.

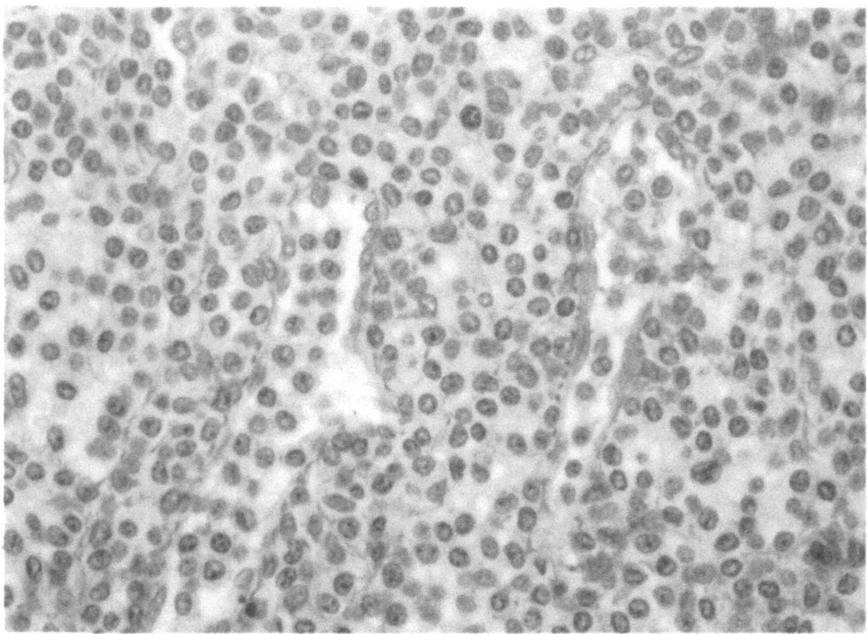

Fig. 13. Photomicrograph of spleen in hairy cell leukemia. The bland appearing leukemic cells infiltrate both cords and sinuses. PAS stain original magnification, ×250

Splenic Infarcts

Splenic infarcts can be generally divided into three types: thromboembolic, mechanical, and those relating to underlying splenic pathology. Because the splenic arterioles are end-arteries, thromboembolic phenomena are fairly common in the spleen. The underlying causes of thromboembolic infarcts include splenic vein thrombosis, portal hypertension, cardiac arrhythmias, and bacterial endocarditis. Also included in this group are infarcts secondary to splenic vasculitis and such conditions as disseminated intravascular coagulation. Mechanical causes of splenic infarction include torsion of the spleen, wandering spleen [41], and trauma. A number of hematologic conditions associated with marked splenic enlargement may also be associated with splenic infarction. These include chronic myeloid leukemia, AMM, and many of the acute and chronic leukemias, as well as the classic example of sickle cell disease.

Other conditions associated with splenic infarction are such conditions as vasculitis, which may either be infectious or associated with polyarteritis nodosa, thrombotic thrombocytopenic purpura, or leukoclastic angiitis [42].

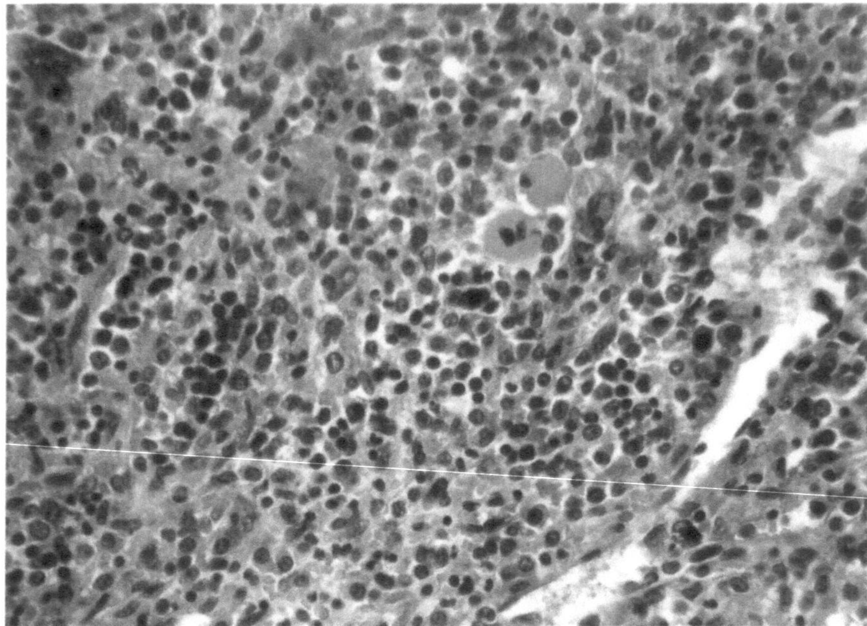

Fig. 14. Agnogenic myeloid metaplasia. Note the cluster of nucleated red blood cells, the megakaryocytes, and the occasional blastic cells (*center*), all manifestations of the trapping of the hematopoietic precursor cells that occur in this disease

Nonhematopoietic Tumors and Cysts

The group of nonhematopoietic disorders includes hemangiomas, hemangiosarcomas (Fig. 15), hamartomas (Fig. 16), and a variety of cysts. Hemangiomas are the most common tumors in the spleen, are usually small and asymptomatic, and are noted incidentally. On occasion, however, they may be large and result in thrombocytopenia, pain, hemorrhage, or even splenic rupture. Their incidence is thought to be about 10% [43].

Hemangiosarcomas may display a wide variety of cytologic differentiation. As a result some have used the term hemangioendothelioma to describe vascular tumors of the spleen that appear more clinically aggressive than hemangiomas, but do not display significant cellular atypia. Use of the term hemangioendothelioma is confusing, however, for it appears that there is little correlation between the degree of cellular atypia and the biologic behavior of hemangiosarcomas. Accordingly, it is preferable to merely use the term hemangiosarcoma.

Hamartomas, cysts, inflammatory pseudotumors, and peliosis are all infrequent disorders involving the spleen that usually require splenectomy for diagnosis. All of these disorders may cause hypersplenism if significantly large and may be associated with pain, bleeding, splenic infarction or rupture. As a result, splenectomy may be therapeutic as well as diagnostic in these disorders.

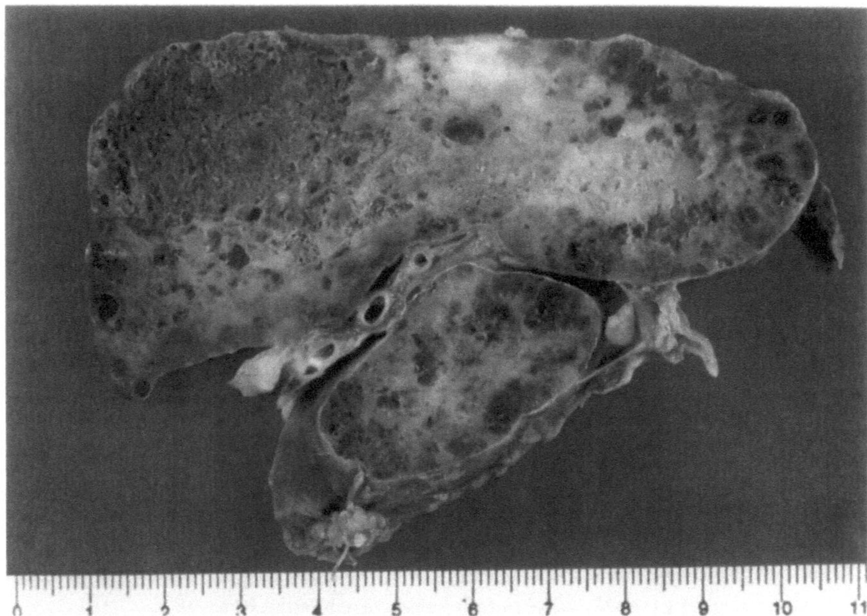

Fig. 15. Cross section of spleen in a case of hemangiosarcoma. Note the virtual total involvement of the organ with no clear-cut margins to the tumor

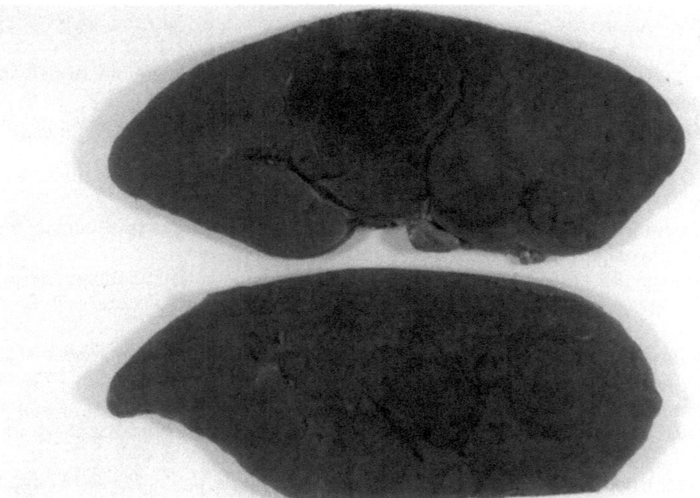

Fig. 16. Cross section of spleen showing two hamartomas. In contrast to hemangiomas and hemangiosarcomas, hamartomas have well-defined borders

Conclusion

The pathology of the spleen encompasses a wide variety of benign and malignant disorders. Although most are hematologic and are similar to those diseases occurring in other hematopoietic organs, many present unique challenges to the clinician and may require splenectomy with pathologic examination to confirm the nature of the disease. It is important for surgeons to recognize that prompt and effective processing of the spleen by the pathologist is frequently necessary in order to document the pathologic processes in that organ. Frequent communication between surgeon and pathologist is therefore necessary to best understand the pathologic processes involving the spleen.

Acknowledgment. I would like to thank Regina D. Bennett for her excellent secretarial support.

References

1. Myers J, Segal RJ (1974) Weight of the spleen. Arch Pathol 98:33–38
2. McCormick WF, Kashgarian M (1965) The weight of the adult human spleen. Am J Clin Pathol 43:332–333
3. Zago MA, Figueiredo MS, Covas DT, Bottura C (1985) Aspects of splenic hypofunction in old age. Klin Wochenschr 63:590–592
4. Ham AW (1963) The structure of the spleen. In: Blaustein A (ed) The spleen. McGraw-Hill, New York, p 1
5. Wadheim BM, Adams PB, Johnson MA (1981) Incidence and location of accessory spleens. N Engl J Med 304:222
6. Hassan MNR, Neiman RS (1985) The pathology of the spleen in steroid treated immune thrombocytopenic purpura. Am J Clin Pathol 84:433
7. Fleming CR, Dickson ER, Harrison EG Jr (1976) Splenosis. Autotransplantation of splenic tissue. Am J Med 61:414
8. Brewster DC (1973) Splenosis. Report of two cases and review of the literature. Am J Surg 126:14
9. Wolf, BC, Luevano E, Neiman RS (1983) Evidence to suggest that the human fetal spleen is not a hematopoietic organ. Am J Clin Pathol 80:140–144
10. Wolf BC, Neiman RS (1985) Myelofibrosis with myeloid metaplasia: pathophysiologic implications between bone marrow changes and progression of splenomegaly. Blood 65:803- 809
11. Wolf BC, Neiman RS (1987) Hypothesis – splenic filtration and the pathogenesis of extramedullary hematopoiesis in agnogenic myeloid metaplasia. Hematol Pathol 1:77–80
12. Casper TJ, Koethe SM, Rodey GE, Thatcher LG (1976) A new method for studying reticuloendothelial dysfunction in sickle cell disease patients and its clinical application: a brief report. Blood 47:183–185
13. Aster RH (1966) Pooling of platelets in the spleen: role in the pathogenesis of "hypersplenic" thrombocytopenia. J Clin Invest 45:645–657
14. Barnard H, Dreef EJ, van Krieken JH (1990) The ruptured spleen. A histological, morphometrical and immunohistochemical study. Histol Histopathol 5:299–304
15. Wolf BC, Neiman RS (1989) Disorders of the spleen, vol 20: major problems in pathology. Saunders, Philadelphia, chap 5, pp 55–63
16. Neiman RS (1977) The incidence and significance of splenic sarcoid-like granulomas. Arch Pathol Lab Med 101:518–521

17. Dacie JV, Brain MC, Harrison CV (1969) Non-tropical idiopathic splenomegaly (primary hypersplenism). A review of ten cases and their relationship to malignant lymphomas. Br J Haematol 17:317–333
18. Neiman RS, Sullivan AL, Jaffe R (1979) Malignant lymphoma simulating leukemic reticuloendotheliosis. A clinicopathologic study of ten cases. Cancer 43:329–342
19. Narang S, Wolf BC, Neiman RS (1985) Malignant lymphoma presenting with prominent splenomegaly: a clinicopathologic study with special reference to intermediate cell lymphoma. Cancer 55:1948–1958
20. Melo JV, Hedge U, Parreira A, Thompson I, Lampert IA, Catovsky D (1987) Splenic B cell lymphoma with circulating "villous" lymphocytes: differential diagnosis with B cell leukemia with a large spleen. J Clin Pathol 40:642–651
21. Rosso R, Neiman RS, Paulli M, Boveri E, Kindl S, Magrini U, Barosi G (1994) Splenic marginal zone cell lymphoma. Report of an indolent variant without massive splenomegaly presumably representing an early phase of the disease. Hum Pathol 26:39–46
22. Harris NL, Aisenberg AC, Myer JE, Ellman L, Elman A (1984) Diffuse large cell (histocytic) lymphoma of the spleen. Clinical and pathologic characteristics of ten cases. Cancer 54:2460–2467
23. Stroup RM, Burke JS, Sheibani K, Ben-Ezra J, Brownell M, Winberg CD (1992) Splenic involvement by aggressive malignant lymphomas of B-cell and T-cell types. A morphologic and immunophenotypic study. Cancer 69:413–420
24. Kadin ME, Glatstein E, Dorfman RF (1971) Clinicopathologic studies of 117 untreated patients subjected to laparotomy for the staging of Hodgkin's disease. Cancer 27:1277–1294
25. Aster RH (1966) Pooling of platelets in the spleen: role in the pathogenesis of "hypersplenic" thrombocytopenia. J Clin Invest 45:645–657
26. Wolf BC, Neiman RS (1989) Disorders of the spleen, vol 20: major problems in pathology, chap 10. Saunders, Philadelphia, pp 115–128
27. Wolf BC, Neiman RS (1989) Disorders of the spleen, vol 20: major problems in pathology, chap 11. Saunders, Philadelphia, pp 129–143
28. Risdall RJ, McKenna RW, Nesbit ME et al (1979) Virus-associated hemophagocytic syndrome. A benign histiocytic proliferation distinct from malignant histiocytosis. Cancer 44:993
29. Risdall RJ, Brunning RD, Hernandez JI, Gordon DH (1984) Bacteria-associated hemophagocytic syndrome. Cancer 54:2968
30. Spiers ASD, Moore D, Cassileth PA et al (1987) Remissions in hairy-cell leukemia with Pentostain (2'-deoxycoformycin). N Engl J Med 316:825
31. Spiers ASD, Baikie AG, Galton DAG et al (1975) Chronic granulocytic leukemia: effect of elective splenectomy on the course of disease. Br Med J 1:175–179
32. Hester JP, Waddell CC, Coltman CA et al (1982) Response of chronic myelogenous leukemia patients to COAP-splenectomy. A Southwest Oncology Group Study. Cancer 54:1977–1982
33. Medical Research Council's Working Party for Therapeutic Trials in Leukemia (1983) Randomized trial of splenectomy in Ph positive chronic granulocytic leukemia including an analysis of prognostic factors. Br J Haematol 54:415–430
34. Italian Cooperative Study Group on CML (1984) Results of a prospective randomized trial of early splenectomy in CML. Cancer 54:333–338
35. Wolf BC, Banks PM, Mann RB, Neiman RS (1988) Splenic hematopoiesis in polycythemia vera: a morphologic and immunohistologic study. Am J Clin Pathol 89:69–75
36. Marsh GW (1966) The use of Cr-labeled heat damaged red cells to study spleen function. II. Splenic atrophy in thrombocythemia. Br J Haematol 12:167–171
37. Benbassat J, Penchas S, Ligumski M (1979) Splenectomy in patients with agnogenic myeloid metaplasia: an analysis of 321 published cases. Br J Haematol 42:207
38. Brenner B, Nagler A, Tatarsky I, Hashmonai M (1988) Splenectomy in agnogenic myeloid metaplasia and post-polycythemic myeloid metaplasia. A study of 34 cases. Arch Intern Med 148:2501–2505

39. Benbassat J, Gilon D, Penchas S (1990) The choice between splenectomy and medical treatment in patients with advanced myeloid metaplasia. Am J Hematol 33:128–155
40. Beguin Y, Fillet G, Bury J, Fairon Y (1989) Ferrokinetic study of splenic erythropoiesis: relationships among clinical diagnosis, myelofibrosis, splenomegaly and extra-medullary erythropoiesis. Am J Hematol 32:123–128
41. Buehner M, Baker MS (1992) The wandering spleen. Surg Gynecol Obstet 4:373–378
42. Wolf BC, Neiman RS (1989) Disorders of the spleen, vol 20: major problems in pathology, chap 15. Saunders, Philadelphia, pp 180–188
43. Husni EA (1961) The clinical course of splenic hemangioma with emphasis on spontaneous rupture. Arch Surg 83:681–688

The Spleen in Infection and Immunity

E. R. STIEHM and MARY WAKIM

> "We must ... look upon the spleen as the great blood filter, purifying the blood in its passage by taking up particles of foreign matter."
> *Galen*, Second Century A.D.

The spleen is to the circulatory system what the lymph nodes are to the lymphatic system. The spleen filters infectious particles and unwanted cells from the bloodstream, is a storage site for blood elements, and initiates immune responses, including the production of immunoglobulin. This chapter will review the anatomy and function of the spleen and discuss the increased susceptibility to infection that occurs with conditions of splenic deficiency.

History

The spleen has been an organ of intrigue and fascination since ancient times. Hippocrates thought it was the source of black bile and melancholy [22]. Galen thought that it filtered humors from the liver and blood and that it was the source of good humor or bad disposition [22].

Splenectomy via cauterization with a hot iron was performed in ancient Greece to enhance athletic performance [26]. Splenectomy has been used since the sixteenth century as a therapeutic treatment of certain medical conditions [26]. In 1952, case reports of overwhelming bacterial infections in patients who had undergone splenectomy began to appear in the literature [13]. Studies of multiple patients followed which demonstrated the danger of overwhelming infection following splenectomy [7, 8, 10, 11, 18, 20, 25–27]. The usual organisms were *Streptococcus pneumoniae* or *Haemophilus influenzae*. Death often is extremely rapid and associated with adrenal hemorrhage. The syndrome of congenital asplenia (Ivemark syndrome) with rapid death was first identified in children with asplenia and congenital heart disease [12]. Splenic insufficiency in sickle cell disease was recognized in 1973 [13] and subsequently has been identified in many other conditions.

Development

Agenesis of the spleen results from damage to the fetus at approximately 30 days of age. At birth, the spleen is deficient in lymphatic components and functional activity; Howell-Jolley and Heinz bodies are regularly found circulating in the newborn peripheral circulation. By 12 months of age, the spleen reaches its maximum size relative to total body weight and has completed its histological differentiation [11]. Spleen size reaches 150 g by early adulthood and then decreases to approximately 100 g in the elderly. Blood flow to the normal spleen is about 3%–4% of the cardiac output (150 ml/min).

Anatomy

The spleen's anatomical structure contributes to its multiple functions. Unlike some animals, the human splenic capsule contains little smooth muscle tissue and contractile ability. The spleen is comprised of white and red pulp. The white pulp contains central arteries surrounded eccentrically by collars of T and B lymphocytes, termed periarteriolar lymphatic sheaths. During antigenic stimulation, these lymphatic sheaths expand to germinal centers and B cell-containing lymphoid nodules [12, 21]. The reticular network of the periarticular sheath traps antigens, permitting them to contact effector lymphocytes [21]. When the quantity of antigen is small, the spleen can concentrate the antigen to provide a high-density stimulus [26].

The red pulp is traversed by numerous thin-walled vascular sinusoids for blood storage. These sinusoids are lined by spleen cells, containing MAd-CAM-1, an adhesion molecule involved in lymphocyte homing, which is expressed on high endothelial venules of Peyer's patches and mesenteric lymph nodes. Lymphocytes migrate from these sites into the white pulp passing through this rim of cells [14]. Within the red pulp are splenic cords, a sponge-like labyrinth of macrophages loosely connected by dendritic processes that filter the blood and remove damaged and antibody-coated cells [21].

Function

The spleen is a major storage site for mononuclear phagocytic cells and platelets (red pulp) and lymphoid cells (white pulp). Lymphocyte and macrophage production normally occurs in the spleen, but this decreases with age. Splenic hematopoiesis normally stops before birth, but may recommence during periods of severe anemia.

Blood passage through the splenic cords results in the removal of unwanted cells and intracellular inclusions. Bacteria, particularly encapsulated organisms, are also removed by the spleen, and this is probably the first site of a primary immunologic response to these organisms. Splenic trapping is particularly important when antibody levels are low or absent, such as in newborns and young infants who lack opsonins. The spleen has greater phagocytic activity per gram of tissue than the liver [26].

Tuftsin, a tetrapeptide that stimulates phagocytic cells and enhances macrophage antigen-specific education of T lymphocytes, is either produced or activated in the spleen. It is a Thr-Lys-Pro-Arg amino acid sequence present in the Fc fragment of the heavy chain of the immunoglobulin molecule. Liu and coworkers [17] postulate that tuftsin also kills tumor cells and inhibits tumor growth.

Splenic phagocytic cells remove aged red cells and particles from the bloodstream as they circulate slowly through the spleen. The spleen is also the site of removal of blood cells coated with IgG and IgM antibody, probably because their interaction with Fc receptors can only occur when circulation is slowed. Damaged or malformed red cells are also removed because they are less deformable and therefore cannot pass through the slits between the endothelial cells of the splenic sinuses.

The spleen enhances antibody and immunoglobulin synthesis. It is probably the first site of synthesis of antibody to encapsulated organisms. IgM synthesis is particularly enhanced, probably because the spleen provides a highly efficient environment for the differentiation of IgM-producing plasma cells [26]. Isotype switching from IgM to IgG also occurs in the spleen. Cyster [6] speculates that autoimmune antibody formation occurs preferentially in the spleen because of abnormal antigen presentation. In addition, it is believed that the spleen is a site of production of coagulation factor VIII [17].

T lymphocytes are taken up directly from the bloodstream because of the special vascular arrangement in the white pulp of the spleen. T cells which have been activated by antigen interact with the B cells in the splenic parenchyma. The spleen may also be a source of suppressor T cell activity. However, Ashsbaugh [1] showed that splenectomy did not impair suppressor T cell activity; thus this activity is not confined solely to the spleen. The spleen may be an important site for generation and/or maintenance of amplifier T cell activity [26].

The spleen may play a major role in thymic involution. In splenectomized animals, thymic weight does not change with age, while it decreases in non-splenectomized animals. Meyer and Meyer [19] speculated that the spleen creates a humoral factor that promotes involution of the thymus.

Deficiency of Splenic Function

Congenital asplenia is often associated with certain cardiac and visceral anomalies in the Ivemark syndrome. Transient hyposplenia (decreased splenic function) occurs in some preterm infants and some elderly patients with idiopathic splenic atrophy. Functional hyposplenia can also be demonstrated in association with a number of conditions, including adult celiac sprue, dermatitis herpetiformis, ulcerative colitis, active rheumatoid arthritis, glomerulonephritis, systemic lupus erythematosus, vasculitis, and Hodgkin's disease [26].

Immunological Results of Splenic Deficiency

Following splenectomy, there is a poor antibody response to particulate antigens, especially those administered intravenously [23]. In vitro IgM synthesis by peripheral blood mononuclear cells of splenectomized patients is diminished, but IgG production is normal. This decrease in B cell function may result from the loss of the intimate anatomical arrangement of macrophages, germinal centers, and marginal zone T cells which are seen in the intact spleen [29].

In splenectomized patients and patients with functional asplenia, opsonic activity and phagocytosis are impaired. Spirer reported that splenectomized children had normal complement levels and increased C3 levels [29]. Corry et al. found that 10% of patients splenectomized for trauma and 16% of sickle cell patients had deficient function of the alternate complement pathway [5].

There are important differences in animals with hereditary asplenia and those with splenectomy. In hereditary asplenic mice, there is absence of T and B cell cooperation because of incomplete differentiation of lymphoid cells [26]. Patients with congenital asplenia have normal levels of IgG, IgA, and IgM, but CD3, CD4, and CD4 to CD8 ratios are significantly decreased [29]. Lymphoproliferative responses to mitogens are also decreased, and Fc-mediated clearance of sensitized autologous erythrocytes is impaired. Decreased reticuloendothelial clearance and decreased T cell function probably play a role in the life-threatening infections that occur in some patients with congenital asplenia syndromes [29].

Infectious Results of Splenic Deficiency

The risk of sepsis is increased 40-fold after splenectomy even in normal subjects. The risk is even higher in splenectomized patients with underlying illnesses or those with congenital or acquired splenic deficiency (Table 1). *Streptococcus pneumoniae* accounts for 50%–75% of the infections. Other organisms causing infection in splenic deficiency, in decreasing order of frequency, are *Hemophilus influenzae, Neisseria meningitidis, β*-hemolytic streptococcus, *Staphylococcus aureus, Escherichia coli*, and pseudomonas. Herpes zoster infections can be severe in splenic deficiency, and parasitic diseases such as babesiosis and malaria may be seen.

Table 1. Relative risk of infection in splenic deficiency states

Risk	Condition
Low	Splenectomy in a normal child after age 10
	Splenectomy for non-malignant hematologic conditions (e.g., ITP, congenital hemolytic anemias)
	Post-traumatic splenectomy in an adult
Medium	Splenectomy in normal child before age 10
	Splenectomy in hemoglobinopathies (i.e., thalassemia)
	Splenectomy in malignant hematologic conditions (i.e., Hodgkin's disease)
	Splenic deficiency of sickle cell anemia
High	Congenital asplenia
	Ivemark syndrome
	Splenic deficiency of prematurity
	Splenectomy in primary or secondary immunodeficiency

ITP, idiopathic thrombocytopenic purpura.

Postsplenectomy infections are often fulminant, with high bacterial titers in the bloodstream. They may begin with mild upper respiratory tract infections and progress rapidly to overwhelming sepsis, often accompanied by disseminated intravascular coagulation. Death may occur within 6–24 h of the onset of symptoms. The occurrence of disseminated intravascular coagulation in postsplenectomy patients led to a study that showed that the generalized Shwartzman phenomenum could be induced at lower doses of endotoxin in splenectomized rabbits [26].

Treatment of Splenic Deficiency

Splenic function decreases progressively in patients with sickle cell disease; by the age of 8, most such patients have complete absence of splenic reticuloendothelial activity. The onset of episodes of bacterial septicemia usually correlates with the appearance of Howell Jolly bodies and rising number of pitted erythrocytes. The risk of serious infections in asplenic patients and those with sickle cell or sickle cell-hemoglobin disease is extremely high before 4–5 years and decreases with age. The risk of sepsis can be decreased by (a) continuous penicillin prophylaxis, particularly in patients less than 5 years of age; (b) pneumococcal and meningococcal vaccines for patients over 2 years of age; (c) provision and maintenance of routine immunizations at the recommended times beginning in infancy; and (d) early and aggressive treatment at the first sign of infection, particularly fever [9, 16].

Butler and coworkers [3] studied the use of pneumococcal polysaccharide vaccine in splenectomized subjects. The overall efficacy for prevention of infections caused by the serotypes included in the vaccine was 57%. In patients with no splenic tissue, the efficacy was 77% and did not decline over 5–

8 years after vaccination. Such patients also responded well to *H. influenzae* vaccination [15].

Penicillin prophylaxis is recommended for all asplenic and functionally asplenic children less than 5 years old. Compliance is improved by repeated warnings about the dangers of overwhelming fatal sepsis [2].

To decrease the likelihood of infection following splenectomy, alternative methods of treatment for certain diseases and avoidance of splenectomy following splenic trauma have been proposed. There is a lower infection rate after splenectomy secondary to trauma when compared to elective splenectomy for some underlying diseases such as idiopathic thrombocytopenic purpura (ITP), thalassemia, Hodgkin's disease, and others. Some splenectomized patients following trauma develop splenosis, or seeding of the peritoneal cavity with splenic fragments, possibly restoring splenic function. This led to the use of autotransplantation and partial splenectomy as a means of avoiding postsplenectomy complications. Szendroi implanted splenic slices between two layers of omental pouch ("Furka's spleen chip") [28]. Follow-up of ten such patients by radionuclide imaging, IgM levels, and tuftsin levels have shown functioning splenic tissue [28]. However, other authors have questioned the ability of splenic tissue that has been autotransplanted, partially resected, or treated by splenic artery ligation to function and protect against infection [4].

Recognition of the infectious risks of splenectomy has stimulated the development of nonoperative protocols for management of solid organ injury [24], as discussed in greater detail by Trunkey (this volume). Medical alternatives to splenectomy for certain disorders such as ITP are available, but in some illnesses splenectomy cannot be avoided.

Conclusion

The spleen's unique anatomical arrangement allows it to play a primary role in initiating the immune response, particularly antibody production, filtering and phagocytizing bacteria and aged red cells, and storage of blood products. Splenic absense, removal, or insufficiency increases the risk of overwhelming bacterial infection. Accordingly, prophylactic antibiotics, appropriate immunizations, and early aggressive treatment of infections are indicated.

References

1. Ashsbaugh D, Prescott B, Baker P (1978) Effect of splenectomy on the expression of regulatory T cell activity. J Immunol 121:1483–1485
2. Buchanan G, Siegel J, Smith S, DePasse B (1982) Oral penicillin prophylaxis in children with impaired splenic function: a study of compliance. Pediatrics 70:926–930

3. Butler J, Breiman R, Campbell J, Lipman H, Broome C, Facklam R (1993) Pneumococcal polysaccharide vaccine efficacy. JAMA 270:1826–1831
4. Clayer M, Drew P, Leong A, Jamieson G (1994) IgG mediated phagocytosis in regenerated splenic tissue. Clin Exp Immunol 97:242–247
5. Corry J, Polhill R, Edmonds S, Johnston R (1979) Activity of the alternate complement pathway after splenectomy: comparison to activity in sickle cell disease and hypogammaglobulinemia. J Pediatr 95:964–996
6. Cyster J, Goodnow C (1995) Pertussis toxin inhibits migration of B and T lymphocytes into splenic white pulp cords. J Exp Med 182:581–586
7. Dyke M, Martin R, Berry P (1991) Septicemia and adrenal haemorrhage in congenital asplenia. Arch Dis Childhood 66:636–637
8. Eraklis A, Filler R (1972) Splenectomy in childhood; a review of 1413 cases. J Pediat Surg 7:382–388
9. Falter M, Robinson M, Kim O, Go S, Taubkin S (1973) Splenic function and infection in sickle cell anemia. Acta Haematol 50:154–161
10. Gerwig M, Witt Kamper A, Liebetrau U, Petrovici JN (1994) Recurrent pneumococcal meningitis after splenectomy. Nervenarzt 65:722–724
11. Heier H (1980) Splenectomy and serious infections. Scand J Haematol 24:5–12
12. Ivemark B (1955) Implications of agenesis of the spleen on the pathogenesis of conotruncus anomalies in childhood: analysis of the heart malformations in spleen agenesis syndrome with fourteen new cases. Acta Paediatr 44 [Suppl]:1–110
13. King H, Schumacher H (1952) Splenic studies. 1. Susceptibility to infection after splenectomy performed in infancy. Ann Surg 136:239–242
14. Kraal G, Schornagel K, Streeter P, Holzman, Butcher E (1993) Expression of the mucosal vascular addressin, MAdCAM-1, on the sinus-lining cells in the spleen. Am J Pathol 147:763–771
15. Kristensen K (1994) Vaccination of splenectomized children, antibody response to haemophilus influenza type b conjugate vaccine. Ugeskr Laeger 156:191–193
16. Lane P (1995) The spleen in children. Curr Opin Pediatr 7:36–41
17. Liu D, Xia S, Tang J, Qin X, Liu H (1995) Allotransplantation of whole spleen in patients with hepatic malignant tumors or hemophilia A. Operative technique and preliminary results. Arch Surg 130:33–39
18. Meeks I, Vander Stark F, Van Oostrom C (1995) Results of splenectomy performed on a group of 91 children. Eur J Pediatr Surg 5:19–22
19. Meyer JA, Meyer JD (1978) Splenectomy and the thymic involution of increasing age. Arch Surg 113:972–975
20. Murdoch I, Anjos R, Mitchell A (1991) Fatal pneumococcal septicemia associated with asplenia and isomerism of the right atrial appendages. Br Heart J 65: 102–103
21. Robbins S, Cotran R, Kumar V (1984) Pathologic basis of disease. Saunders, Philadelphia, pp 697–703
22. Rosse W (1987) The spleen as a filter. New Engl J Med 317: 704–706
23. Rowley D (1950) The effect of splenectomy on the formation of circulating antibody on the splenectomized human being following intravenous injection of heterologous erythrocytes. J Immunol 65:515–521
24. Rutledge R, Hunt J, Lentz C, Fakhry S, Meyer A, Baker C, Sheldon G (1995) A statewide, population-based time-series analysis of the increasing frequency of nonoperative management of abdominal solid organ injury. Ann Surg 222:311–326
25. Singer D (1973) Postsplenectomy sepsis. In: Rosenberg HS, Bolande RP (eds) Perspectives in pediatric pathology, vol 1. Yearbook Medical, Chicago, pp 285–311
26. Spirer Z (1980) The role of the spleen in immunity and infection. Adv Pediatr 27:55–88
27. Styrt B (1990) Infection associated with asplenia: risks, mechanisms, and prevention. Am J Med 88:33N–42N
28. Szendroi T, Hajdu Z, Miko I, Baayo J, Bokk A, Barnak G, Furka I (1993) Autologous spleen transplantation. Orvos Hetilap 134:125–128
29. Wang J, Hseih K (1991) Immunologic study of the asplenia syndrome. Pediatr Infect Dis J 10:819–22

Spleen Imaging

M. S. KOMAIKO

"Anyone can learn to turn on an x-ray current, but it requires special training over a period of years to become an expert in the use of that valuable agent."
Franklin H. Martin, 1934

General Considerations

Prior to the advent of cross-sectional imaging modalities such as ultrasonography (US), computed tomography (CT), and magnetic resonance imaging (MRI), imaging of the spleen was limited primarily to plain film radiography, liver/spleen radionuclide scintigraphy, angiography, and splenoportography. Splenoportography is no longer performed, and arteriography is rarely used for diagnostic purposes. Liver/spleen scintigraphy is used primarily in the evaluation of patients with cirrhosis. CT and, to a lesser extent, US are the modalities of choice for splenic imaging. MRI is currently reserved for those cases unexplained by conventional US or CT studies [1, 2].

Imaging evaluation of the spleen may be required to determine the presence or absence of normal splenic tissue, to evaluate the clinically enlarged spleen, to determine the cause of the left upper quadrant discomfort, or to evaluate involvement of the spleen with adjacent as well as systemic pathologic processes.

Normal Anatomy

A detailed description of the normal anatomy is described elsewhere in this textbook. A length of 13 cm, AP diameters of 7 cm, and thickness of 4 cm are the upper limits of normal for splenic size. A more accurate means of determining splenic volume is the splenic index, which is the result of the product of the length, width, and height expressed in centimeters. This volume is normally not greater than 480 cm^3 [3].

The lateral surface of the spleen typically has a smooth or lobulated convex margin, and the hilar surface is usually concave [4]. Clefts and notches are frequent and, on occasion, may simulate splenic laceration (Fig. 1). The absence of an associated history of trauma and the lack of perisplenic fluid aid in making this distinction.

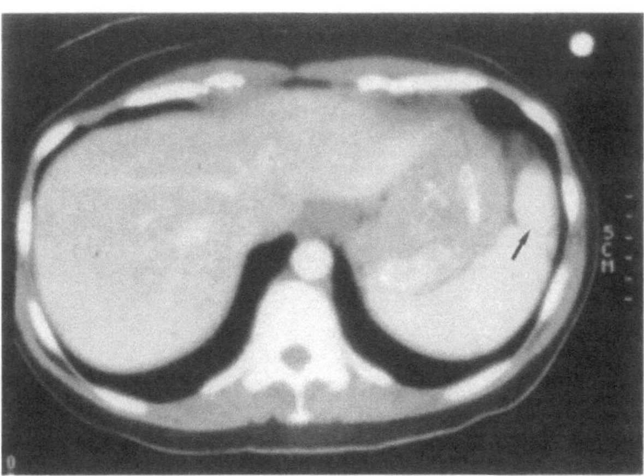

Fig. 1. Splenic cleft (*arrow*); a normal variant. Note absence of adjacent fluid

The parenchyma of the normal spleen appears uniform in density with US, MRI, and nonenhanced CT examinations. The CT attenuation values of the spleen without intravenous (i.v.) contrast enhancement are slightly less than that of the normal liver. However, with rapid i.v. infusion of iodinated contrast material, the splenic parenchyma may exhibit an inhomogeneous pattern of attenuation, which reflects variable blood flow within different compartments of the spleen. This appearance may mimic a focal or diffuse abnormality. Delayed images will confirm uniform enhancement if the spleen is normal. Miles et al. [5] demonstrated that transient splenic inhomogeneity is more pronounced in patients with liver disease. More subtle apparent abnormalities may also be seen in the normal liver with rapid i.v. infusion of contrast and inadequate delays in CT imaging. Therefore, imaging should be delayed at least 40 s from the onset of the rapid i.v. infusion (2–3 cc/s) of contrast, if this potential pitfall is to be avoided.

Congenital Variations

A pronounced degree of lobulation may occasionally mimic a mass on cross-sectional imaging, plain films, or i.v. pyelography (Fig. 2). Accessory splenic tissue is identified in approximately 10–30% of cases at autopsy, with the size varying from millimeters to several centimeters in diameter. Most frequently these are located within the hilar region of the spleen [6]. Accessory splenic tissue often enlarges after splenectomy and, if the location is atypical, may mimic a mass (Fig. 3). A liver/spleen radionuclide scan is a useful diagnostic test to confirm functioning splenic tissue in the region of concern [7].

Asplenia is associated with congenital absence of the spleen and bilateral right-sidedness, as well as numerous cardiac abnormalities. Polysplenia is associated with several splenculi within the abdomen and bilateral left-sidedness, as well as with numerous systemic vascular and cardiac abnormalities

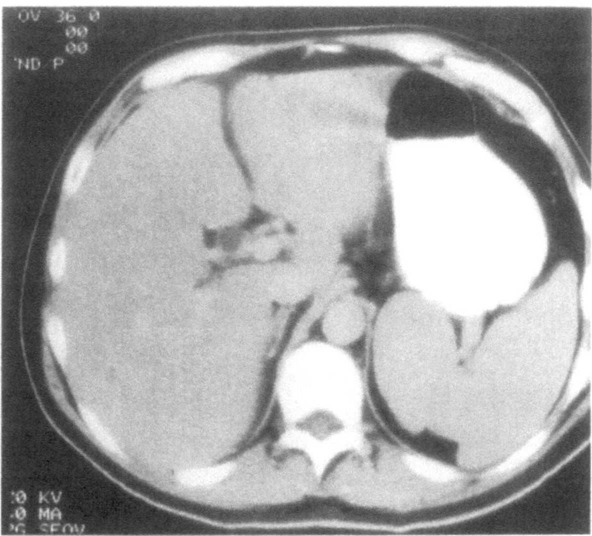

Fig. 2. Splenic lobulations; a normal variant

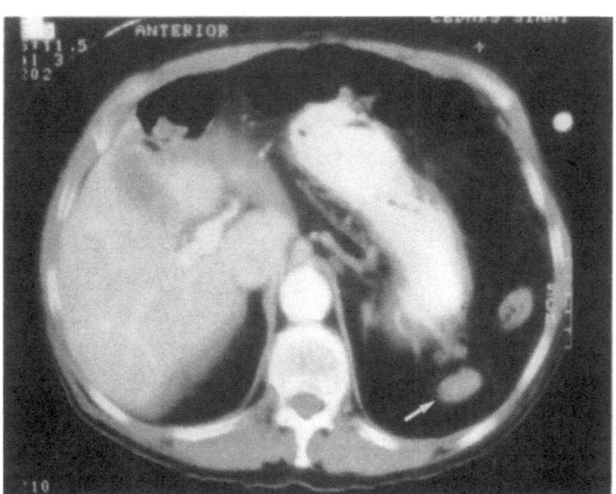

Fig. 3. Accessory splenic tissue (*arrow*) in a post-splenectomized patient

(Fig. 4). With both entities, the liver is often midline, with indistinct separation of its lobes. Interruption of the inferior vena cava with continuation of the cava through the azygous or hemiazygous venous systems may be present.

"Wandering spleen" refers to a normal spleen which is highly mobile, resulting in rotation to the center of the abdomen. This is due to a lack of fixed splenorenal attachments. Although most often discovered as an asymptomatic mass in the mid or lower abdomen, it may cause pain if associated with torsion. CT suggests the diagnosis if a mass is present within the mid or lower abdomen

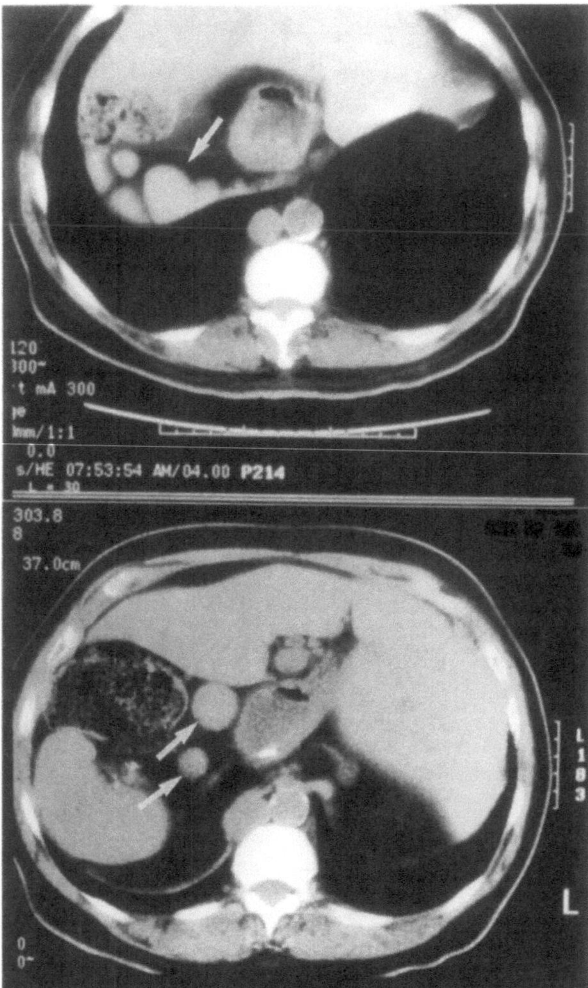

Fig. 4a,b. Polysplenia. Multiple splenculi (*arrows*) and situs inversus

and there is absence of splenic tissue within the anticipated left upper quadrant location. Cross-sectional imaging studies may also demonstrate splenic vessels coursing into this structure; in association with the lack of a spleen in its typical location, this would strongly suggest the diagnosis of wandering spleen [8, 9]. Nuclear scintigraphy with ^{99m}Tc sulfur colloid will provide a definitive diagnosis, presuming that torsion does not totally obstruct the arterial flow of a tracer into the organ. Because the pancreatic tail lies with the long splenic mesentery, it also may become involved when splenic torsion occurs.

Abnormalities of the Spleen

Splenomegaly

There are numerous etiologies of splenomegaly. Although the diagnosis of splenic enlargement is often apparent clinically, imaging modalities may be of value in confirming this impression. A specific cause of enlargement cannot be determined from plain films unless there is an associated systemic disease which results in bone changes, such as with hemolytic anemias. If the enlargement results from cirrhosis, associated portal hypertension with ascites, varices, and a colloid shift (liver/spleen scintigraphy) to the spleen and bone marrow may be seen [10]. Other common causes of splenomegaly include lymphoma, acquired immunodeficiency syndrome (AIDS), and chronic myelogenous leukemia (Fig. 5). Splenomegaly may occur in as many as 60% of patients with sarcoidosis, with the parenchyma appearing inhomogeneous following contrast infusion secondary to small nodular lesions. Spontaneous rupture of the spleen may occur as a complication of splenomegaly, especially in patients with mononucleosis or leukemia.

Splenic Calcification

Calcifications in the spleen are common, with old granulomatous disease representing the most frequent etiology. They are usually punctate and may be associated with calcifications in the lung and liver (Fig. 6). The character of the calcifications can assist in determining the diagnosis of splenic pathology. Linear or curvilinear calcifications are often vascular if located along the course of a splenic artery or within the splenic hilum. Similar calcifications within the spleen suggest calcification within the walls of a cyst or hematoma. A hydatid cyst may demonstrate characteristic wall calcification and intracystic components associated with daughter cysts.

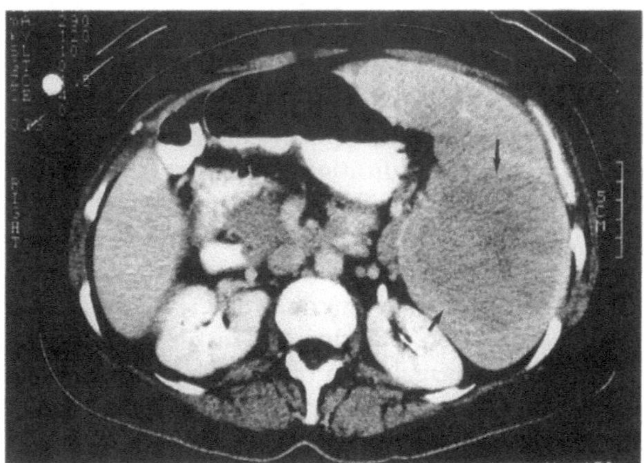

Fig. 5. Splenomegaly in a patient with lymphoma. A mass (*arrows*) secondary to focal lymphomatous involvement is present

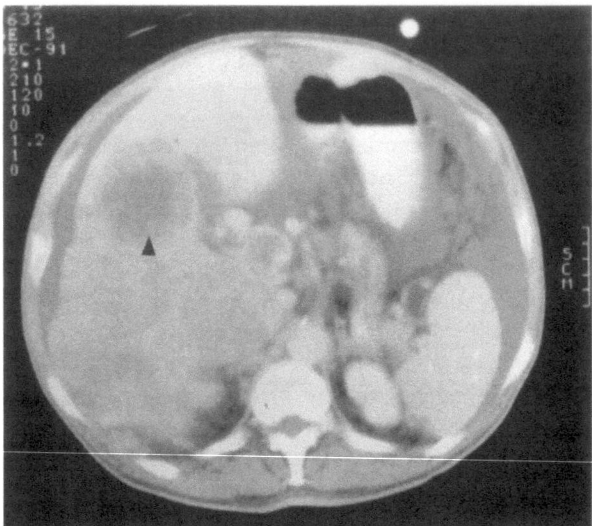

Fig. 6. Punctate calcification in spleen presumably secondary to old granulomatous disease in a patient with metastatic colonic carcinoma. Ascites and hepatic metastasis (*arrowhead*) are present

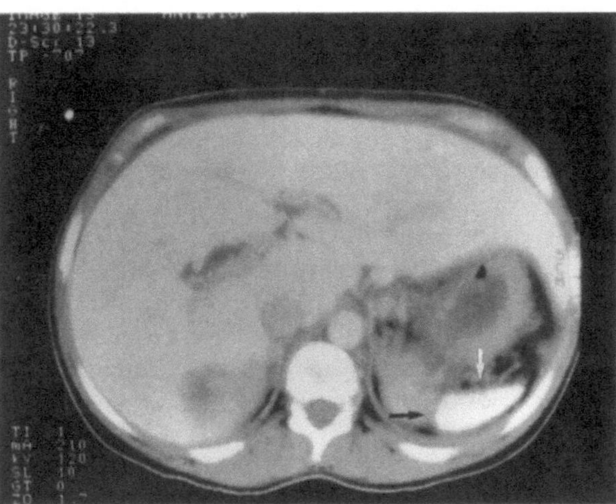

Fig. 7. Contracted and calcified spleen (*arrows*) in a patient with homozygous sickle-cell disease

Hemoglobinopathies, most commonly homozygous sickle-cell disease, can lead to splenic calcification and, eventually, marked contraction secondary to repeated infarctions (Fig. 7). Numerous infections may result in secondary calcification. Splenic calcifications from *Pneumocystis carinii* infections have been reported. Recent articles suggest that other infectious processes, such as those resulting from mycobacteria, can result in a similar appearance [11]. Calcifications on occasion are associated with splenic infarction or neoplasms. An unusual form of rim calcification surrounding the spleen may result from diffuse infection, hemorrhage, or splenic sequestration.

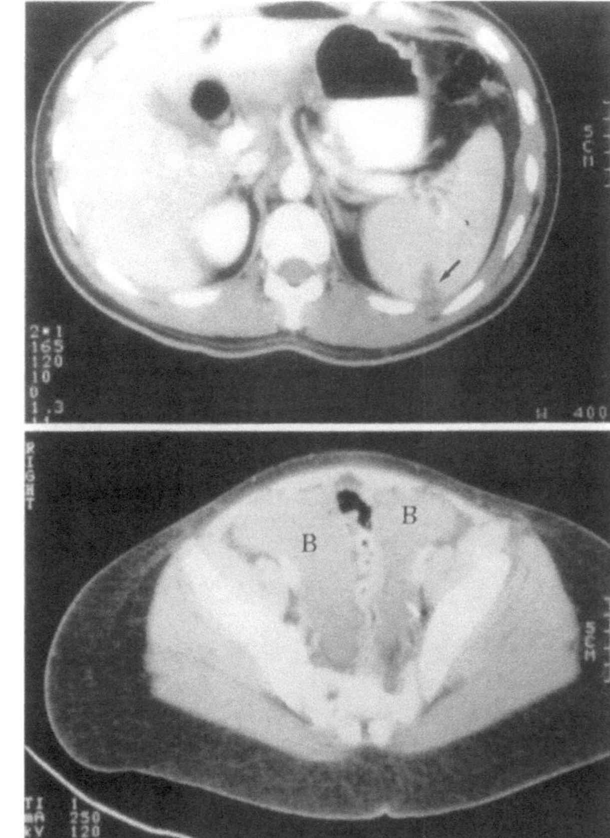

Fig. 8a. Wedge-shaped peripheral laceration (*arrow*) in a patient with recent trauma. An infarction could have a similar CT appearance. **b** Blood (*B*) within pelvis in same patient

Splenic Trauma

The spleen is the abdominal organ most frequently injured with blunt abdominal trauma. If there is preexisting disease with associated splenomegaly, there is increased susceptibility of the spleen to blunt trauma [12–15]. Although radionuclide scintigraphy, angiography, and US imaging are capable of diagnosing splenic trauma, CT is considerably more sensitive and specific in determining splenic injury. Accuracy rates as high as 91% and sensitivity and specificity exceeding 95 % have been reported. At the present time, CT is the imaging modality of choice for the evaluation of splenic trauma. CT is also of considerable value in determing the presence of fluid within the peritoneal cavity, as well as in defining the associated injuries to the liver, pancreas, kidney, and mesentery (Fig. 8a,b). Although CT is extremely sensitive in determining the presence of a splenic injury, the traumatized spleen may on occasion appear normal on the initial CT examination (Fig. 9a,b). It is postulated that in such cases an initial splenic fracture has a

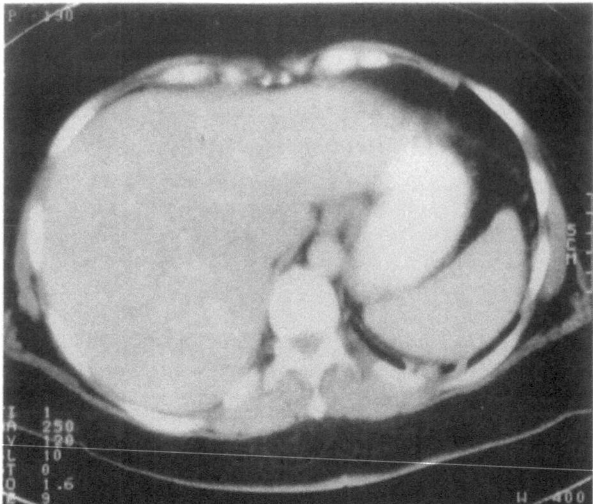

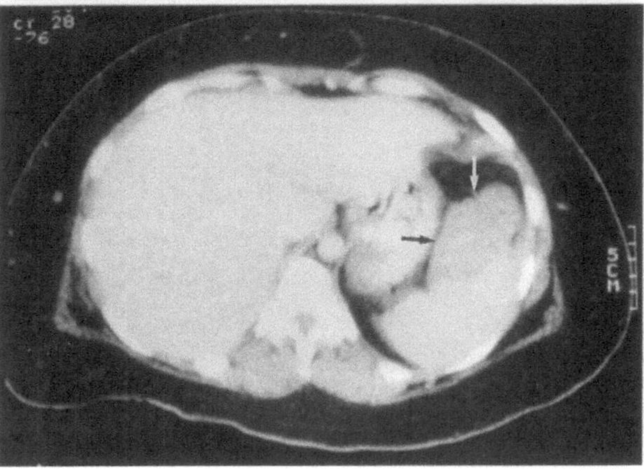

Fig. 9a. Normal-appearing spleen in a patient immediately following trauma. b Parasplenic hematoma (*arrows*) compressing anterior surface of spleen in same patient, 48 h after initial CT examination

density similar to that of the adjacent normal parenchyma, but there is no associated subcapsular or perisplenic hemorrhage. The hyperosmolar effect of hemorrhage may result in expansion of the small initial tear and the appearance of the delayed splenic rupture. McIndoe has defined delayed splenic rupture as hemorrhage occurring more than 48 h after trauma, with the incidence varying from 0.3 to 20% of all blunt splenic injuries. If there is delayed bleeding, 70% occurs within the first 2 weeks after the initial injury [16, 17].

Associated left lower rib fractures are present in approximately 44% of cases. Fractures visualized on plain films obtained in the ER should suggest the possibility of splenic injury. Enlargement of the spleen and perisplenic fluid may result in displacement of the gastric air bubble medially. There is also a 10% incidence of associated left kidney injury and a 2% incidence of injury to the left hemidiaphragm.

Fig. 10. Focal areas of high density show acute hemorrhage (*arrow*) within spleen on noncontrast study

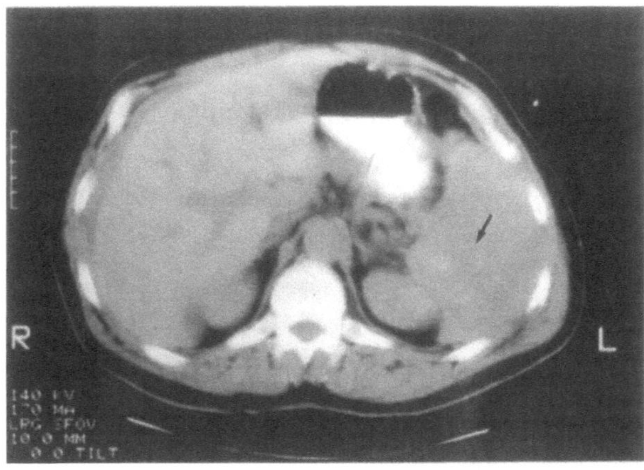

CT examinations of the traumatized patient are usually performed during rapid i.v. infusion of contrast material. As stated previously, the normal spleen may appear extremely inhomogeneous if imaging is performed without at least a 40-s delay following contrast infusion. In addition, lobulations and clefts within the normal spleen can mimic trauma, but there is no associated perisplenic fluid in these cases. A prominent left lobe of the liver may also mimic a perisplenic hematoma. Although a laceration or intrasplenic hematoma is generally visible with a noncontrast CT exam, these abnormalities are usually more conspicuous when i.v. contrast material is used. An acute intrasplenic hematoma is typically more dense than the adjacent normal parenchyma without the use of i.v. contrast, and some authors have suggested that examinations of the spleen be performed initially without contrast so as to increase the sensitivity in detecting injury (Fig. 10).

Numerous CT grading systems of splenic trauma have been developed in the attempt to determine which patients should be treated conservatively and which will require surgery. These systems were initially based only on the severity of the splenic injury, but subsequent authors also considered the presence, volume, and location of fluid within the peritoneal cavity and perisplenic region [18–20]. Mirvis et al. [18] demonstrated that 35% of patients initially graded by CT as having severe splenic injuries were treated successfully without surgery; 29% graded with mild injuries required delayed celiotomy or emergency rehospitalization. More recent papers have also concluded that CT cannot reliably be used to determine the need for surgical intervention or to predict clinical outcome.

Because intra-abdominal fluid may extend along the left pericolic gutter, into the retroperitoneum, or into the pelvis, CT imaging of the entire abdomen and pelvis is routinely performed in patients with suspect splenic trauma. An intrasplenic contusion or hemorrhage maybe appear as an irregular area of low attenuation on the initial contrast-enhanced CT examination. Splenic lacerations may be single or multiple with irregular margins and fre-

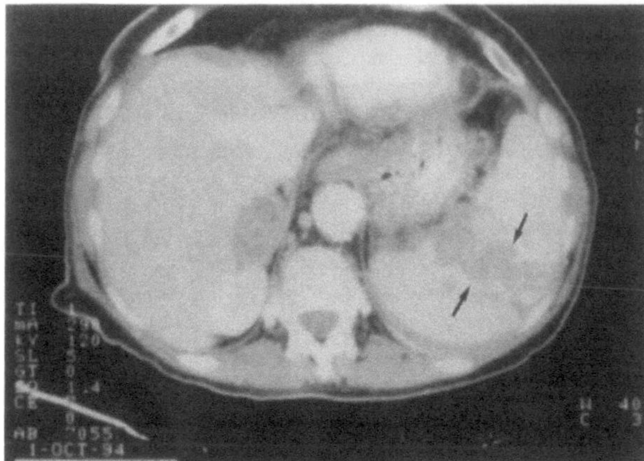

Fig. 11. Splenic fracture (*arrows*). Small amount of fluid adjacent to spleen posteriorly. Larger amounts of blood are present on more caudad imaging sections

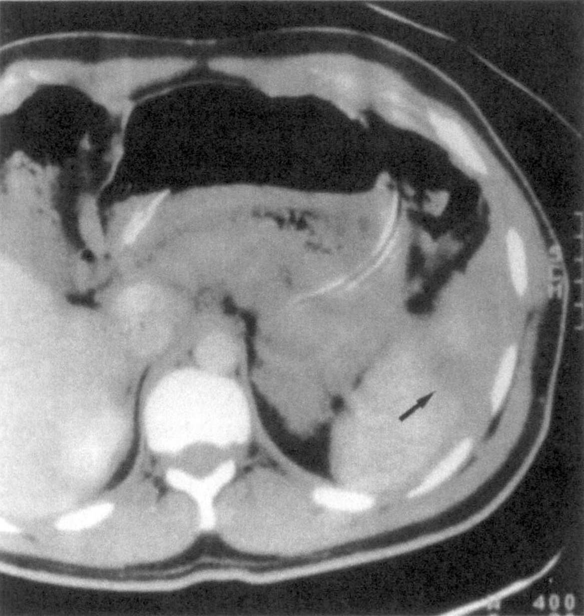

Fig. 12. Wedge-shaped laceration (*arrow*) with perisplenic and/or subcapsular fluid

quently extend to the capsule. An associated subcapsular or intrasplenic hematoma is common. A laceration which traverses two capsular surfaces has been defined as a fracture (Fig. 11). A subcapsular hematoma appears as a crescentic fluid collection which flattens or indents the normally convex lateral margin. The distinction between a subcapsular hematoma and a contiguous perisplenic hematoma is often difficult to make by means of CT imaging (Fig. 12). On occasion, a perisplenic hematoma may be present adjacent to an otherwise normal appearing spleen. This "sentinel clot" has an inhomogeneous appearance with high attenuation values (greater than 60 Hounsfield units) [21]. If there are recurrent episodes of perisplenic hemorrhage, the clot may have an onionskin appearance.

Although the CT grading systems of splenic trauma do not directly correlate with the need for surgery or with the subsequent development of delayed rupture, there is evidence that CT may be used to monitor healing of splenic injuries. CT-demonstrated mild to moderate splenic injuries heal completely by 6 weeks, with more severe injuries requiring 6 months or longer to heal. A sequential decrease in perisplenic and intrasplenic hematoma or healing laceration can be documented, and this information may be of value in determining when patients can return to normal activities [22].

Progressive enlargement of the spleen seen on serial CT exams is not necessarily an abnormal sign. The traumatized spleen may initially contract as a result of decreased intravascular volume or in response to adrenergic stimuli. The increase in spleen size seen on subsequent examinations may simply indicate a return to normal [23].

On occasion, the severely damaged spleen may result in fragments of splenic tissue implanting in the peritoneal cavity and referred to as splenosis. These may enlarge following splenectomy.

As stated above, CT is the primary imaging modality used in cases of abdominal trauma. If US is performed, it may demonstrate a laceration, intrasplenic hematoma or fluid within the peritoneal cavity. Angiography is rarely used to evaluate splenic injury, but it may be of limited value if splenic artery embolization is contemplated [24].

Nontraumatic Lesions of the Spleen

Cysts

Splenic cysts frequently are classified as parasitic, congenital, or pseudocysts. Urrutia et al. [25] have classified cystic splenic masses as congenital, inflammatory (including pyogenic, echinococcal, and fungal abscesses), vascular (including infarction and peliosis), post traumatic, and neoplastic, with a smaller percentage resulting from old infarctions. US, CT, and MRI are equally sensitive in determining the presence of splenic cysts, although thin internal septations may not be visualized with CT.

Parasitic splenic cysts are almost always the result of infections caused by the *Echinococcus granulosus* tapeworm. A peripheral rim-type calcification is frequent but may also be seen with other forms of splenic cysts. However, the presence of multiple daughter cysts within a larger cyst and associated ring-like calcifications within the liver or lung may help in differentiating from other etiologies (Fig. 13).

True cysts, which are also called congenital or epidermoid cysts, have an inner and epithelial lining and are relatively uncommon. They tend to be

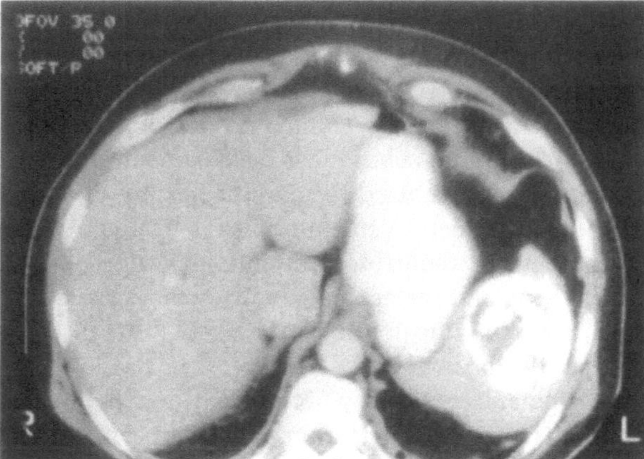

Fig. 13. Calcified ecchinococcal cyst. Dense central calcification also present with walls of daughter cysts

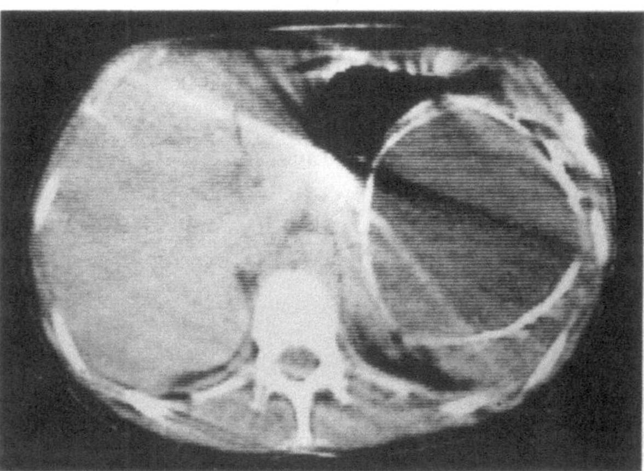

Fig. 14. Epidermoid cyst with peripheral rim calcification

unilocular and asymptomatic unless their large size or a secondary infection/ hemorrhage results in left upper quadrant discomfort. The cysts typically are of uniform water density with a thin wall, and this does enhance during the infusion of (i.v.) contrast (Fig. 14). Although recent hemorrhage can often be determined with CT or MRI, an infected cyst is difficult to distinguish from a sterile cyst unless there is evidence of contained gas.

Pseudocysts or false cysts lack an epithelial lining and account for 80% of splenic cysts. Pseudocysts most commonly result from hematomas and less often are secondary to infarction or infection. Pancreatitis may result in fluid accumulating adjacent to the spleen and, on rare occasion, in fluid tracks from the splenic hilum along the course of the splenic artery or vein, producing an intrasplenic pseudocyst (Fig. 15). Pancreatic enzymes may erode small intrasplenic vessels, resulting in hemorrhage, and cases of rupture secondary to this process have been documented [26]. The presence of associated inflammatory changes and pseudocysts within the region of the

Fig. 15. Fluid within splenic hilum (*white arrow*) and within peripheral subcapsular splenic space (*black arrow*) secondary to pancreatitis

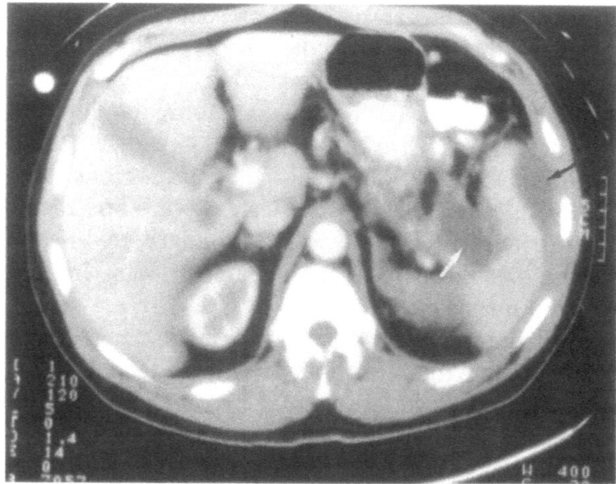

Fig. 16. Intrasplenic pseudocyst (*arrow*) and pancreatic tail (pseudocyst, *arrowheads*) secondary to pancreatitis

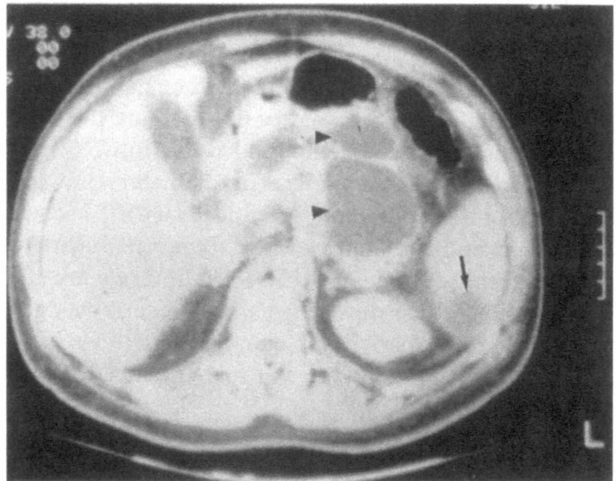

pancreas would suggest pancreatitis as the etiology of an associated splenic cyst (Fig. 16). As with true cysts, pseudocysts tend to be unilocular. However, septations, peripheral calcification, and debris may occur.

Splenic Abscess

The vast majority of abscesses are associated with general septicemia and hematogenous spread of infection. Trauma and infarction, resulting in splenic damage, increase the susceptibility to infection. Multiple abscesses are most common in immunocompromised patients, and the spleen may be the only site of infection in this population. Fungal infections are frequent and associated splenomegaly is often present. Although the abscesses may reach several centimeters in size, they are typically small and may be associated with involvement of the liver and kidneys.

Patients with AIDS more commonly develop abscesses associated with mycobacteria or *P. carinii*. Radin [27] reported that 21% of his AIDS patients with abnormal abdominal CT examinations demonstrated low-attenuation splenic lesions; 87% of the lesions were less than 1 cm in diameter, and the vast majority of these were secondary to infection with mycobacteria. Lesions greater than 2 cm in diameter were more commonly the result of *P. carinii* infection.

Splenomegaly secondary to infection in the immunocompromised patient may occur with or without associated focal lesions. Following treatment, previously visualized lesions may become imperceptible or may calcify. Early papers described splenic calcifications in patients with *P. carinii* infection, but subsequent studies have demonstrated this finding with other infectious causes.

Abscesses can be visualized with US, CT, and MRI and scintigraphy, but the imaging findings are nonspecific. A mass of low density (CT) can also result from a sterile cyst, infarction, hematoma, lymphoma, Kaposi's sarcoma, or peliosis. Unfortunately, neither gallium-67 citrate- nor indium-111-labeled white blood cell studies are of value in making the distinction between sterile and infected splenic fluid collections.

Lesions larger than 1 cm in diameter can also be identified with liver/ spleen scintigraphy. Sonographically (US), lesions are either hypoechoic or anechoic and are more easily appreciated with the use of high frequency transducers [28] (Fig. 17). The CT findings are those of a focal lesion of low attenuation which does not enhance centrally during infusion of i.v. contrast material; some peripheral enhancement may be present. These lesions tend to be more apparent on contrast-enhanced CT examinations (Fig. 18). The

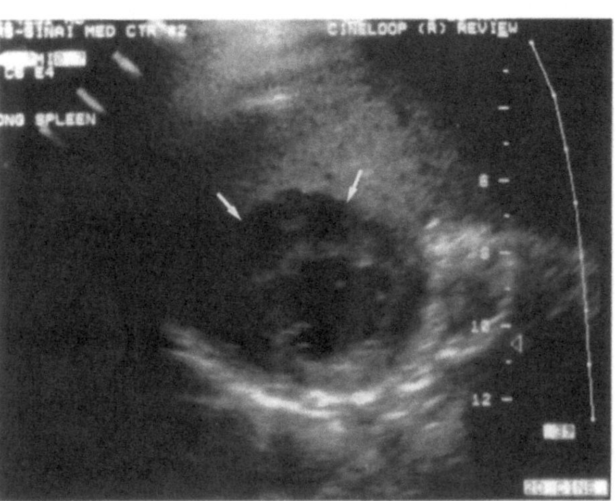

Fig. 17. Splenic abscess. Longitudinal ultrasonography of spleen demonstrating a large hypoechoic mass containing fluid (*arrows*)

Fig. 18. Splenic abscess. Splenic mass of low attenuation in a septic diabetic patient. Although consistent with an abscess, similar findings can be present with trauma, infarction, or tumor

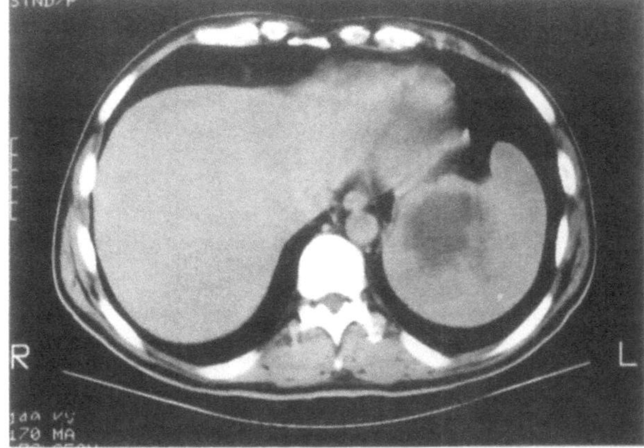

Fig. 19. Microabscesses in liver and spleen in a patient with AIDS. *Candida* was cultured from patient's blood

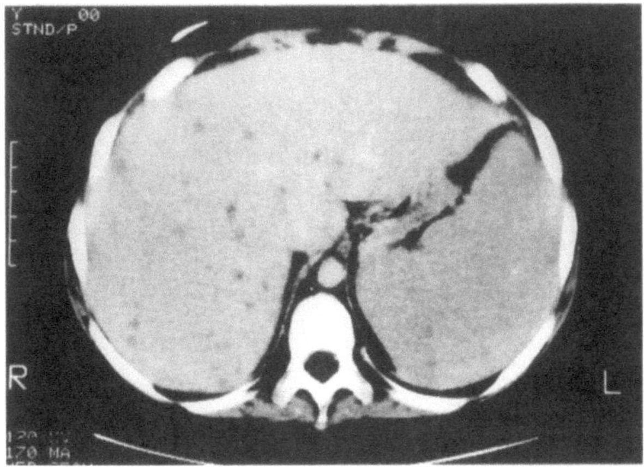

more common appearance of splenic abscesses in the immunocompromised patient is that of multiple small lesions with the above characteristics (Fig. 19). Foci of increased echogenicity (US) or calcification (CT) may appear during the course of a patient's disease. On the rare occasion, gas may be present within an abscess, resulting in bright internal echoes (US). The contents of the abscess may also appear inhomogeneous as a result of more solid components early in the infection [29].

Splenic Infarction

Splenic infarctions are relatively common and may be asymptomatic. Infarction can be either arterial or venous in origin, venous infarction most commonly being the result of thrombosis of splenic sinusoids in patients with massive splenomegaly. The splenic arterial branches are end arteries that do

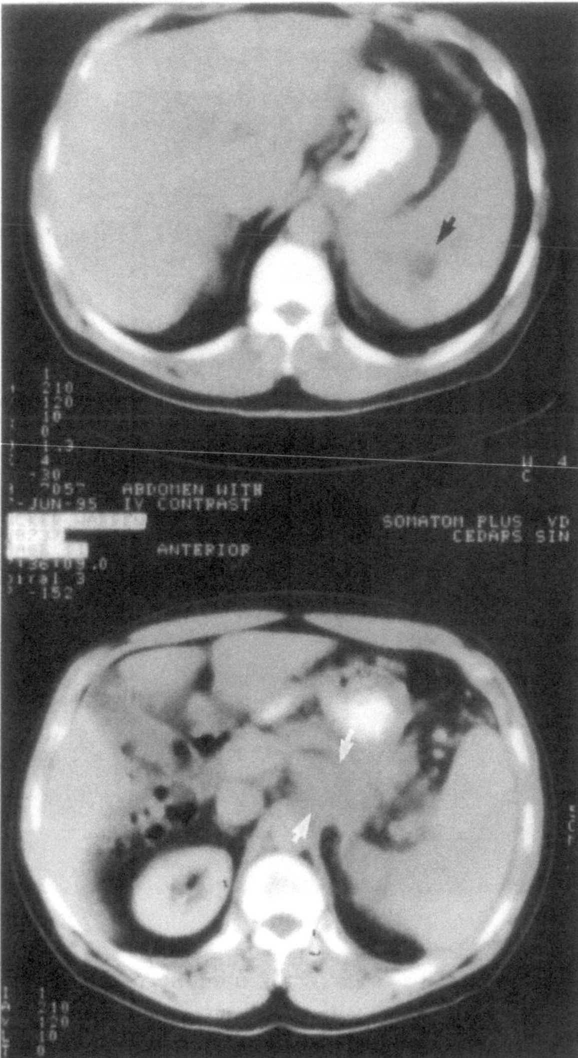

Fig. 20a. Focal splenic infarction with oval configuration (*black arrow*).
b Pancreatic tail carcinoma (*white arrow*) in same patient

not communicate, and occlusions therefore result in infarction. Arterial embolization is the most frequent cause. The spleen may or may not be enlarged, and involvement may be focal or diffuse. Infarctions may also occur in patients with splenic artery aneurysm, hemolytic anemia, leukemia, and collagen vascular disorders. Central inflammatory or neoplastic involvement of the splenic hilum may result in infarction (Fig. 20a,b).

Although infarction can be visualized with liver/spleen scintigraphy, US, and MRI, it is usually diagnosed on the basis of its CT characteristics [30]. A single small lesion may be present, or the entire spleen may be involved

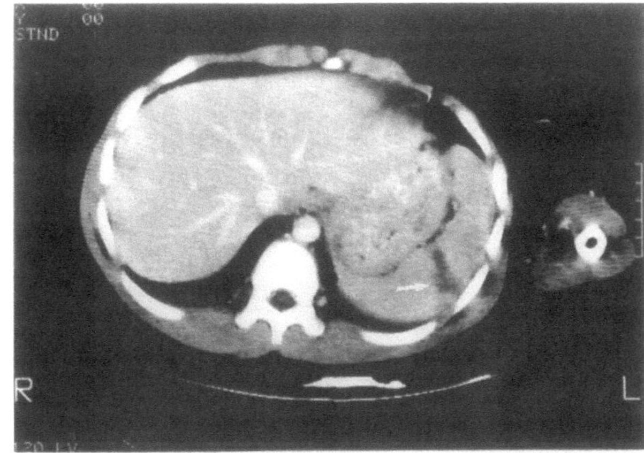

Fig. 21. Wedge-shaped infarction (*arrow*) in a patient without history of recent trauma. Note similarity to splenic laceration. No fluid was present adjacent to spleen or elsewhere within peritoneal cavity

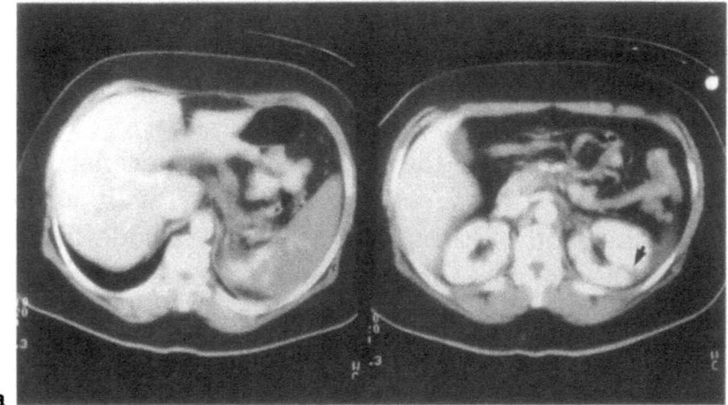

Fig. 22a. Diffuse splenic infarction with decreased contrast enhancement. **b** Small wedge-shaped renal infarction (*arrow*) in same patient

(Figs. 21, 22a,b). In general, infarction is more easily visualized during rapid i.v. infusion of contrast material. However, the CT findings are not specific for an infarction and may on occasion appear similar to abnormalities resulting from inflammation, neoplasm, or trauma.

The CT appearance depends on the time of imaging relative to the acute event. In the first few days an infarction may be either low or high in attenuation (depending on the presence of associated hemorrhage) [31]. Extensive infarction may cause a diffuse mottling or a decrease in attenuation during the infusion of i.v. contrast medium (Fig. 23). Although usually wedge-shaped in configuration, infarctions may also be oval or geographic in appearance. Between 5 and 10 days following an event, the infarcts appear more well defined or even cystic if there is extensive associated necrosis. In the chronic phase (2–4 weeks) infarctions tend to gradually decrease in size and become less apparent. They may heal completely or result in a residual contour defect secondary to scarring. Sonographically, they often appear as areas of decreased echogenicity with poorly defined margins and more cystic if there is extensive necrosis. MRI signal characteristics are highly variable, depending on the presence of hemorrhage and the age of the infarct.

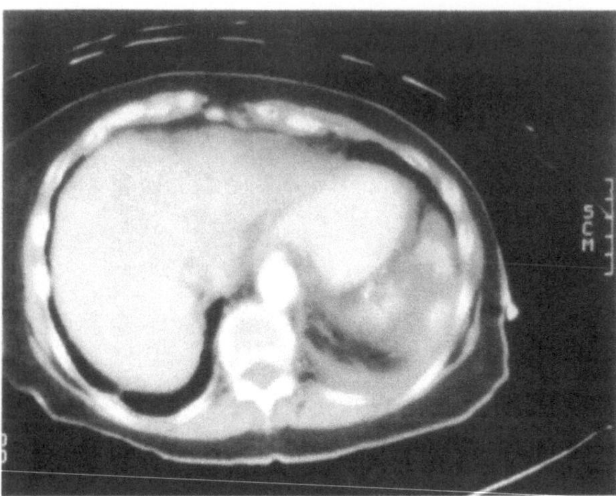

Fig. 23. Extensive infarction with small areas of contrast enhancement. A severely shattered spleen secondary to trauma could have a similar appearance

Benign Splenic Neoplasms

Hemangiomas are the most common primary neoplasms of the spleen, although they are very rare. They are usually asymptomatic and are discovered incidently. Other benign lesions include fibromas and lymphangiomas. On occasion, the spleen may enlarge as a result of these neoplasms. The imaging findings are nonspecific and can vary from predominantly solid to cystic.

Hemangiomas sometimes contain central punctate calcifications, and contrast CT examinations may demonstrate increased vascularity with progressive enhancement of the central portion of the lesion. As in the liver, hemangiomas often appear hyperechoic with US. The lesions tend to be of high signal intensity on T2-weighted MRI images; the signal intensity on T1-weighted images varies with the presence of associated hemorrhage [32, 33].

Malignant Splenic Neoplasms

Angiosarcoma

Primary angiosarcomas are rare and have a very poor prognosis. There are frequent metastases to the liver, and spontaneous rupture may occur. They may be associated with toxic or radiation exposure but may also develop without such an association. The imaging findings are variable with US, MRI, and CT. Multiple nodules or a solitary large complex mass with solid or cystic features have been described. Contrast enhancement with CT is variable and nonspecific.

Fig. 24. Metastasis to spleen (*arrow*) secondary to ovarian carcinoma. Splenic hilar cystic metastases (*arrowhead*) are also present

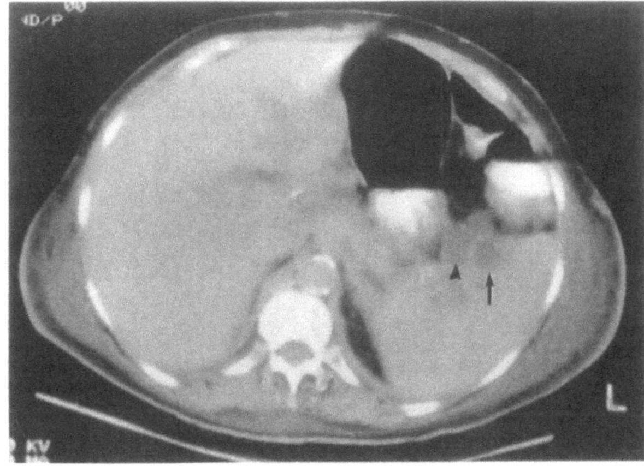

Metastases

Splenic involvement in metastatic disease is relatively uncommon, seen in approximately 7% of patients with widespread malignancy [34]. Approximately 50% of splenic metastases are due to melanoma. The spleen may be enlarged or normal in size. Lesions are solitary or multiple and demonstrate variable imaging features with solid and cystic characteristics (Fig. 24). Lesions tend to be hypoechoic with US, and the degree of contrast enhancement with CT or MRI is variable. Therefore, a CT or US examination demonstrating no abnormalities in the spleen does not exclude metastatic involvement of the spleen.

Lymphoma

Lymphomatous involvement of the spleen as a manifestation of a generalized lymphoproliferative disorder is the most common splenic neoplasm, involving the spleen in both Hodgkin's and non-Hodgkin's lymphoma. Primary splenic lymphoma is relatively uncommon. Enlargement of the spleen can be evaluated with US, CT, and MRI, as well as with liver/spleen scintigraphy. CT is most commonly used in evaluating and staging patients with suspected or known lymphoma because of its ability to determine associated lymphadenopathy. Although CT is reliable in detecting splenomegaly, it is unreliable in detecting or excluding lymphomatous involvement of the spleen. Rolfes and Ros [7] determined that approximately one third of their patients with lymphoma and splenomegaly did not have pathological involvement of the spleen. Conversely, one third of their patients with lymphoma without associated splenomegaly demonstrated lymphomatous involvement of the spleen pathologically. However, if massive splenomegaly is encountered in a patient with non-Hodgkin's lymphoma, it is likely that there is lymphomatous involvement of the spleen.

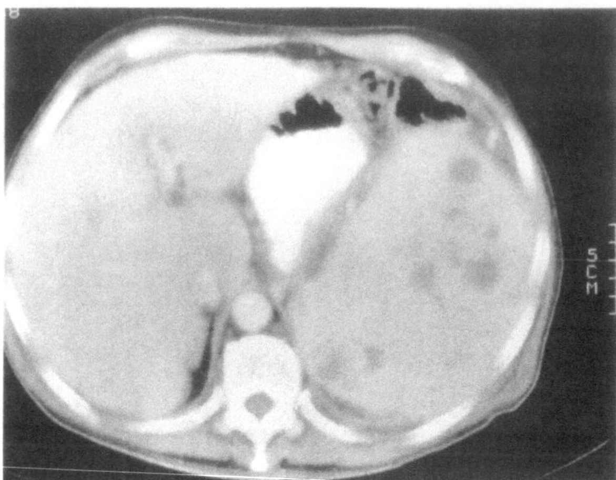

Fig. 25. Lymphomatous involvement of spleen resulting in splenomegaly and multiple focal lesions. Splenomegaly and focal lesions with other etiologies can have a similar appearance

The imaging features of splenic lymphoma are variable. The spleen may appear normal or enlarged, with or without small or large masses (Fig. 25). Because CT has not been proven to be an accurate modality for detecting splenic lymphoma, there was initial enthusiasm over the potential of MRI for distinguishing between the normal spleen and infiltrating splenic lymphoma [35]. Unfortunately, studies to date have demonstrated overlapping T1 and T2 values of infiltrating splenic lymphoma and normal spleen. The presence of adenopathy in association with splenomegaly yields a higher accuracy in a diagnosis of lymphoma (Fig. 26a,b). However, as described previously, patients with AIDS and other diseases also demonstrate splenic lesions, splenomegaly, and lymphadenopathy with or without associated infection.

The spleen may appear uniform in echogenicity (US), density (CT), or signal (MRI). Nodules less than 1 cm in diameter are often not detected by the above-mentioned imaging modalities. However, as nodules enlarge or become cystic in appearance, they are more easily visualized. Typically, lesions appear hypoechoic (US), low in density without contrast enhancement (CT), and slightly hypointense on T1-weighted and hyperintense on T2-weighted (MRI) images (Figs. 27, 28).

When necrosis or secondary infection occurs, lesions may become cystic and must then be differentiated from other etiologies described previously in the section on cystic lesions.

Both CT and MRI studies using newer contrast agents such as superparamagnetic iron oxide (MRI) demonstrate promise in evaluating splenic lymphoma.

Leukemia

Marked splenomegaly may be present, and there is often associated lymphadenopathy. The spleen usually appears homogeneous without discrete focal

Fig. 26. a Lymphomatous mass in spleen (*white arrow*). **b** Enlarged upper abdominal lymph nodes (*black arrows*) in same patient

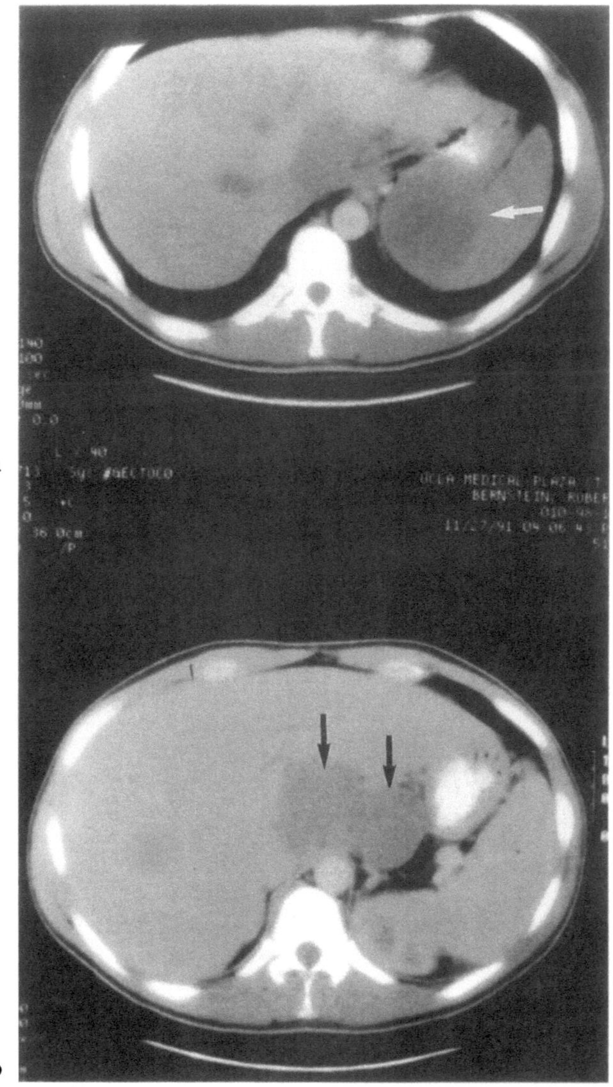

lesions. As in the case of other causes of marked splenomegaly, associated spontaneous rupture may occur.

Miscellaneous Conditions

Portal Hypertension

Portal hypertension is a frequent cause of splenomegaly. It is often associated with a shrunken and lobulated cirrhotic liver with a prominent caudate lobe.

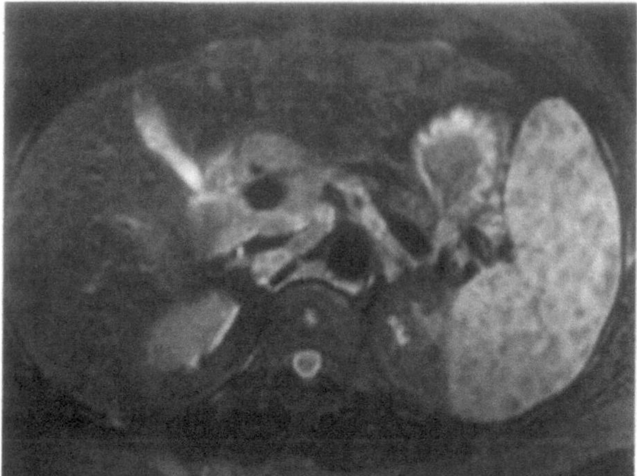

Fig. 27. Axial T2-weighted MRI image demonstrating a focal mass in spleen secondary to lymphoma. (Courtesy of Dr. Jeffrey Silverman)

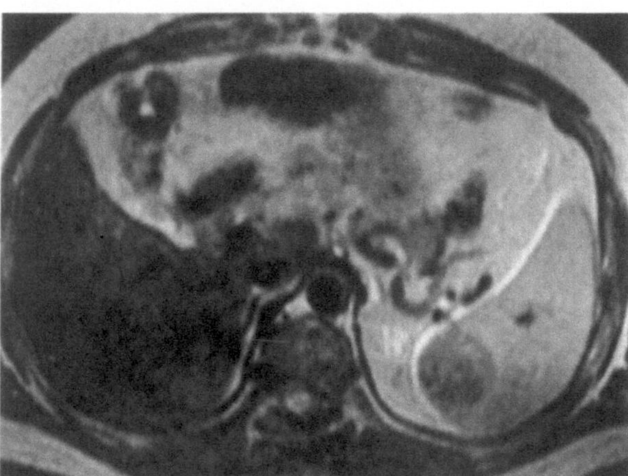

Fig. 28. Axial T2-weighted MRI image demonstrating multiple small focal lesions secondary to lymphoma. Microabscesses usually appear more bright with this sequence

Secondary ascites and varices can be demonstrated with US, CT, and MRI (Fig. 29). A redistribution of sulfur colloid to the bone marrow and spleen is seen in cirrhotic patients examined with liver/spleen scintigraphy (Fig. 30).

Amyloidosis

There are two patterns of splenic involvement with amyloidosis: a nodular form resulting in discreet low-attenuation masses and a diffuse infiltrating form resulting in a diffuse low-density spleen with poor contrast enhancement. Splenomegaly is uncommon (4–13%), but spontaneous rupture may occur.

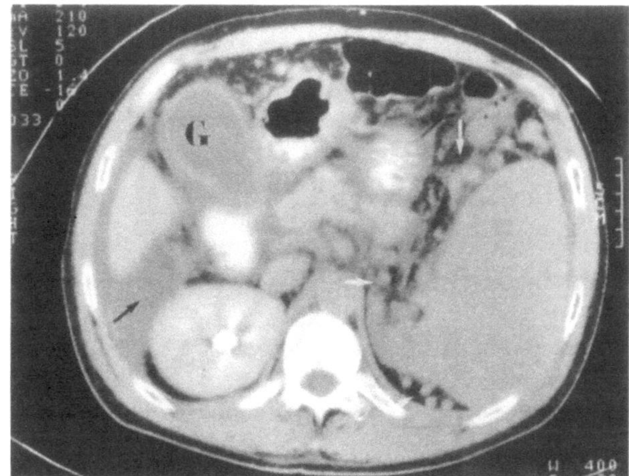

Fig. 29. Cirrhosis with portal hypertension resulting in splenomegaly, venous collaterals (*white arrow*), ascites (*black arrow*), and a small liver. (*G* Gallbladder)

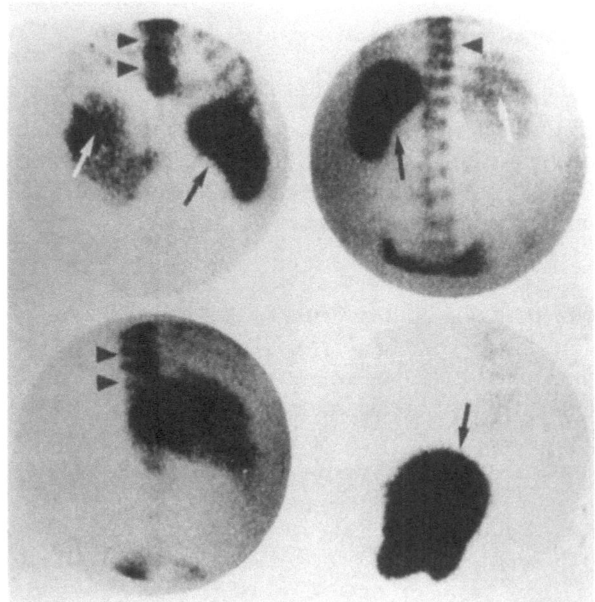

Fig. 30. Cirrhosis with portal hypertension. Technetium-99m sulfur colloid liver-spleen scan demonstrating increased tracer uptake in an enlarged spleen (*black arrow*) and bone marrow (*arrowheads*), and a contracted inhomogeneous liver (*white arrow*). (Courtesy of Dr. Alan Waxman)

Thorotrastosis

Thorotrast was a previously used angiographic contrast material which resulted in particles phagocytosed by the reticuloendothelial cells of the liver, spleen, and bone marrow. Splenic involvement is manifested by a homogeneous or punctate pattern of markedly increased density associated with contraction of the spleen secondary to fibrosis.

Extramedullary Hematopoiesis

Involvement of the spleen is relatively infrequent in adults and is associated with myeloproliferative disorders such as chronic hemolytic anemias and myelofibrosis. Although diffuse enlargement is more common, focal masses (in the liver or spleen) may also develop.

Acute Splenic Sequestration

Acute splenic sequestration develops primarily in infants and young children with homozygous sickle-cell anemia. There is sudden splenic enlargement with a concomitant drop in hematocrit. The imaging characteristics are those of multiple low-density (CT) or bright T1 and T2 (MRI) lesions at the periphery of an enlarged spleen, presumably secondary to hemorrhage (Fig. 31).

Hemochromatosis

An increased deposition of iron in the reticuloendothelial systems of the liver and spleen occurs with the secondary form of the disease and in multiple organs in the primary form. The CT features are those of a diffuse increase in density of the liver and spleen. MRI demonstrates a markedly reduced signal in the involved organs.

Percutaneous Biopsy Procedures

Lesions of unknown origin within the spleen can be biopsied with US or CT guidance and the aspirated material sent for appropriate cultures and cyto-

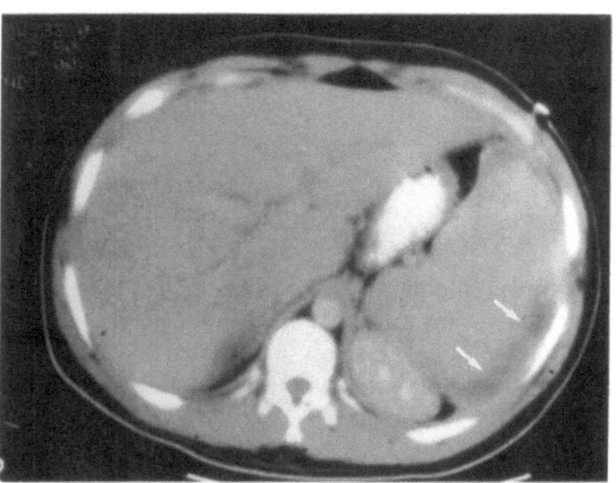

Fig. 31. Acute splenic sequestration resulting in splenomegaly and a peripheral crescent of fluid (*arrows*), presumably secondary to hemorrhage

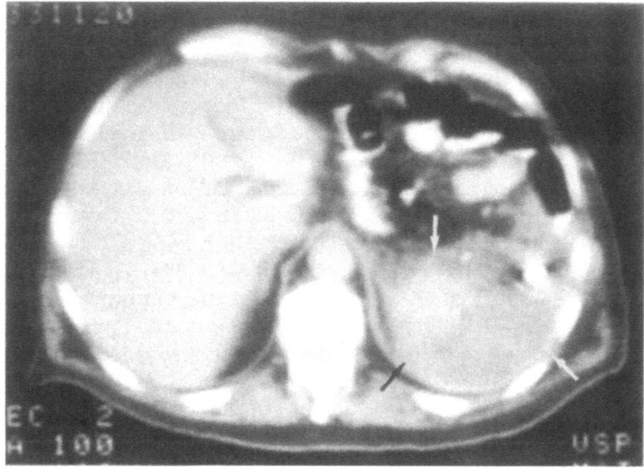

Fig. 32. Post splenectomy, complex left subdiaphragmatic fluid collection (*arrows*). The posterior region of low attenuation may indicate liquefying hematoma and/or abscess formation

logic evaluation. The risk is relatively low with "skinny" needles but, in general, this procedure is infrequently requested. One should take care to avoid traversing the pleural surface or bowel.

Post-splenectomy Hematomas and Abscesses/Drainage Procedures

As with percutaneous biopsies, one should avoid traversing the pleural surface with large catheters when draining subdiaphragmatic fluid collections. The success rate in percutaneously draining acute hematomas is relatively low because of the presence of associated clot (Fig. 32). Some improvement in drainage might result from the placement of larger catheters (14-F) and the injection of thrombolytic agents such as urokinase.

Percutaneous drainage of subphrenic abscesses is associated with a high success rate and often obviates open surgical drainage [36]. McNicholas et al. [36] recently suggested that there is only a slightly increased complication rate and a similar success rate using a transpleural approach, but most interventional radiologists would avoid the pleural space if possible.

Angiographic Embolization

Transcatheter embolization has been used to treat stable trauma patients with arterial extravasation. More recently, this procedure has been performed prior to laparoscopic splenectomy to decrease the vascularity of the spleen. It has also been performed in patients with splenomegaly associated with a consumptive (primarily platelet) disorder and in an attempt to perform partial splenectomy in patients with massive splenomegaly such as that associated with Gaucher's disease. There are case reports of patients with symptoms secondary to splenomegaly who, because of medical contraindications to surgery, might benefit from the procedure.

References

1. Chintapalli KN, Schnitker JB (1994) Spleen imaging. Appl Radiol 23:29–37
2. Freeman JL, Jafri SZ, Roberts JL, Mezwa DG, Shirkhoda A (1993) CT of congenital and acquired abnormalities of the spleen. Radiographics 13: 597–610
3. Koehler RE (1989) Spleen. In: Lee JK, Sagel SS, Stanley RJ (eds) Computed body tomography with MRI correlation, 2nd edn. Raven, New York, pp 521–541
4. Dodds DJ, Taylor AJ, Erickson SJ, Stewart ET, Lawson TL (1990) Radiologic imaging of splenic anomalies. AJR 155: 805–810
5. Miles KA, McPherson SJ, Hayball MP (1995) Transient splenic inhomogeneity with contrast-enhanced CT: mechanism and effect of liver disease. Radiology 194: 91–95
6. Federle MP (1992) The spleen. In: Moss AA, Gamsu G, Genant HK (eds) Computed tomography of the body with magnetic resonance imaging, 2nd edn. Saunders, Philadelphia, pp 1059–1090
7. Rolfes RJ, Ros PR (1990) The spleen: an integrated imaging approach. Crit Rev Diagn Imaging 30: 41–83
8. Taylor AJ, Dodds WJ, Erickson SJ, Stewart ET (1991) CT of acquired abnormalities of the spleen. AJR 157: 1213–1219
9. Herman TE, Siegel MJ (1991) CT of acute splenic torsion in children with wandering spleen. AJR 156: 151–153
10. Spencer RP (1979) Spleen imaging. In: Gottschalk L, Potchen EJ (eds) Diagnostic nuclear medicine. Williams and Wilkins, Baltimore
11. Radin DR, Baker EL, Kiatt EC (1990) Visceral and nodal calcification in patients with AIDS-related *Pneumocystis carinii* infection. AJR 154: 27–31
12. Do HM, Cronan J (1991) CT appearance of splenic injuries managed nonoperatively. AJR 157: 757–760
13. Lawson, DE, Jacobson, JA, Spizarny DL, Pranikoff TP (1995) Splenic trauma: value of follow-up CT. Radiology 194: 97–100
14. Federle MP (1995) Splenic trauma: is follow-up CT of value? Radiology 194: 23–24
15. Wolfman NT, Bechtold RE, Scharling EF, Meredith JW (1992) Blunt upper abdominal trauma: evaluation by CT. AJR 158: 493–501
16. Pappas D, Mirvis SE, Crepps JT (1987) Splenic trauma: false-negative CT diagnosis in cases of delayed rupture. AJR 149: 727–728
17. McIndoe AH (1931) Delayed hemorrhage following traumatic rupture of the spleen. Br J Surg 20: 249–268
18. Mirvis SE, Whitley No, Gens DR (1989) Blunt splenic trauma in adults: CT-based classification and correlation with prognosis and treatment. Radiology 171: 31–39
19. Umlas SL, Cronan JJ (1991) Splenic trauma: can CT grading systems enable prediction of successful nonsurgical treatment? Radiology 178: 481–487
20. Becker CD, Spring SP, Glättli A, Schweizer W (1993) Blunt splenic trauma in adults: CT findings to be used to determine the need for surgery? AJR 162: 343–347
21. Orwig D, Federle MP (199?) Localized clotted blood as evidence of visceral trauma on CT: the sentinel clot sign. AJR 153: 747–749
22. Benya EC, Bulas BI, Eichelberger MR, Sivit CJ (1995) Splenic injury from blunt abdominal trauma in children: follow-up evaluation with CT. Radiology 195: 685–688
23. Goodman LR, Aprahamian C (1990) Changes in splenic size after abdominal trauma. Radiology 176: 629–632
24. Sclafani FJA, Weisberg A, Scalea TM (1991) Blunt splenic injuries: nonsurgical treatment with CT, arteriography and transcatheter arterial embolization of the splenic artery. Radiology 181: 189–196
25. Urrutia N, Nergo PJ, Ros LH, Tores GM, Ros PR (1996) Cystic masses of the spleen: radiologic-pathologic correlation. Radiographics 16: 107–129
26. Fishman EK, Soyer P, Bliss BF, Bluemke DA, Devine N (1995) Splenic involvement in pancreatitis: spectrum of CT findings. AJR 164: 631–635

27. Radin R (1995) HIV infection: analysis of 259 consecutive patients with abnormal abdominal CT findings. Radiology 197: 712–722
28. Murray JG, Patel MD, Le S, Sandhu JS, Feldstein VA (1995) Microabscesses of the liver and spleen in AIDS: detection with 5-megaHertz sonography. Radiology 197: 723–727
29. Bathar EJ, Hilton S, Naidich D, Megibow A, Levine R (1985) CT of splenic and perisplenic abnormalities in septic patients. AJR 141: 53–56
30. Goerg C, Schwerk WB (1990) Splenic infarction: sonographic patterns, diagnosis, follow-up and complications. Radiology 174: 803–807
31. Balcar I, Seltzer SE, Geller S (1984) CT patterns of splenic infarction: a clinical and experimental study. Radiology 151: 723–729
32. Ros PR, Moser RP, Dachman AH, Murari PJ, Olmsted WW (1987) Hemangioma of the spleen: radiologic-pathologic correlation in ten cases. Radiology 162: 73–77
33. Disler DG, Chew FS (1991) Splenic hemangioma. AJR 157:44
34. Rabuschka LS, Kawashima A, Fishman EK (1994) Imaging of the spleen: CT with supplemental MR examinations. Radiographics 14: 307–302
35. Kawashima A, Fishman E (1994) Benign splenic lesions. In: Gore RM, Levine MS, Laufer I (eds) Textbook of gastrointestinal radiology. W.B. Saunders, Philadelphia, pp 2251–2299
36. McNicholas MJ, Mueller PR, Lee MJ, Echeverri J, Gazelle GS, Boland GW, Dawson SL (1995) Percutaneous drainage of subphrenic fluid collections that occur after splenectomy. AJR 165: 355–359

Section II: Splenic Diseases

Benign Neoplasms of the Spleen

L. Morgenstern

> "We were then struck by the appearance of the cyst, its colour, the nature of the tissue which constituted its walls ... and soon no further doubt was possible; the investigation of the points of attachment ... the manual exploration of the dome of the diaphragm and of the left hypochondrium ... all proved that it was the spleen which was involved ..."
>
> *Jules Péan*, 1867, describing the first successful splenectomy for splenic cyst

Introduction

Benign tumors of the spleen are not frequently encountered by the surgeon. Indications for surgical intervention with these tumors are equally rare within the broad spectrum of splenic diseases. This chapter stresses those benign tumors and tumor-like lesions of the spleen which are likely to be encountered in current surgical practice.

Classification

The following classification is adapted from the latest *Atlas of Tumor Pathology*, published by the Armed Forces Institute of Pathology [1]:

I. Vascular lesions
    A. Hemangioma
    B. Littoral cell angioma
    C. Lymphangioma
    D. Peliosis of the spleen
    E. Hemangioendothelioma
    F. Angiomyolipoma
    G. Bacillary angiomatosis
    H. Hemangiopericytoma

II. Tumor-like lesions of the spleen
    A. Inflammatory pseudotumor
    B. Mycobacterial spindle cell pseudotumor

 C. Hamartoma
 D. Cysts
   1. True cysts
     a. Epithelial cyst
     b. Parasitic cyst
   2. False cysts

Hemangioma

Hemangioma is the most common benign primary neoplasm of the spleen. Most frequently it is but an incidental finding following removal of the spleen for other reasons (Fig. 1). Occasionally, as in the liver, it may be palpated as a surface lesion during surgical exploration. Otherwise, it is encountered by the surgeon if it has become symptomatic or has been discovered on an imaging examination.

Hemangiomas of the spleen may be solitary or multiple. They have been reported rarely in children [2, 3] but, curiously, most often occur in young and middle-aged adults.

The solitary hemangiomas are bluish-red, well-circumscribed nodules within the splenic parenchyma which may vary in size from several millimeters to several centimeters. Microscopically, the most common type is the cavernous hemangioma, a conglomerate of cystic, endothelium-lined, blood-filled spaces. Hemangiomas may sclerose and calcify. It is the larger lesions which may give rise to the complications which are indications for surgical removal.

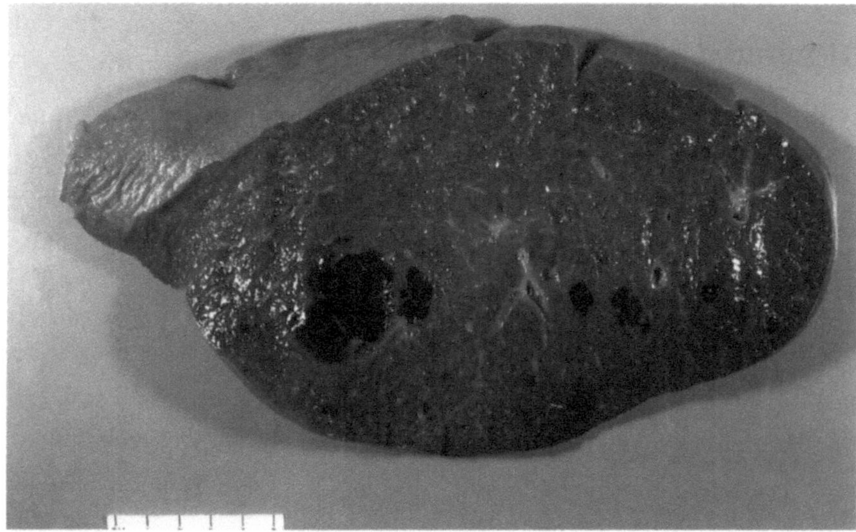

Fig. 1. Multiple hemangiomas in a normal-sized spleen. Incidental finding

Alternatively, the angiomatous process may involve the whole spleen as diffuse hemangiomatosis. Such spleens may become quite large and be detectable as splenomegaly in addition to other concurrent symptoms. The splenomegaly may be only one manifestation of a widespread systemic vasoproliferative disorder involving the skin, bones, liver, and other organs.

The most common and most life-threatening complication of splenic hemangioma or hemangiomatosis, before it became possible to diagnose earlier by imaging, was rupture. Currently, excellent radiologic-pathologic correlation is possible with a CT scan [4], which reduces the incidence of rupture as a presenting symptom.

The hematologic manifestations of hemangiomas or hemangiomatosis include consumption coagulopathy, thrombocytopenia, and microangiopathic anemia. Disseminated intravascular coagulation may also be associated with larger hemangiomas and is known as the Kasabach-Merritt syndrome, seen in older children and adults with marked splenomegaly due to the tumor.

In addition to imaging procedures, fine-needle aspiration biopsy (FNAB) has been used [5, 6] as a diagnostic tool. FNAB does not carry the risk of ordinary needle biopsy of the spleen, a maneuver that has fallen into disrepute.

The treatment for splenic hemangioma when symptomatic has traditionally been total splenectomy. It is reasonable to expect that partial splenectomy may be done in the future for localized, accessible lesions in which the diagnosis is reasonably secure. Diffuse splenic hemangiomatosis is treated by splenectomy. Correction of hematologic deficiencies such as thrombocytopenia and anemia must be considered in the preoperative preparation of such patients.

A variant of the usual pathologic picture of splenic hemangioma is littoral cell angioma [7, 8], characterized by anastomosing vascular channels and other histologic features that differ from those of the ordinary cavernous hemangioma. It is also a benign lesion but may be mistaken for angiosarcoma.

Lymphangioma

Lymphangiomas are less common than hemangiomas. The clinical spectrum of lymphangiomas and lymphangiomatosis has recently been described by Morgenstern et al. [9].

The solitary focal lesion which is most common among the lymphangiomas and the easiest to recognize is the subcapsular lymphangioma (Fig. 2). It appears as a soft, compressible, multicystic lesion on the splenic surface and is rarely large. Such lesions are so characteristic as not to require biopsy and certainly are no indication for splenectomy.

As with hemangiomas, lymphangiomas within the splenic parenchyma may be solitary or multiple. There is a lack of agreement among pathologists about whether the lymphangioma is a true neoplasm or a hamartoma. Pathologic characteristics and clinical manifestations, closely allied to those of

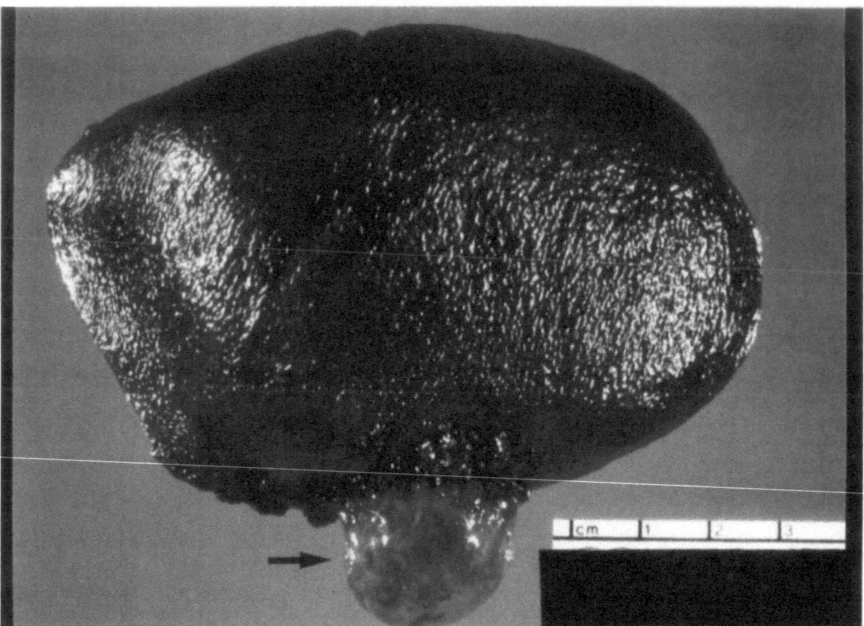

Fig. 2. Typical subcapsular lymphangioma

hemangioma, favor the origin as being vasoformative rather than developmental abnormalities.

Solitary lesions may be large, giving rise to splenomegaly and presenting an indication for resection. Multifocal lesions may be multiple and large, with islands of residual splenic parenchyma, resulting in splenomegaly. Also, nearly the entire splenic parenchyma may be replaced by a diffuse lymphangiomatosis, which may involve the spleen alone or a number of other viscera as well [10–13]. Involved along with the spleen may be the liver, kidneys, and bone, and there may be extravisceral involvement in the mediastinum, retroperitoneum, axilla, and neck. Cystic hygroma in these extravisceral sites in infants may presage visceral involvement in later years. The syndrome of multicentric, multisystem involvement has been reported with much greater frequency with lymphangiomatosis than with hemangiomatosis.

As with hemangiomas, hypersplenic syndromes, consumptive coagulopathy, and even portal hypertension have been reported. Rupture with hemorrhage has also been encountered [14]. Malignant transformation has been described [15] but is not yet accepted as an entity.

The indication for surgical intervention is splenomegaly, with or without multisystem involvement or hematologic complications. However, there have been reports of successful partial splenectomy in lesions which were amenable to such a procedure [16, 17]. If the diagnosis is reasonably certain, partial splenectomy is a thoroughly plausible procedure for localized lesions of this nature.

Peliosis

Although peliosis of the spleen is not a neoplastic lesion, it is included here because of its superficial resemblance to vascular neoplasms. The lesion consists of blood-filled cysts or spaces distributed either in patches or diffusely and involving the whole spleen. Such spleens may be markedly enlarged, as reported by Chopra et al. [18], or the lesions may be only microscopic. The latter type are usually encountered only incidentally. Previously thought to be found only in association with similar hepatic involvement, splenic peliosis has been described more recently to occur alone.

The etiology and pathogenesis of peliosis are far from certain. It has been reported in association with malignancies and in tuberculosis and in recipients of anabolic steroids or oral contraceptives.

Major intraperitoneal hemorrhage from rupture of one or more cysts may occur. As with the vasoformative neoplastic lesions, splenic peliosis with splenomegaly can also result in the hypersplenic syndromes.

Although this lesion is rare, it is important that the surgeon be aware of and recognize the condition. As an indication for surgical intervention it is considerably less frequent than the vascular neoplasms which it mimics.

Hemangioendothelioma

Hemangioendothelioma of the spleen, also known as epithelioid hemangioendothelioma, is a neoplasm thought to be intermediate between hemangioma and angiosarcoma. Its existence as a benign, primary neoplasm has been questioned, with many pathologists believing that all such lesions are angiosarcomas. Nevertheless, it has been described as occurring in both children and adults as a borderline lesion with mild cellular atypia and other histological features which distinguish it from the ordinary hemangioma [19, 20].

The clinical presentation may be with splenomegaly, although those reported lesions thought to be benign have been small (6 cm or less). It is more than likely that the larger lesions are angiosarcomas.

Of importance to the surgeon is the knowledge that a diagnosis of hemangioendothelioma, although implying benignity, should suggest the possibility of a malignant vascular neoplasm. This lesion is extremely rare.

As with the other vascular tumors, rupture with intraperitoneal hemorrhage has been reported in one case [21]. Segmental splenectomy of the lower pole was performed as an emergency procedure.

Hemangiopericytoma

Hemangiopericytoma may occur rarely in the spleen as a primary tumor, either as an incidental finding or large enough to cause splenomegaly. As in the soft tissue sites, its malignant potential is questionable.

Bacillary Angiomatosis

Bacillary angiomatosis is a reactive proliferative response to infection with certain species of *Rickettsia* (*R. quintana*, *R. henselae*) occurring in the spleen and lymph nodes. As such, it is similar to the lymph-node lesions of cat-scratch fever. The proliferative reaction is so intense as to resemble tumor-like nodules of proliferating vessels in a background of neutrophils, fibrous stroma, and dead bacilli. It must be distinguished from the more lethal lesions which it mimics, namely angiosarcoma or Kaposi's sarcoma.

Clinically, bacillary angiomatosis is a disorder found in immunodeficiency states, particularly AIDS. In addition to splenomegaly, other manifestations may be generalized lymphadenopathy and multiple skin nodules of the same histologic character.

This condition should not be an indication for surgical intervention if the diagnosis has been established by biopsy of extrasplenic sites. It is responsive to antibiotic therapy and should be so treated. Erythromycin has been an effective agent.

Inflammatory Pseudotumors

Inflammatory pseudotumors have been found in nearly every major organ system, including gastrointestinal, genitourinary, endocrine, skeletal, and central nervous system sites. Its occurrence in the spleen, first reported in 1984 and thought to be very rare, has recently been the subject of an increasing number of case reports [22–25].

The lesion is a reactive, inflammatory mass within the splenic parenchyma, often very well circumscribed, exhibiting a wide variety of reactive inflammatory cells, proliferating spindle cells, and a broad spectrum of reparative and inflammatory cellular components. Usually solitary, measuring from several centimeters to over 11 cm, the lesions may also be multiple.

The clinical presentation is variable. Occurrence is more frequent in the fifth and sixth decades, often with nonspecific symptoms, leading to investigations which disclose a splenic mass lesion. Definitive diagnosis is made after the spleen is removed.

The splenic mass cannot be differentiated from other neoplastic masses on imaging studies. The typical CT picture is that of a circumscribed, hypoechoic, heterogeneous mass lesion.

The etiology of inflammatory pseudotumors has not been clearly established. There is some correlation with infectious agents, but the current consensus is that they are an exaggerated immunologic response to one of a variety of stimuli. Their predilection for one organ site or another is unexplained.

Differential diagnoses which are considered in light of the symptom complexes and demonstration of a splenic mass lesion include lymphoma or other malignant splenic lesions. The surgical indication is splenectomy. If the underlying condition is benign, splenectomy is curative.

Mycobacterial Spindle Cell Pseudotumors

In the same family of inflammatory pseudotumors of the spleen is the more specific mycobacterial spindle cell pseudotumor [26]. These are inflammatory tumor-like masses found in HIV-positive patients in response to mycobacterial infection. In light of the underlying disease, splenectomy contributes little to improving the prognosis.

Hamartomas

Hamartomas are not neoplasms, but focal developmental anomalies arising within the normal spleen. The normal cellular elements are in random disarray, rather than functionally organized, within circumscribed nodules which are solitary (Fig. 3) or multiple (Fig. 4). The Greek term *hamartos* means error. Alternative terms for hamartoma are splenoma, splenadenoma, and nodular hyperplasia, illustrating the confusion that exists with regard to their etiology.

Hamartomas are most frequently encountered at autopsy or in spleens removed for other conditions. Their association with hematologic and neoplastic states in the spleen has been stressed by Steinberg et al. in a comprehensive review of the subject entitled "The spleen in the spleen syndrome" [27].

Hamartomas of the spleen achieve surgical significance in relatively rare circumstances. Solitary or multiple splenomas may be discovered incidentally during imaging studies done for various reasons. Since there is no way of validating a diagnosis based on imaging studies alone, surgical intervention is indicated. FNAB has been attempted [28] but is not dependable because of the diverse cellular elements which may be retrieved. There have also been instances of rupture of a hamartoma with intraperitoneal hemorrhage, necessitating emergency laparotomy and splenectomy [29].

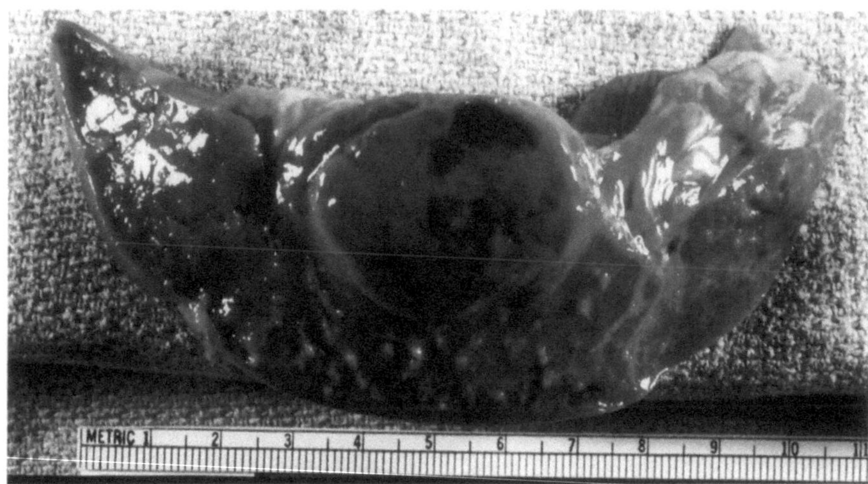

Fig. 3. Solitary hamartoma near splenic hilum. Splenic mass was discovered on CT scan for other complaints. Splenectomy was diagnostic

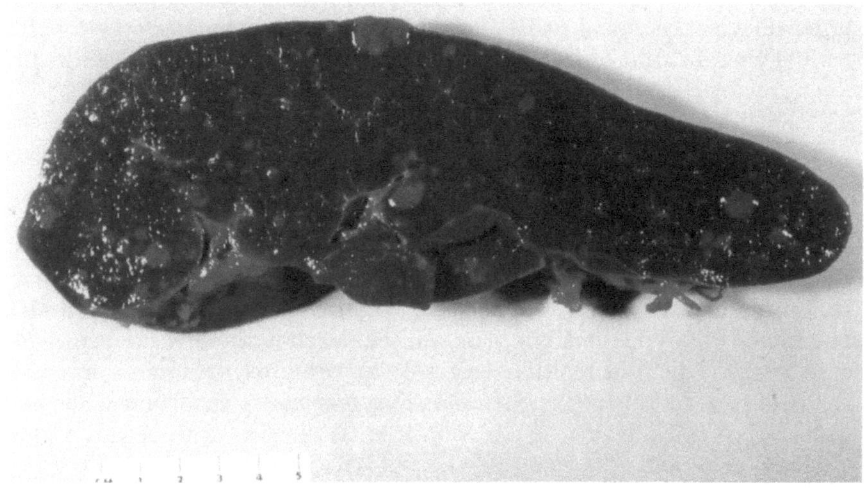

Fig. 4. Multiple hamartoma manifested clinically by splenomegaly and hypersplenism

Another hamartomatous condition which mandates surgical intervention is diffuse hamartomatosis of the spleen [30]. Such spleens may be markedly enlarged and give rise to all the symptoms and signs of hypersplenism [31]. Splenectomy is curative.

At operation the hamartoma may present as a mass bulging from the splenic surface. If the location is polar, partial splenectomy is possible. Such a case was reported by Havlik et al. [32].

Splenic Cysts

Nonparasitic Cysts

Nonparasitic splenic cysts (NPSC) occur in all age-groups, from infancy to old age. There is even a report of antenatal diagnosis [33]. The vast majority of NPSC probably result from a developmental anomaly, during which primitive mesothelium becomes entrapped within the splenic parenchyma. Mesothelium has a great metaplastic potential, which accounts for the variable nature of the cyst lining. Thus the lining may resemble mesothelium or differentiate into transitional or epidermoid epithelium. The most common lining is epidermoid.

Classifications of NPSC have generally divided them into "true" cysts, which bear an epithelial lining, and "false" or "traumatic" cysts, in which no lining can be demonstrated. This is a spurious differentiation, since the lining is often easily stripped from the fibrous cyst wall and is demonstrable only by a careful search. Cystic lesions secondary to trauma, evolving from subcapsular hematomas, have an entirely different appearance, clearly resembling the evolution of hematomas at other locations in the body. In the now vast literature on the conservative management of splenic trauma, including nonoperative treatment, splenorrhaphy, and partial resection, there is no correlation whatsoever with any increased incidence of splenic cysts. More often than not, no history of trauma can be elicited, even though ostensibly no lining has been demonstrated.

The most common presenting symptom of NPSC is left upper quadrant discomfort, usually vague in nature. The most common presenting sign is splenomegaly. On imaging studies, NPSC have a characteristic appearance (Fig. 5). They are round, well-circumscribed, hypoechoic or hypodense masses which are clearly cystic. The absence of variation in density within the cyst or irregularity of the wall differentiates NPSC from other cystic lesions, such as degenerating primary or secondary neoplasms.

Cysts which are 4 cm or less in size should be observed for symptoms or for increase in size on imaging studies, preferably not involving radiation. Ultrasound is perfectly suitable for following cyst size. Cysts which exceed 4 cm in size or are symptomatic should be resected, although some physicians might take issue with this arbitrary criterion. Some judgement must be used in recommending resection of cysts larger than 4 cm if they are asymptomatic, the likelihood of infection or rupture being small. Fine-needle aspiration cytodiagnosis of epidermoid cysts has been reported [34].

When surgical intervention is indicated for NPSC, the preferred treatment is cystectomy or partial splenectomy [35]. This is one of the clearest indications for such a spleen-conserving surgical approach. Many reports in the literature attest to the success of this method.

There are two alternative approaches to resection of the cyst. Complete excision of the cyst can be accomplished only with partial splenectomy, by resecting a small rim of splenic parenchyma that is contiguous with the cyst.

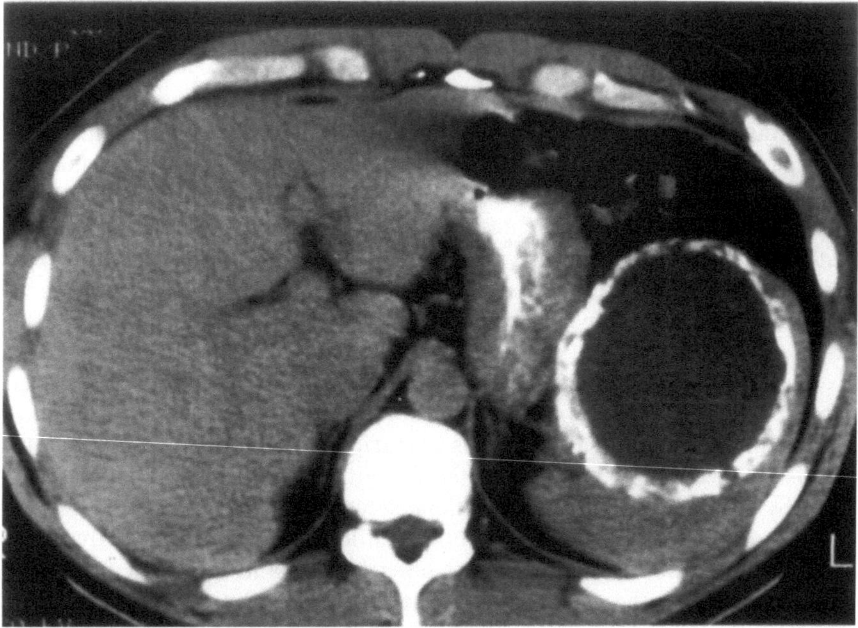

Fig. 5. CT scan demonstrating typical nonparasitic splenic cyst. This cyst showed calcification of the cyst wall

Cysts arising from either pole of the spleen, as they most commonly do, lend themselves to this approach (Fig. 6). Cysts involving the hilum may sometimes be safely excised in this way, but with greater risk.

The alternative to cystectomy with partial splenectomy has been termed "splenic decapsulation" or "partial cystectomy." Instead of resecting through splenic parenchyma a small rim of the cyst wall is left, and the major portion of the cyst is resected; splenic parenchyma is not traversed at all. Hemostasis in the cyst wall rim is accomplished with a hemostatic suture or other suitable techniques. Although little follow-up information is as yet available regarding this method of partial splenectomy, no recurrences have been reported in the cases published [36, 37].

Resected cysts are remarkably similar in appearance (Fig. 7). The wall is characteristically trabeculated and may show zones of calcification. Contents of the cyst vary from clear serous fluid to murky greenish, brownish, or yellow fluid. The cysts may reach remarkably large sizes of 20 cm or more, displacing contiguous organs such as the stomach, colon, and kidney.

Splenic cysts have also been resected laparoscopically, by either of the two methods described above. Partial cystectomy seems more suited to the laparoscopic approach, although partial splenectomy with cystectomy using the surgical stapler has also been described [38].

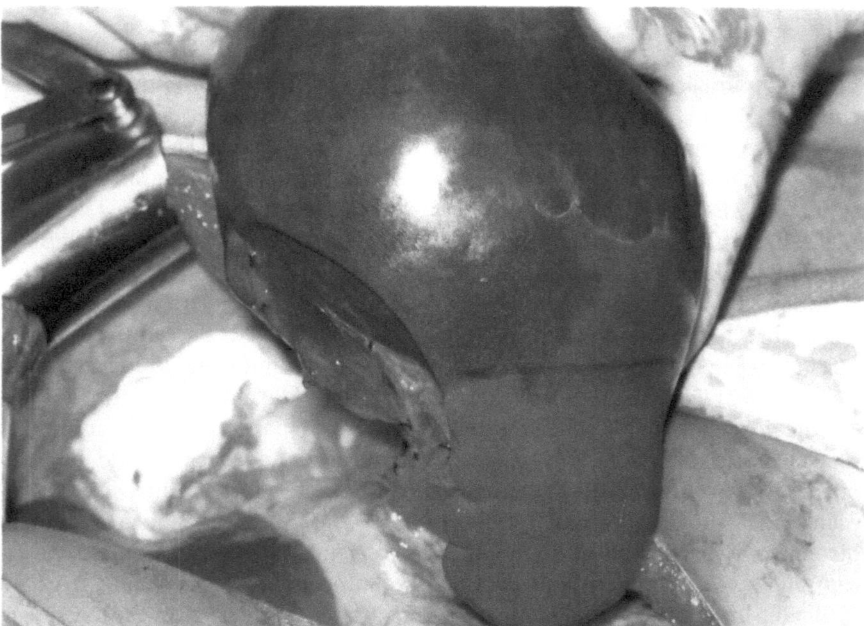

Fig. 6. Giant nonparasitic cyst of upper pole resected by partial splenectomy. Line of demarcation after ligation of segmental vessels indicates level of resection

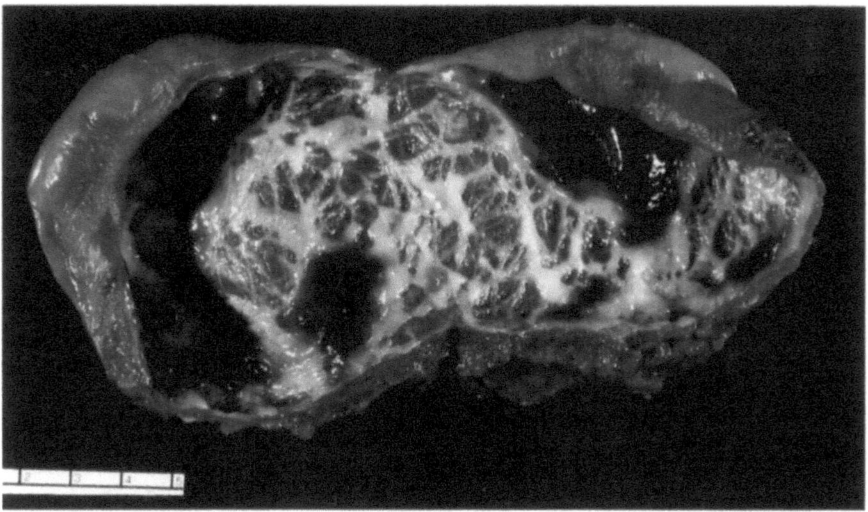

Fig. 7. Classic appearance of interior of nonparasitic splenic cyst. Glistening white trabeculation is typical

Parasitic Cysts

The only parasitic cyst of the spleen of surgical importance is the echinococcus or hydatid cyst. The most common species involved is *Echinococcus granulosus*, whose larval forms encyst in the viscera, principally in the liver but rarely in the spleen (2–3%). Diagnosis of hydatid disease of the spleen should be suspected in endemic areas, such as the Near East, New Zealand, Australia, and the western United States. The complement-fixation test of Ghedini-Weinberg is the most reliable serologic test.

Although at least one partial splenectomy for echinococcus cyst of the spleen has been reported [39], the suitability of such a procedure is highly questionable. In view of the possibility of occult, multicentric loci of infection in the spleen, the preferred treatment is splenectomy.

Since excision of the spleen without rupture or parenchymal disruption is especially important in this disease, the surgical approach should be with maximal exposure. The best exposure is with a left subcostal incision of generous size, allowing careful mobilization of the spleen by sharp and blunt dissection. During and after mobilization the perisplenic area should be exceptionally well isolated with packs to contain any spillage, should it occur. If, during mobilization, it is apparent that pressure or traction on the spleen may rupture a cyst, the contents of the cyst should be aspirated and replaced with 20% saline twice, to kill the contained scoleces. The cyst should then be emptied and the spleen carefully resected, keeping the area well walled off with packs at all times.

Considering the fragile nature of the cysts and the dire consequences of rupture, laparoscopic splenectomy is not advisable. Laparoscopic aspiration of the cyst is to be strictly avoided.

References

1. Warnke RA, Weiss LM, Chan JKC, Cleary ML, Dorfman RF (1995) Atlas of tumor pathology: tumors of the lymph nodes and spleen. Armed Forces Institute of Pathology, Washington DC
2. Panuel M, Ternier F, Michel G, Scheiner C, Bourliere B, Faure F, Guys JM, Devred P (1992) Splenic hemangioma – report of three pediatric cases with pathologic correlation. Pediatr Radiol 22: 213–216
3. Hoeger PH, Helmke K, Winkler K (1995) Chronic consumption coagulotherapy due to an occult splenic hemangioma: Kasabach-Merritt syndrome. Eur J Pediatr 154: 365–368
4. Ros PR, Moser RP Jr, Dachman AH, Murari PJ, Olmsted WW (1987) Hemangioma of the spleen: radiologic-pathologic correlations in ten cases. Radiology 162: 73–77
5. Barbazza R, DeMartini A, Mognol M, Banzi A, D'Agata G (1990) Fine needle aspiration biopsy of a splenic hemangioma: a case report with review of the literature (review). Haematologica (Pavia) 75: 278–281
6. Goerg C, Schwerk WB, Goerg K (1991) Splenic lesions: sonographic patterns, follow-up, differential diagnosis. Eur J Radiol 13: 59–66
7. Falk S, Stutte HJ, Frizzera G (1991) Littoral cell angioma: a novel splenic vascular lesion demonstrating histiocytic differentiation (review). Am J Surg Pathol 15: 1023–1033

8. Rosso R, Paulli M, Gianelli U, Boveri E, Stella G, Magrini U (1995) Littoral cell angiosarcoma of the spleen: case report with immunohistochemical and ultrastructural analysis. Am J Surg Pathol 19: 1203–1208

9. Morgenstern L, Bello JM, Fisher BL, Verham RP (1992) Clinical spectrum of lymphangiomas and lymphangiomatosis of the spleen. Am Surg 58: 599–604

10. Asch MJ, Cohen AH, Moore TC (1974) Hepatic and splenic lymphangiomatosis with skeletal involvement: report of a case and review of the literature. Surgery 76: 334–339

11. Schneiderman H, Gruhn J (1983) Metachronous axillary and splenic lymphangiomatosis: demonstration of immunoreactive factor VIII-related antigen. Am J Clin Pathol 79: 625–627

12. Avigad S, Jaffe R, Frand M, Izhak Y, Rotem Y (1976) Lymphangiomatosis with splenic involvement. JAMA 236: 2315–2317

13. Bardeguez A, Chatterjee M, Tepedino M, Sicuranza B (1990) Systemic cystic angiomatosis in pregnancy: a case presentation and review of the literature. Am J Obstet Gynecol 163: 42–45

14. Nirmala Devi N, Ramakrishana Pillai PG (1974) Cystic lymphangioma of the spleen – a case report. Indian J Pathol Bacteriol 17: 60–62

15. Feigenberg Z, Wysenbeek A, Avidor E, Dintsman M (1983) Malignant lymphangioma of the spleen. Isr J Med Sci 19: 202–204

16. Khan AH, Bensoussan AL, Ouimet A, Blancharg H, Grignon A, Ndoye M (1986) Partial splenectomy for benign cystic lesions of the spleen. J Pediatr Surg 21: 749–752

17. Quandalle P, Rousseau B, Mascaut A, Wurtz A (1987) La splénectomie partielle dans les lésions bénignes non traumatiques de la râte. J Chir (Paris) 124: 326–330

18. Chopra S, Edelstein A, Koff RS, et al (1978) Peliosis hepatis in hematologic disease. Report of two cases. JAMA 240: 1153

19. Kaw YT, Duwaji MS, Knisley RE, Esparza AR (1992) Hemangioendothelioma of the spleen. Arch Pathol Lab Med 116: 1079–1082

20. Suster S (1992) Epithelioid and spindle-cell hemangioendothelioma of the spleen: report of a distinctive splenic vascular neoplasm of childhood. Am J Surg Pathol 16: 785–792

21. Cerda J, Luque Mialdea R, Soleto J, Martin-Crespo R, Aguilar F (1994) Segmentary splenectomy of the lower tip because of spontaneous rupture of a splenic hemangioendothelioma in a new-born child – a case report. Eur J Pediatr Surg 4: 113–115

22. Safran D, Welch J, Rezuke W (1991) Inflammatory pseudotumors of the spleen. Arch Surg 126: 904–908

23. Glazer M, Lally J, Kanzer M (1992) Inflammatory pseudotumor of the spleen: MR findings. J Comput Assist Tomogr 16: 980–983

24. Inada T, Yano T, Shima S, Ishikawa Y, Irie S, Ishida M, Nakamura Y, Ishibashi K, Kageyama H (1992) Inflammatory pseudotumor of the spleen (review). Intern Med 31: 941–945

25. Dalal BI, Greenberg H, Quinonez GE, Gough JC (1991) Inflammatory pseudotumor of the spleen: morphological, radiological, immunophenotypic, and ultrastructural features. Arch Pathol Lab Med 115: 1062–1064

26. Suster S, Moran CA, Blanco M (1994) Mycobacterial spindle-cell pseudotumor of the spleen. Am J Clin Pathol 101: 539–542

27. Steinberg JJ, Suhrland M, Valensi Q (1991) The spleen in the spleen syndrome. The association of splenoma with hematopoietic and neoplastic disease: compendium of cases since 1864. J Surg Oncol 47: 193–202

28. Kumar PV (1995) Splenic hamartoma: a diagnostic problem on fine needle aspiration cytology. Acta Cytol 39: 391–395

29. Morgenstern L, McCafferty L, Rosenberg J, Michel SL (1984) Hamartomas of the spleen. Arch Surg 119: 1291–1293

30. Iozzo RV, Haas JE, Chard RL (1980) Symptomatic splenic hamartoma: a report of two cases and review of the literature. Pediatrics 66: 261–265

31. Beham A, Hermann W, Vennigerholz F, Schmid C (1989) Hamartoma of the spleen with haematological symptoms. Virchows Arch [A] 414: 535–539

32. Havlik RJ, Touloukian RJ, Markowitz RI, Buckley P (1990) Partial splenectomy for symptomatic splenic hamartoma (review). J Pediatr Surg 25: 1273–1275
33. Stiller RJ, Haynes de Regt R, Choy OG (1991) Antenatal diagnosis of fetal splenic cyst: a case report. J Reprod Med 36: 320–322
34. Nerlich A, Permanetter W (1991) Fine needle aspiration cytodiagnosis of epidermoid cysts of the spleen: report of two cases. Acta Cytol 35: 567–569
35. Morgenstern L, Shapiro SJ (1980) Partial splenectomy for nonparasitic splenic cysts. Am J Surg 139: 278–281
36. Salky B, Zimmerman M, Bauer J et al (1985) Splenic cyst – definitive treatment by laparoscopy. Gastrointest Endosc 31: 213–215
37. Touloukian RJ, Seashore JH (1987) Partial splenic decapsulation: a simplified operation for splenic pseudocyst. J Pediatr Surg 22: 135–137
38. Üranus S, Kronberger L, Kraft-Kine J (1994) Partial splenic resection using the TA-stapler. Am J Surg 168: 49–53
39. Nangalia R, Al-Salem AH (1993) Splenic salvage in hydatid disease. Ann Saudi Med 13: 88–90

Malignant Splenic Lesions

F. J. GILES and S.W. LIM

> "... enlargement of the spleen in leukocythaemia appears to be only a part of a general disease affecting the glandular system as a whole ... in splenotomy for such a disease there is a predisposition to haemorrhage with which surgery is incompetent to deal."
> *Sir Berkeley Moynihan, 1920*

Introduction

The involvement of the spleen by human malignancy varies depending on the specific neoplasm. Lymphoproliferative and myeloproliferative disorders comprise a majority of the splenic malignancies. Clinically relevant primary and metastatic carcinoma to the spleen is rare. This chapter covers the initial work-up of the spleen that is suspicious for neoplastic involvement. It then reviews the individual causes of malignant splenic lesions (see Table 1). Presentation, evaluation, and management for each major entity are discussed, and the roles of splenectomy and radiation therapy are specifically addressed.

Epidemiology

Splenomegaly is the most common presentation of a spleen involved by malignancy, but not all enlarged spleens are pathologic. Ebaugh and McIntyre [20] evaluated 2200 college students and found that 63 (2.9%) had palpable spleens. At a 10-year follow-up there was no evidence of lymphoreticular malignancy. In a study of patients referred for scintigraphy because of spleno-with palpable spleens, 16.4% of 110 cases were found to be normal [3]. The main underlying diagnoses in that series were hepatic cirrhosis (37%) and lymphoma or leukemia (16%).

Table 1. Malignant splenic lesions

I.   Lymphoproliferative disorders
     Non-Hodgkin's lymphoma
     Hodgkin's disease
     Chronic lymphocytic leukemia
     Hairy cell leukemia
     Acute lymphoblastic leukemia
     Waldenström's macroglobulinemia
     Plasmacytoma
II. Myeloproliferative disorders
     Chronic myelogenous leukemia
     Myelofibrosis (agnogenic myeloid metaplasia)
     Polycythemia vera
     Essential thrombocythemia
III. Vascular tumors
     Benign
     Hemangioma
     Hamartoma
     Lymphangioma
     Malignant
     Hemangiosarcoma
     Lymphangiosarcoma
IV. Metastatic tumors
     Breast, lung, melanoma, cervix, etc.
V.   Others
     Lipoma
     Malignant fibrous histiocytoma
     Fibrosarcoma
     Leiomyosarcoma
     Malignant teratoma
     Kaposi's sarcoma

Diagnosis

When a patient presents with idiopathic splenomegaly, a broad differential, including malignant and nonmalignant causes, should be considered. When screening specifically for malignancy, one should ask the patient about fever, night sweats, weight loss, adenopathy, weakness, and malaise. A thorough physical exam includes careful palpation of all lymph-node groups. Screening tests include a complete blood count with review of the smear, a chemistry panel, and lactate dehydrogenase.

Diagnostic imaging techniques, if needed, include ultrasonography, computerized tomography, and radioisotope scanning. Ultrasonography is a simple and noninvasive technique, but it lacks the sensitivity to alone provide a specific diagnosis. Often, adjuvant clinical or pathologic data are required to confirm the diagnosis. In a study of 172 patients with abnormal splenic echotexture, 73 were found to have neoplastic involvement based on sonographic appearance, clinical data, and short-term ultrasound follow-up [25]. Of the 73 patients, 60 had non-Hodgkin's lymphomas. Eighteen had normal spleen size. Patients with Hodgkin's disease exhibited focal (11/21) and diffuse (10/21) splenic lesions, whereas high-grade non-Hodgkin's lymphomas were focal and larger than 3 cm in 16 of 20 patients. The low-grade non-Hodgkin's lymphomas caused both diffuse and focal lesions, with 17 of 19 patients having lesions less than 3 cm in diameter. Ninety-seven percent of the lymphomatous lesions were hypoechoic. Other neoplasms found were two cases of ovarian cancer and one case of medullary carcinoma of the thyroid that exhibited hyperechoic lesions. Lesions that progressed and regressed with cytotoxic therapy were small cell lung cancer, malignant melanoma, and lymphoepithelial carcinoma. Metastatic colon, pancreatic, and breast cancers were also found.

Because the normal spleen is usually hypoechoic, hyperechoic lesions are generally thought to be benign. Siler et al. [78] reported nine patients with hyperechoic malignant lesions. These lesions were caused by acute lymphocytic leukemia (3), chronic myelogenous leukemia (3), chronic lymphocytic leukemia, Hodgkin's disease, and metastatic adenocarcinoma (one case each).

Scintigraphy is a noninvasive test and provides an accurate determination of spleen size. With massive splenomegaly it can detect focal splenic defects. However, spleen scanning is not of benefit in the staging of lymphoma since it will not detect microinfiltrates. Computer tomography may provide additional information about the spleen while also imaging the remainder of the abdomen. MRI does not generally add to the information from CT. The ultimate diagnosis of an abnormal spleen often relies on other clinical, laboratory, or pathologic data.

When the noninvasive workup fails to provide a diagnosis, splenectomy is the gold standard for the pathologic diagnosis of splenic abnormalities. Of ten diagnostic splenectomies performed at Cork Regional Hospital over an 11-year period, there were eight malignancies; five patients had lymphoma, two had Hodgkin's disease, and one patient had hairy cell leukemia [16]. The two nonmalignant cases were splenic congestion and a normal spleen. King et al. [43] reported six patients with massive splenomegaly without peripheral adenopathy who were diagnosed by splenectomy as having lymphoma.

Several studies have been published that report the use of fine-needle or core biopsies of the spleen. A large series of over 1000 cases was reported by Soderstrom [82]. Recently Zeppa et al. [104] analyzed a series of 140 consecutive fine-needle aspiration biopsies (FNAB) of the spleen. They used 22-gauge spinal needles in adults with a subdiaphragmatic approach. Thirty-two cases were found to be malignant. Lymphomas and leukemias were diagnosed during the staging of known primaries in 18 cases, whereas in nine cases the results of the splenic FNAB provided the first diagnosis. To improve diagnostic accuracy, Lindgren et al. [47] used a spring-trigger Tru-Cut needle to obtain core biopsies from 32 patients. The reported side effects were slight to moderate pain (16/32 patients) and bleeding requiring transfusion (4/32). One patient required splenectomy because of bleeding. Suzuki et al. [88] reported a series of eight patients who had core biopsies performed as part of staging for non-Hodgkin's lymphoma. They reported no complications from the procedure using a 21-gauge Surecut needle.

Despite the low reported incidence of complications with these procedures, fine-needle and core biopsy have not gained wide acceptance due to continued concern regarding complications, primarily hemorrhage. If malignancy is suspected, splenectomy may be the more useful procedure, being relatively safe along with providing more tissue for diagnosis.

Specific Malignancies

Lymphoproliferative Disorders

The lymphoproliferative disorders comprise a large proportion of malignant splenic disease. The spleen normally loses hematopoietic function by the end of the fetal period. It then functions mainly as an immune organ, comprised primarily of lymphocytes. Because of this, the spleen may exhibit the full spectrum of lymphoid malignancies.

Non-Hodgkin's Lymphoma

The incidence of non-Hodgkin's lymphoma (NHL) is increasing in the United States. There will be an estimated 57 000 cases in 1996 [64]. Most patients with NHL will present with lymphadenopathy or signs of systemic or localized disease. Splenic involvement is seen in approximately 30–40% of patients with NHL at laparotomy [42, 48, 85] and in 50%–80% at autopsy [72, 85]. The spleen as a site of primary presentation is rare. Narang et al. [63] reported a series of 31 patients who were diagnosed with lymphoma after presenting with prominent splenomegaly. The diagnosis was made by splenectomy, either for diagnostic or for therapeutic purposes. Other staging procedures were performed on these patients, including lymph-node biopsies from areas including the splenic hilum, liver biopsy, and bone marrow biopsy. Thirty of the 31 cases were of the small lymphoid (small lymphocytic and small cleaved cell) types, and one was a lymphocytic lymphoma. Although initially referred as cases of primary splenic malignancy, the majority of these patients were found to have widespread involvement.

Imaging modalities such as ultrasonography and computerized tomography are used to evaluate the spleen in patients with NHL. As discussed above, spleens with NHL commonly exhibit diffuse hypoechogenicity, but cases of hyperechogenicity on ultrasound examination have been reported [78]. Computerized tomography can accurately define the size of the spleen in three dimensions. By determining the product of the length, width, and thickness of the spleen, a "splenic index" is calculated [87]. The splenic index has been shown to correlate well with the presence of malignancy. In a group of 23 patients with autopsy data, none of three patients with an index of less than 480 had splenic involvement by NHL. The remaining 20 patients, with indices of greater than 480, had splenic involvement at the time of death. In the total group of 33 patients (including laparotomy patients), the splenic index had an accuracy of 100% in predicting the histologic state of the spleen. In this study, hepatic involvement also indicated splenic involvement. This study supports the use of CT without surgical intervention to define splenic involvement by NHL.

On pathologic examination, each type of lymphoma has been found to have a specific pattern of infiltration of the red and white pulp [96]. The low-grade lymphomas had a specific pattern of infiltration dependent on their Kiel classification (Fig. 1). The high-grade lymphomas behave as solid tumors randomly distributed in the spleen (Fig. 2). Based on this study, the authors conclude that the spleen is compartmentalized and that the routes of circulation of lymphocytes in the spleen are based on homing mechanisms. This difference may be beneficial for further classification of NHL in the spleen.

Therapy of NHL usually consists in multiagent chemotherapy. Because of the use of systemic therapy, surgical-staging splenectomy is rarely employed in patients with NHL. Splenectomy may be indicated for therapeutic purposes such as improvement of anemia, leukopenia, thrombocytopenia, or symptoms of local discomfort. Lehne et al. [46] performed a retrospective

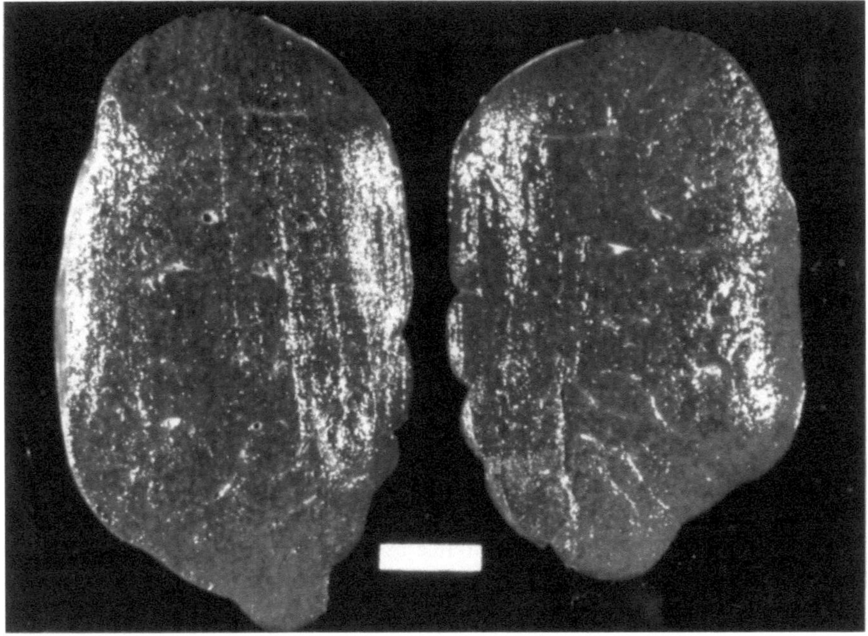

Fig. 1. Spleen diffusely involved by low-grade non-Hodgkin's lymphoma. Note fine white miliary pattern. (Courtesy of Dr. Jonathan Said)

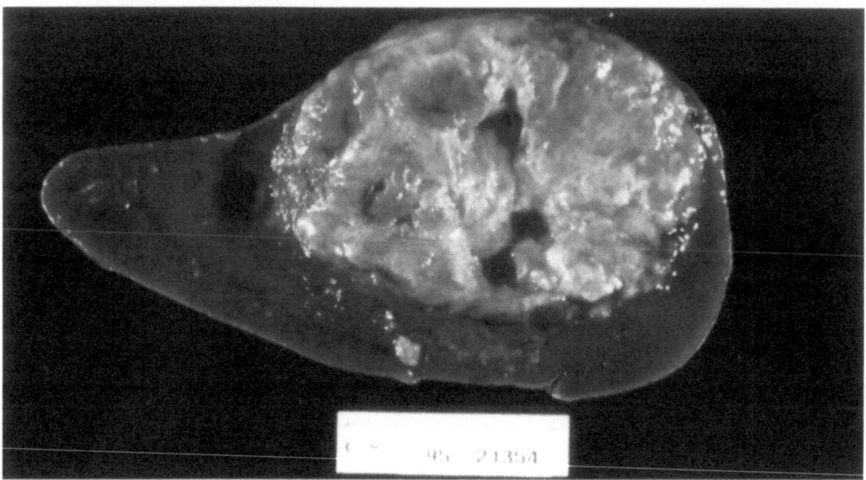

Fig. 2. Characteristic solitary tumor-like involvement of the spleen by a high-grade non-Hodgkin's lymphoma. (Courtesy of Dr. Jonathan Said)

analysis of 35 patients who had had NHL and had undergone splenectomy at one institution over a 10-year period. The indications were diagnostic in five patients and therapeutic in 30 (to relieve hypersplenism in 20 and to relieve abdominal discomfort or reduce tumor burden in five patients each). Correction of at least one cytopenia within 1 month post-op was seen in 18 of 25 (72%) patients. The response rates for leukopenia, thrombocytopenia, and anemia were 83, 68, and 50%, respectively. Infection was the most common complication, occurring in seven patients (20%), with one death due to septicemia. Three patients had postoperative fever, one patient had a hematoma in the splenic bed, and there was one death due to a myocardial infarction. The authors concluded that splenectomy could be performed with acceptable mortality and morbidity even in patients with advanced disease. Splenectomy may induce significant reversal of hematologic abnormalities in patients with non-Hodgkin's lymphoma.

Primary Splenic Lymphoma

Primary splenic lymphoma (PSL) is thought to originate in the spleen and accounts for less than 1% of cases of NHL in most series [1, 11]. The criteria for defining PSL, and even its existence as a distinct entity, are controversial. Most authors define PSL as a lymphoma with the predominant involvement in the spleen, indicating its origin. The staging system described by Ahmann et al. [1] defines group I as showing involvement only of the spleen, group II as having involvement of the spleen and splenic hilar lymph nodes, and group III as having involvement of the spleen, liver, abdominal lymph nodes, and bone marrow. Small lymphocytic lymphoma (well-differentiated lympho-cytic lymphoma) is the most common histologic type [45, 63, 84]. In a retro-spective review [22], the histologic and immunohistochemical studies did not reveal any difference between PSL and disseminated malignant lymphomas with splenic involvement with regard to morphological features, immunophe-notype, host cell infiltrates, or proliferation activity. PSL was initially re-ported as having a poor prognosis, but recent reports indicate a good prog-nosis for patients with group-I PSL [5] and even potential cure with sple-nectomy alone for low-grade patients [11]. The overall 5-year survival in two small series was 31 and 43% [1, 41]. The role of adjuvant therapy following splenectomy has not been defined.

Marginal Zone Lymphoma of the Spleen

Splenic marginal zone lymphoma (SMZL) is a recently described entity [75]. In one review of 13 cases, the mean age was 61.8 years [57]. All patients pre-sented with splenomegaly, nine had some abdominal discomfort. Cytopenia was present in six of the 13 cases, and 11 showed peripheral blood lympho-cytosis. None had peripheral adenopathy at the time of splenectomy. Macro-scopically, the spleen had a micronodular white miliary pattern in all cases (Fig. 3). Microscopically there was a marginal zone pattern of infiltration, distinct from the mantle zone. Immunohistochemically, the tumor cells were usually CD20+, KiB3+, Bcl2+, CD11c–, and CD5–. SMZL is often misdiag-

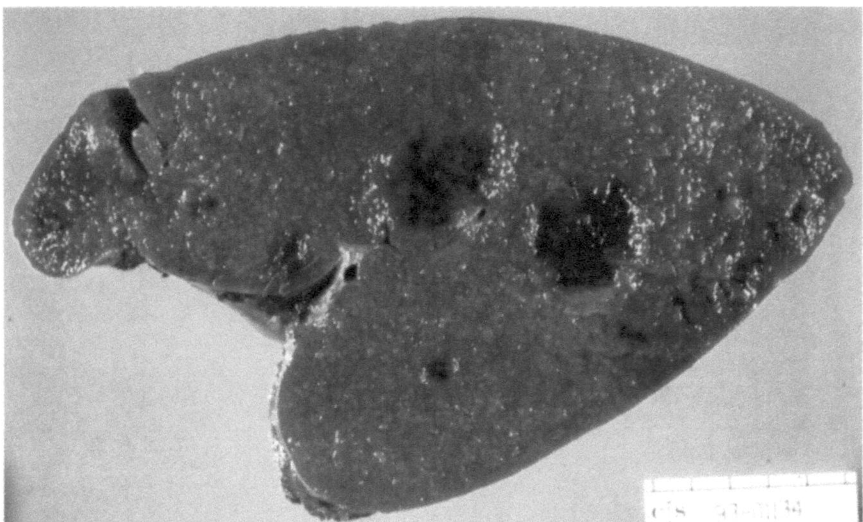

Fig. 3. Spleen with marginal zone lymphoma with nodular expansion of the white pulp. This patient also had autoimmune hemolytic anemia with splenic congestion and hemor-rhage, indicated by darker splenic regions. (Courtesy of Dr. Jonathan Said)

nosed as other entities such as chronic lymphocytic leukemia, immunocyto-
ma, mantle-cell lymphoma, monocytoid B-cell lymphoma, lymphoma with
epithelioid reaction, and splenic lymphoma with villous lymphocytes.

Patients with advanced marginal zone lymphoma, stage III and IV, have a
clinical course similar to that of patients with Working Formulation categories A–E who are treated with CHOP [23]. The clinical course of patients
with SMZL is often protracted, with a good clinical response to splenectomy
[57]. Further series are needed to fully characterize the clinical course and
define the best therapy.

Hodgkin's Disease

Hodgkin's disease (HD) is highly curable and has become the model for the
development of diagnostic and therapeutic techniques in oncology. There
will be an estimated 7500 cases of HD in the United States in 1996 [64]. The
disease presents above the diaphragm in 90% of cases, usually with mediastinal or cervical adenopathy. Patients may also present with B-symptoms,
i.e., fever, night sweats, and a greater than 10% weight loss over 6 months.

The diagnosis is made by biopsy and the finding of Reed-Sternberg cells
in the pathologic specimen (Fig. 4). HD is traditionally categorized as lym-

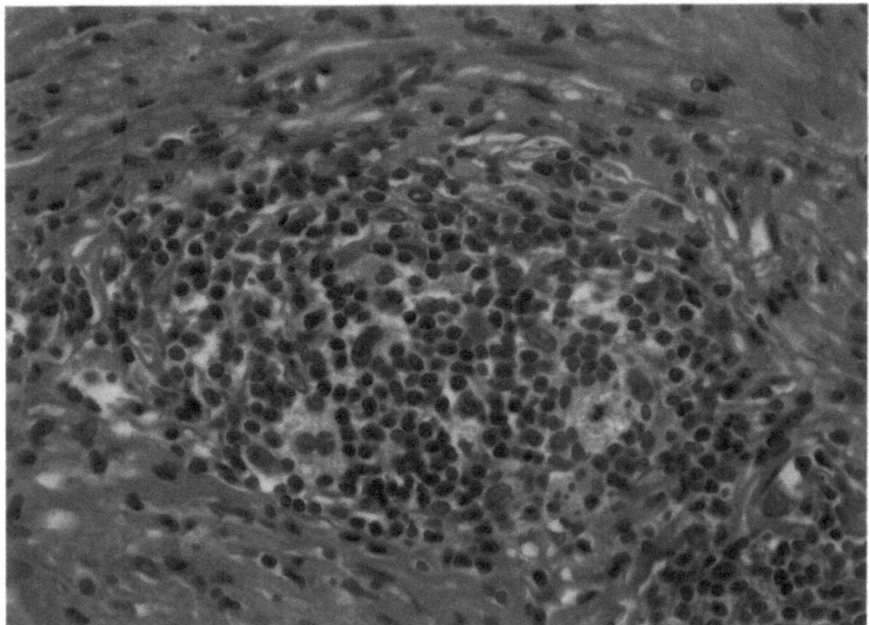

Fig. 4. Micrograph of a spleen with the pathognomonic lacunar Reed-Sternberg cell. (Courtesy of Dr. Jonathan Said)

phocyte predominant, nodular sclerosing, mixed cellularity, or lymphocyte depleted. This simple classification belies the fact that HD is an enigmatic and heterogeneous disorder; even the cell of origin is still being debated. The lymphocyte-predominant category may actually represent a B-cell non-Hodgkin's lymphoma [13].

Patient characteristics that portend a worse prognosis in HD include B-symptoms, age greater than 45 years, mediastinal width greater than 45% of the greatest chest wall diameter, involvement of bone marrow, liver, or multiple extranodal sites, high lactate dehydrogenase, and a high sedimentation rate [86]. The extent of splenic involvement has also been found to be a prognostic factor. Patients with fewer than five splenic nodules do well with radiation therapy alone, compared with those who have extensive splenic involvement [36].

Despite the fact that it is not completely understood, HD is a very treatable disorder. For limited-stage disease (stages I and II), radiation therapy may be curative [35]. Multiagent chemotherapy with regimens such as MOPP and ABVD have proven very effective in advanced-stage disease [18]. In some patients, multimodality therapy may be indicated. The choice of treatment modality is based on clinical and pathologic staging. Pathologic staging may involve laparotomy, which includes splenectomy, liver biopsy, and abdominal lymph-node sampling.

The role of laparotomy in HD is continuing to evolve. Marble et al. [52] reviewed 156 splenectomies performed for all indications at one institution between 1979 and 1991. Patients were divided into two groups, those undergoing splenectomy from 1979 to 1985 (period I) and those undergoing splenectomy from 1986 to 1991 (period II). More splenectomies were performed for hematologic disorders, cytopenias, and anemias in period II than in period I. In contrast, splenectomies for Hodgkin's disease decreased from period I to period II. Currently, laparotomy is performed in HD only if radiation therapy is the planned treatment and the finding of abdominal disease would alter the management, calling for chemotherapy. The use of staging laparotomy has diminished with the advent of improved radiographic techniques, less toxic multiagent chemotherapy regimens, and better prognostic indices.

Recent reports have examined the possibility of replacing staging laparotomy with noninvasive radiographic studies or prognostic indices. Two studies of pediatric patients with HD revealed that imaging studies and positive and negative prognostic models correlated well with findings at laparotomy but had high false-positive and false-negative rates [10, 56]. This limited their capacity for predicting the presence of abdominal disease in an individual patient. A report from the Children's Cancer Study Group found that CT and gallium were specific but not sensitive [33]. Laparotomy allowed a smaller radiation field in 29 of 49 patients, and the classification of patients as having stage-IV disease was determined only by pathologic staging in five cases.

Muscat et al. reviewed 94 patients who had undergone staging laparotomy for HD [61]. Lymphangiograms were performed in 86 patients and abdominal CT in 53. Both tests had an accuracy of 76%, but the results of laparotomy required a change in the staging for 28% of the patients, with a subsequent change in the clinical management for 18%. Staging laparotomy continues to be a valuable diagnostic technique for a certain subset of HD patients.

The upstaging of a patient with HD may not be as important clinically in early-stage cases. The EORTC compared clinical staging and irradiation alone with indicated treatment determined by staging laparotomy in patients with a favorable prognosis [14]. A total of 262 adult patients with favorable prognostic factors were randomly assigned to clinical staging and subtotal nodal irradiation versus staging laparotomy and irradiation or chemotherapy, depending on the pathologic findings. Favorable prognosis was defined as clinical stage I or II, no bulky mediastinal disease, and either no B-symptoms with an ESR of less than 50 mm or B symptoms and an ESR of less than 30 mm. Six-year freedom from progression rates were similar in the clinical- and laparotomy-staged arms. The survival rates were 93% and 89%, respectively. The poorer survival in the laparotomy arm was attributed to laparotomy-related deaths. The authors concluded that staging laparotomy is unnecessary for patients with a favorable prognosis.

Several reviews have attempted to determine the accuracy of noninvasive techniques for staging patients with HD. The splenic index, the product of the length, width, and thickness of the spleen as measured by CT, correlates well with splenic weight [32, 87]. Although splenic weight is the strongest factor correlating with splenic involvement by HD, it is not a sensitive predictor. In a study reported by Sombeck et al. [83], the positive predictive value of abdominal and splenic involvement was poor, being 20% and 43%, respectively. The respective negative predictive values were 93% and 77%. Magnetic resonance imaging also appears to have no advantage over CT [71, 81].

Complications of splenectomy in HD patients are well documented. Short- and long-term complications include overwhelming postsplenectomy infection, small bowel obstruction, atelectasis, abscess, and wound dehiscence [39]. Splenectomy in patients with HD may predispose them to higher rates of secondary malignancy despite their being cured of the original disease. Tura et al. looked at the incidence of acute nonlymphocytic leukemia in 503 HD patients [95]. It was 0.69% in 145 nonsplenectomized patients and 5.86% in 358 splenectomized patients. This confirms earlier reports [40, 97], though a review of patients from the British National Lymphoma Investigation did not reveal an increased leukemic risk in HD patients who had undergone splenectomy [89].

The relatively new technique of laparoscopic splenectomy has been shown to decrease some of the complications of splenectomy [4, 67, 73]. This technique appears to be well tolerated and safe, though the series of patients with HD is small. Laparoscopic splenectomy may reduce the short- and long-term complications, but it still does not address the potentially increased risk of leukemia.

Chronic Lymphocytic Leukemia

Chronic lymphocytic leukemia (CLL) is the most frequent of the chronic leukemias. It commonly affects individuals in their sixth or seventh decade. Presenting symptoms include fatigue, lymphadenopathy, and organomegaly. The diagnosis is often made incidentally on routine complete blood cell count and with the finding of mature-appearing lymphocytes on a peripheral smear (Fig. 5). CLL is staged using the Rai classification that employs splenomegaly as a prognostic factor [68]. Rai stage 0 is lymphocytosis greater than 50 000, stage I is the presence of lymphadenopathy, stage II is the presence of either hepatomegaly or splenomegaly, stages III and IV involve anemia (less than 11 g/dl) and thrombocytopenia ($<10^5/mm^3$) respectively.

Therapy of CLL depends on the stage. Stage-I disease, because of its long median survival, may be watched without intervention. Systemic chemotherapy is the treatment of choice, often with alkylators such as chlorambucil or cyclophosphamide. Newer agents such as the purine analog fludarabine show great promise.

The role of splenic irradiation has been addressed in several studies. Roncadin et al. reported treating 38 patients with CLL with 10 Gy in 100-cGy fractions over a period of 10 weeks [74]. Seventy-eight percent had a hematologic response, defined as normalization of the differential leukocyte count

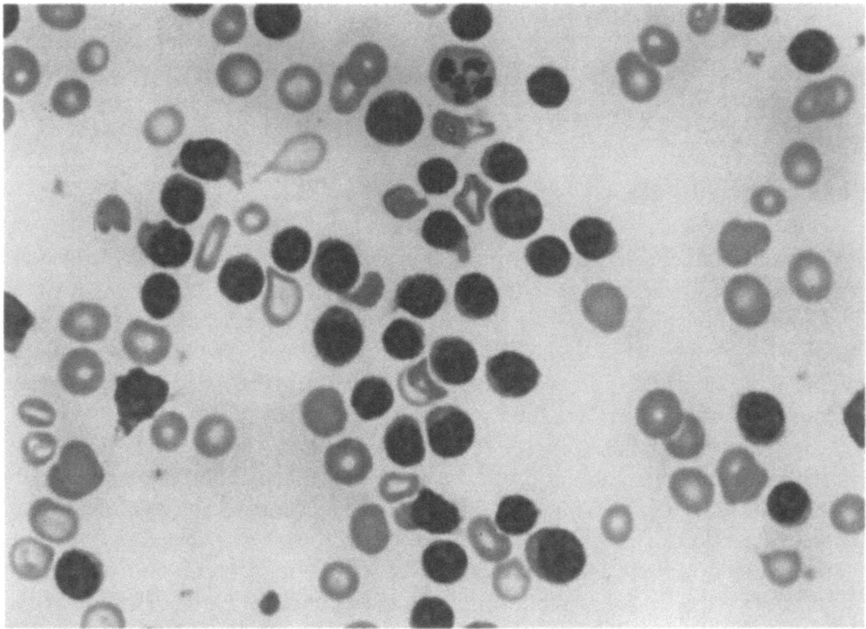

Fig. 5. Peripheral smear of a patient with chronic lymphocytic leukemia. Neoplastic cells appear as mature lymphocytes. (Courtesy of Drs. Stephen Lee and Susanne Spira)

or the total blood count and resolution of bone marrow infiltration. There were no complete responses. More than 50% reduction in splenomegaly was obtained in 63% of the patients. There were no reports of toxicity.

Guiney et al. [31] performed a retrospective study of splenic irradiation in CLL. There were 31 courses given for splenomegaly and 19 (61%) responses. Reduction in spleen size was usually seen within the first 2 weeks, and previous chemotherapy was associated with a poorer response. The total dose ranged from 125 to 2400 cGy and no dose–response relationship was detected. The treatment-related toxicity was hematologic, including both symptomatic leukopenia and thrombocytopenia.

In general, splenic irradiation appears to have a role in the management of CLL. It is indicated when the patient has discomfort from an enlarged spleen, progressive anemia, or thrombocytopenia, and when the patient is not a candidate for other therapy.

Splenectomy also appears to have a role in the management of patients with CLL. A recent trial incorporated splenectomy when patients progressed following therapy with chlorambucil [66]. It reported an 85% and 100% resolution of thrombocytopenia and anemia, respectively. Though it also reported a 34% complication rate, with fever, infection, pulmonary embolism, and one death. Delpero et al. [17] reported their experience with splenectomy for splenomegaly and hypersplenism in 62 patients with CLL and non-Hodgkin's lymphoma who failed initial therapy. There was an 89% response rate. The morbidity was 29% with one death, similar to that reported by Pegourie-Bandelier et al. [66]. Splenectomy is indicated for patients with disease that progresses despite systemic chemotherapy, to alleviate symptoms of splenomegaly and hypersplenism, though there is morbidity and a risk of mortality.

Hairy Cell Leukemia

Hairy cell leukemia is an uncommon lymphoproliferative disorder. It is a disease that usually affects middle-aged and older men and presents with pancytopenia and splenomegaly [24, 26]. This disorder is characterized by the finding of "hairy cells," cells with narrow cytoplasmic projections in the peripheral circulation (Fig. 6), bone marrow, spleen, liver, and other organs. These cells are tartrate-resistant and acid phosphatase positive.

Until recently, splenectomy was the treatment of choice for HCL. Following splenectomy, hematologic improvement has been reported in up to 90% of patients [38, 98]. Patients with greater than 85% marrow cellularity had a shorter duration of response with removal of the spleen [70].

The role of splenectomy has decreased with the introduction of effective systemic agents such as alpha-interferon, pentostatin (2′-deoxycoformycin), and 2-chlorodeoxyadenosine (2-CDA). A single 7-day course of 2-CDA achieves a complete remission in 80–90% of patients [92]. In view of these effective chemotherapies, splenectomy should be performed only on patients

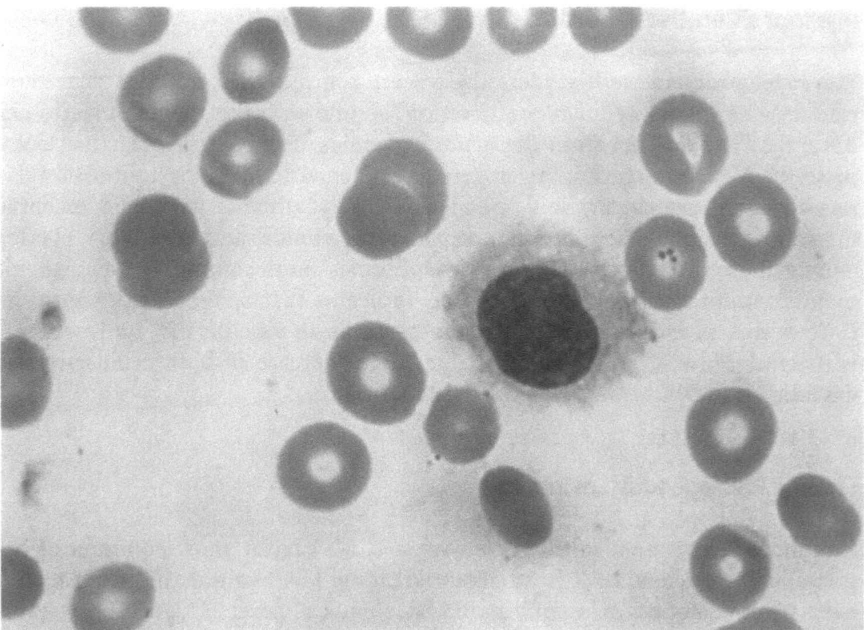

Fig. 6. Micrograph of hairy cell leukemia. Note villous membrane projections. (Courtesy of Drs. Stephen Lee and Susanne Spira)

failing to respond to systemic therapy who have massive splenomegaly or splenic rupture.

Other Lymphoid Malignancies

Waldenström's macroglobulinemia (WM) is a rare disorder that affects approximately 1500 patients per year in the United States. WM patients tend to be older, with a median age of 63 years, and 55% are male. Splenomegaly or lymphadenopathy occurs in 20%–40% of patients [19]. The hyperviscosity syndrome due to IgM occurs in approximately 15% of patients. Other presenting abnormalities include lytic bone lesions, hypercalcemia, anemia, and Bence Jones proteinuria.

Therapy, when indicated, is with an alkylating agent such as cyclophosphamide. Treatment with the nucleoside analogs fludarabine and 2-CDA is promising. If the patient is experiencing hyperviscosity symptoms, plasmapheresis is indicated. There have been case reports of patients responding to splenectomy [62, 70]. These patients had massive splenomegaly and a rapid and durable response to splenectomy, with hematologic improvement and a reduction in IgM. Splenectomy should be considered for patients with massive splenomegaly and macroglobulinemia who are refractory to systemic chemotherapy.

Myeloproliferative Disorders

The myeloproliferative disorders (MPD) are a group of conditions characterized by the clonal cellular proliferation of one or more hematopoietic cell lines; they are distinct from the acute leukemias. The four diseases that comprise the MPD are chronic myelogenous leukemia (CML), myelofibrosis (also known as agnogenic myeloid metaplasia), polycythemia vera, and essential thrombocythemia. There is often considerable clinical and laboratory overlap among these disorders. CML and myelofibrosis most commonly have splenic manifestations. Radionuclide scanning indicates that splenic enlargement in CML is due to increased cellularity rather than to vascularity [106], whereas with myelofibrosis, enlargement is due to an increase in both cellularity and vascularity.

Chronic Myelogenous Leukemia

Chronic myelogenous (myeloid) leukemia (CML) is the most common of the granulocytic leukemias. It is an acquired clonal MPD originating from malignant transformation at a multipotential stem cell level [15]. CML accounts for 15% of all leukemias and 25%–30% of adult leukemias, with the age-specific incidence rising sharply in the sixth decade to a peak of 15 patients per 100 000 U.S. population in the eighth decade. The total annual incidence in the United States is approximately 3800 new cases each year. Sixty percent of patients are male, and the median age at time of CML diagnosis is 49 years[34]. The etiology of CML is unknown, although an increase in incidence has been associated with exposure to ionizing radiation.

The diagnosis of CML is made on the basis of the findings of leukocytosis with the full spectrum of myeloid differentiation and basophilia (Fig. 7). The Philadelphia chromosome, a reciprocal translocation of genetic material between chromosomes 9 and 22, is pathognomonic for this disease. Common presenting symptoms of chronic-phase CML include fatigue (65% of patients), abdominal fullness (35% of patients), and weight loss (20% of patients) [34]. Less common but frequent presenting symptoms are diminished exercise tolerance, night sweats, bone pain, and easy bruising.

Splenomegaly is the most common physical finding on initial examination, being detected in 55%–70% of patients, and the magnitude of splenomegaly correlates well with the total body granulocyte mass and the blood granulocyte count. The enlarged spleen is firm and not tender (unless splenic infarction has occurred). The spleen is of prognostic significance along with hemoglobin concentration, leukocyte count, and clinical grade [54]. The degree of splenomegaly is an indication of chronic-phase duration; thus gross splenomegaly predicts a shorter time to blast crisis. Patients with large spleens extending more than 15 cm below the costal margin survived for significantly shorter periods than did patients with smaller spleens [94, 105]. Hepatomegaly is less frequently present (30%–50% of patients) and rarely massive.

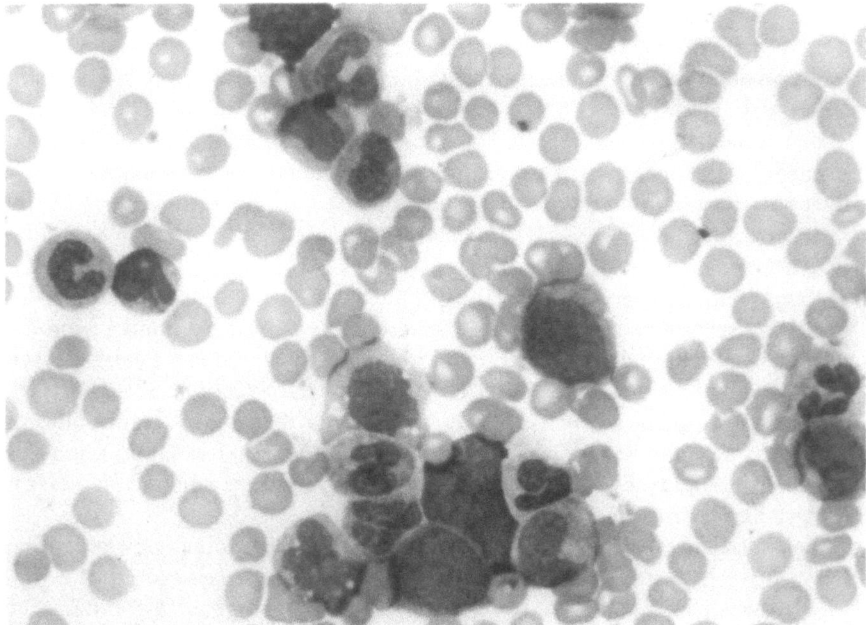

Fig. 7. Peripheral smear of a patient with chronic myelogenous leukemia. This micrograph shows the spectrum of myeloid differentiation. (Courtesy of Drs. Stephen Lee and Susanne Spira)

For most CML patients, disease progression is divisible into three stages: the chronic phase, in which hematologic progression is generally predictable and uniform; the accelerated phase, or beginning of transformation to an acute leukemia-like illness; and the terminal blast crisis, in which blast forms predominate in marrow and blood and may be evident in most other organs.

Alpha-interferon alone in adequate doses is the current optimal regimen for all patients with chronic-phase disease. Where adequate doses cannot be either given or maintained, an alpha-interferon-cytotoxic combination regimen is indicated. Patients who achieve a durable complete cytogenetic response should have autologous marrow stored. Patients who are less than 30 years of age and have a fully matched sibling donor should be offered allogeneic bone marrow transplantation. Patients over 30 years of age for whom an allogeneic bone marrow transplant donor is available may well benefit from an initial trial of alpha-interferon therapy. If a major cytogenetic remission is achieved, allogeneic bone marrow transplantation can be deferred until cytogenetic relapse occurs. Critical challenges posed by current data are how to define the relative roles of allogeneic bone marrow transplantation and alpha-interferon and – for the great majority of patients for whom allogeneic bone marrow transplantation plays no role – to design affordable alpha-interferon-based regimens with increased efficacy and less toxicity.

Experimental bone marrow transplant-related therapies which may offer advances in CML include matched unrelated donor BMT, autologous BMT, BMT involving in vitro marrow purging, CD34-positive stem cell selection, and negative selection of Ph1-positive cells in BMT [2, 6, 53, 55, 76]. The potential use of oncogene-targeted therapy (anti-sense oligonucleotides or conjugated toxins) for in vitro purging or in vivo therapy is exciting, as is investigation of agents that inhibit cytokines involved in the pathogenesis of CML, including interleukin-1 (IL-1) receptor antagonists or IL-1-soluble receptors [91, 102].

Since splenomegaly may persist despite systemic therapy, treatment may therefore be directed at the spleen. Prior to the use of busulfan in the early 1950s, splenic irradiation was commonly used to reduce the size of the spleen and restore the leukocyte count to normal. Wagner et al. [101] performed 24 courses of treatment in 17 patients with CML or myelofibrosis with total doses of 15–1650 rads. There was a significant reduction in subjective pain, and 16 of 26 courses given for splenomegaly resulted in at least a 50% reduction in spleen size.

Splenectomy performed early in the course of CML, during chronic phase, has not been shown to delay the onset of blastic transformation or to prolong survival [37, 54]. Early splenectomy also did not decrease the need for transfusion of red blood cells or improve quality of life. Neither has splenic irradiation or splenectomy been shown to be of benefit prior to allogeneic bone marrow transplantation for CML [28, 29].

Splenectomy may be useful as a palliative procedure in advanced CML, benefiting 10%–15% of such patients [27]. Significant hematologic and clinical improvement can be achieved, but the blastic evolution is not substantially altered. Infectious and thrombotic complications are frequently reported in patients treated by splenectomy, particularly those with preoperative platelet counts greater than $500\,000/mm^3$ [103]. These patients may require maintenance hydroxyurea to reduce the platelet count both preoperatively and postoperatively. With the advent of systemic therapy, including potentially curative bone marrow transplantation, splenic irradiation and splenectomy have been relegated to a palliative role for those in whom initial therapy has failed.

Myelofibrosis

Myelofibrosis (MF) is a rare disorder. The incidence is approximately $0.5/10^5$, with the median age at diagnosis being 60 years. There is a slight male predominance. This disease remains incurable and the median survival is 5 years.

Clinically, MF is characterized by bone marrow fibrosis, pancytopenia, leukoerythroblastosis, extramedullary hematopoiesis, and hepatosplenomegaly. Isoenzyme studies indicate a clonal proliferation of stem cell-derived hematopoietic cells. The bone marrow fibrosis is a result of a nonclonal proliferation of fibroblasts, probably mediated by transforming growth factor (TGF)-β, epidermal growth factor, and platelet-derived growth factor [93].

The most common presentation of myelofibrosis is anemia and splenomegaly. The peripheral blood may exhibit a leukoerythroblastic picture, with tear-drop and nucleated RBCs, and immature WBC forms (Fig. 8). As the disease progresses, splenomegaly and cytopenia become increasingly symptomatic. Transformation to acute leukemia occurs in about 8% of patients [93]. Poor prognostic factors are a short period of time (<13 months) between first symptoms and diagnosis, anemia (hemoglobin <10 g/dl), leukocyte count $>12\times10^9$/l, and peripheral blood granulocyte precursors >10% [51, 100]. Spleen size was not found to be a prognostic factor [51, 99, 100]. Splenectomy has been found to affect survival only on univariate analysis [100].

Therapy for patients with MF is supportive. Corticosteroids and androgens such as danazol have been use to improve anemia. Hydroxyurea may be used to improve organomegaly, leukocytosis, and thrombocytosis.

Splenectomy is most commonly performed in patients with MF who have massive splenomegaly and transfusion-dependent anemia. Splenectomy has been shown to improve hematologic parameters and quality of life, but not to prolong survival [7, 12, 60]. In a review of the published literature [9], Benbassat et al. found that anemia was improved in 60%, painful splenomegaly in 97%, thrombocytopenia in 56%, and portal hypertension in 83% of cases.

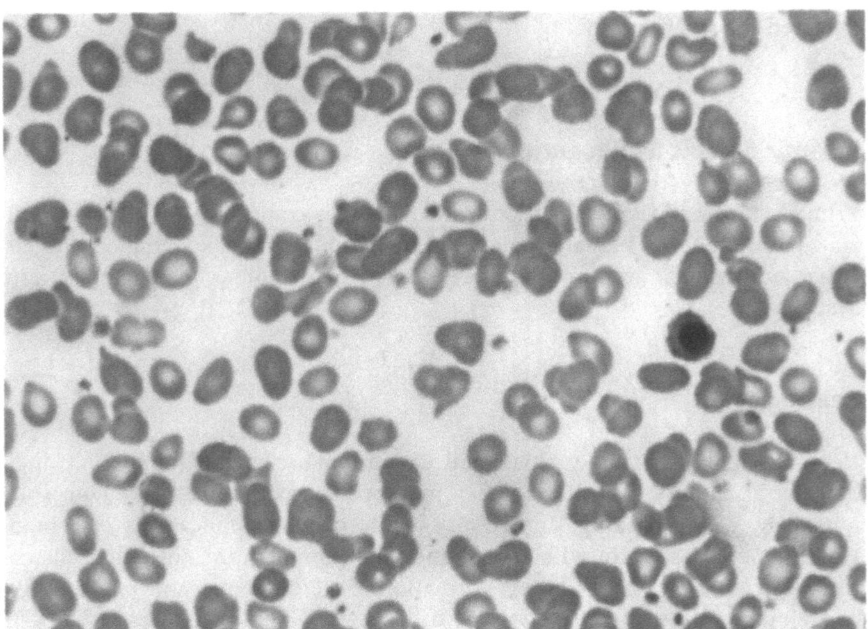

Fig. 8. Peripheral blood smear from a patient with myelofibrosis revealing leukoerythroblastic features – teardrop-shaped RBCs and nucleated RBCs. (Courtesy of Drs. Stephen Lee and Susanne Spira)

Major post-splenectomy complications include hemorrhage, subphrenic abscess, bowel infarction, and extreme thrombocytosis. Minor complications reported were fever, pleural effusion, pneumonia, wound infection, and deep vein thrombosis. In the long-term thrombotic and hemorrhagic complications (16.9%) and massive liver enlargement with hepatic dysfunction (24%) occur [7]. There is no pre-splenectomy characteristic that best predicts adverse events. In a retrospective series, the operative risk of splenectomy for both mortality (8.4%) and morbidity (39.3%) was unpredictable [7]. A review of the literature showed splenectomy in MF was associated with an operative mortality of between 7 and 18% (average 13.4%), an average early morbidity of 45.3%, and an average late morbidity of 16.3% [9]. This review also did not reveal an affect on survival post splenectomy.

Splenic irradiation may be used to reduce symptomatic splenomegaly and hypersplenism and is indicated in patients who are not suitable candidates for surgery [30, 65]. The pancytopenia that occurs with splenic irradiation is due to the destruction of proliferating precursors in the splenic tissue and sinusoids [44]. Low doses of radiation, i.e., 450–600 rads, produced few serious side effects [30, 65].

In patients with MF, splenectomy may provide significant relief of anemia, thrombocytopenia, and pain, but it does not affect the ultimate outcome. It carries significant morbidity and mortality compared with the procedure performed in non-MF patients, and must be weighed against potential benefit. Splenic irradiation provides another treatment modality for patients unsuited for splenectomy.

Intrinsic Splenic Malignancies

Primary tumors of the spleen are rare. They are comprised mainly of vascular tumors such as hemangiomas, lymphangiomas, and hemangiosarcomas. Other nonvascular tumors include fibrosarcoma, lipomas, hamartomas, and cysts.

Hemangiomas

Hemangiomas are usually small and asymptomatic, being found only incidentally at autopsy [21]. Rarely, they may present symptomatically with splenomegaly, pain, vomiting, and dyspnea. Infrequent complications of hemangiomas include rupture with intra-abdominal hemorrhage, thrombus formation, and infection with abscess formation. Severe anemia and consumptive coagulopathy have also been described [77].

Hemangiosarcoma

Hemangiosarcoma of the spleen is a rare disorder, only approximately 60 cases having been reported. Splenic rupture occurs in approximately 30% of patients [58, 80]. Thorotrast and polyvinyl chloride have been implicated as causative agents in this tumor [58]. Treatment is surgical, and adjuvant therapy with either radiation or chemotherapy has not been shown to be effective.

Lymphangioma

Lymphangiomatosis is a rare disorder characterized by the proliferation of lymphatic channels. It may involve osseous and nonosseous tissue including the spleen. Pleural and lung involvement indicates a poor prognosis [69]. Many cases occur in young children.

Hamartomas

Splenic hamartomas are benign primary neoplasms that are usually found incidentally following splenectomy or at autopsy. Microscopically, they are characterized by the presence of slit-like vascular channels, variably infiltrated with lymphocytes [79]. Because of this, splenic hamartomas may be confused histologically with Hodgkin's disease involving the spleen and must be distinguished from a malignant process.

Cysts

Splenic cysts can be classified as primary and secondary. Primary, or true, cysts usually have a squamous epithelial lining and are thought to be congenital. Secondary, or false, cysts are more common than primary cysts and do not have a true lining. The etiology of the secondary cyst is unknown, but some have suggested a relationship to trauma.

Other Splenic Tumors

Other tumors that have occasionally been reported include lipomas, primary splenic malignant fibrous histiocytomas, and primary plasmacytomas. Kaposi's sarcoma, with it's increasing incidence secondary to the emergence of AIDS, may also involve the spleen.

Metastatic Splenic Lesions

Clinically evident metastasis to the spleen is uncommon compared with the incidence of spread to other organs. If the spleen is involved, it is usually in the setting of widespread metastasis. Autopsy studies of patients with cancer revealed splenic involvement in only 7% [59]. Breast cancer, lung cancer, and malignant melanoma are the most common sources. Klein et al. [90] reported four patients in whom splenomegaly was the first clinical sign of metastatic disease. These patients had cervical cancer, endometrial cancer, lung cancer, and malignant melanoma. All four underwent splenectomy and received either adjuvant radiation or chemotherapy. Two patients lived more than 2 years, the third lived more than 1 year, and the fourth was alive 12 years following splenectomy. The authors recommended aggressive therapy, with splenectomy and combined-modality treatment in these patients. Theories to explain the paucity of splenic metastases have involved the spleen being an immune organ, but they have yet to be proven.

Complications

The combination of anemia, leukopenia, and thrombocytopenia caused by splenomegaly of any etiology is termed hypersplenism. As described in the specific disease sections, either splenic irradiation or splenectomy may often have a dramatic effect. Splenectomy or splenic irradiation may also improve the pain or discomfort due to an enlarged spleen.

Splenic rupture is a rare complication of hematologic malignancies. Bauer et al. [8] reviewed 53 cases of splenic rupture. These patients had acute leukemia, chronic leukemia, and lymphoma. Nearly all presented with pain and were initially considered to have other various diagnosis. In only ten cases was the preoperative diagnosis of splenic rupture made. Other common presenting features included tachycardia (75%), fever (74%), and hypotension (66%). Forty-eight percent of patients died without an operation. Of the 52% who had surgery, 78% survived the procedure. Early surgery is crucial in the management of the patient with a suspected splenic rupture due to hematologic malignancies.

The incidence of morbidity and mortality is higher following splenectomy than after other types of abdominal surgery and depends on the underlying disease [107]. Patients with MF have a higher rate of complications compared with patients with Hodgkin's disease who undergo splenectomy as part of a staging laparotomy. Common complications include infection, such as wound infection, pneumonia, and abscess, hemorrhage, and thromboembolic phenomena. Patients with myeloproliferative disorders have the highest rates of complications, primarily bleeding [49, 50]. Spleen size may be predictive of intraoperative bleeding.

Conclusion

Despite the prevalence of human cancers, clinically important involvement of the spleen is relatively uncommon. The myeloproliferative and lymphoproliferative disorders account for the majority of malignant splenic diseases. In general, primary and metastatic malignant splenic lesions are rare.

There are several means of examining the spleen, such as physical examination and radiographic techniques. Radiographic modalities, ultrasonography, CT, and MRI adequately determine splenic size and texture but are often not specific enough to diagnose an abnormality without additional clinical or pathologic data. Fine-needle aspiration and core biopsy, though reported in large series as safe, have not gained wide use outside of large academic medical centers. These techniques are hampered by the paucity of diagnostic tissue and lingering concern about hemorrhagic complications.

Splenectomy and splenic irradiation in malignant splenic diseases have been investigated. Due to the improvement of systemic therapies, in most situations splenectomy or splenic irradiation is currently reserved for the palliative management of symptoms of pain or hypersplenism. An exception to this is staging laparotomy with splenectomy in patients with Hodgkin's disease, though its role in this disorder continues to evolve. Splenectomy carries a higher rate of morbidity and mortality in patients with neoplastic disease than in patients who undergo this procedure for nonmalignant entities.

In the future, more research is needed to improve diagnostic modalities, including radiographic and pathologic techniques. More accurate prognostic indices may enable physicians to better direct conventional therapy for these patients. Also needed is improvement in therapies for cancer, such as new chemotherapy agents and biological response modifiers. The role of high-dose chemotherapy with stem cell transplantation in most of these malignant diseases is being actively investigated. Laparoscopic splenectomy is a promising technology. Although there is a lack of large reported series with this procedure, laparoscopic splenectomy may potentially reduce the morbidity and mortality that are commonly associated with splenectomy in patients with malignant splenic disease.

References

1. Ahmann DL, Kiely JM, Harrison EG, Payne WS (1966) Malignant lymphoma of the spleen. Cancer 16: 461–469
2. Andrews RG, Singer JW, Bernstein ID (1989) Precursors of colony-forming cells in humans can be distinguished from colony-forming cells by expression of the CD33 and CD34 antigens and light scatter properties. J Exp Med 169: 1721–1731
3. Arkles LB, Gill GD, Molan MP (1986) A palpable spleen is not necessarily enlarged or pathological. Med J Aust 145: 15–17
4. Arregui ME, Barteau J, Davis CJ (1994) Laparoscopic splenectomy: techniques and indications. Int Surg 79: 335–341

5. Audouin J, Diebold J, Schvartz H, Le Tourneau A, Bernadou A, Zittoun R (1988) Malignant lymphoplasmacytic lymphoma with prominent splenomegaly (primary lymphoma of the spleen). J Pathol 155: 17–33

6. Barnett MJ, Eaves CJ, Phillips GL, Hogge DE, Klingemann HG, Lansdorp, PM, Nantel SH, Reece DE, Shepherd JD, Sutherland HJ, et al (1992) Autografting in chronic myeloid leukemia with cultured marrow. Leukemia 6 [Suppl 4]: 118–119

7. Barosi G, Ambrosetti A, Buratti A, Finelli C, Liberato NL, Quaglini S, Ricetti MM, Visani G, Tura S, Ascari E (1993) Splenectomy for patients with myelofibrosis with myeloid metaplasia: pretreatment variables and outcome prediction. Leukemia 7: 200–206

8. Bauer TW, Haskins GE, Armitage JO (1981) Splenic rupture in patients with hematologic malignancies. Cancer 48: 2729–2733

9. Benbassat J, Gilon D, Penchas S (1990) The choice between splenectomy and medical treatment in patients with advanced agnogenic myeloid metaplasia. Am J Hematol 33: 128–135

10. Breuer CK, Tarbell NJ, Mauch PM, Weinstein HJ, Morrissey M, Neuberg, D, Shamberger RC (1994) The importance of staging laparotomy in pediatric Hodgkin's disease. J Pediatr Surg 29: 1085–1089

11. Brox A, Bishinsky JI, Berry G (1991) Primary non-Hodgkin lymphoma of the spleen. Am J Hematol 38: 95–100

12. Cabot EB, Brennan MF, Rosenthal DS, Wilson RE (1978) Splenectomy in myeloid metaplasia. Ann Surg 187: 24–30

13. Carde P (1992) Hodgkin's disease. I: Identification and classification. Br Med J 305: 99–102

14. Carde P, Hagenbeek A, Hayat M, Monconduit M, Thomas J, Burgers MJ, Noordijk EM, Tanguy A, Meerwaldt JH, Le Fur R, et al (1993) Clinical staging versus laparotomy and combined modality with MOPP versus ABVD in early-stage Hodgkin's disease: the H6 twin randomized trials from the European Organization for Research and Treatment of Cancer Lymphoma Cooperative Group. J Clin Oncol 11: 2258–2272

15. Champlin RE, Golde DW (1985) Chronic myelogenous leukemia: recent advances. Blood 65: 1039–1047

16. Cronin CC, Brady MP, Murphy C, Kenny E, Whelton MJ, Hardiman C (1994) Splenectomy in patients with undiagnosed splenomegaly. Postgrad Med J 70: 288–291

17. Delpero JR, Houvenaeghel G, Gastaut JA, Orsoni P, Blache JL, Guerinel, G, Carcassonne Y (1990) Splenectomy for hypersplenism in chronic lymphocytic leukaemia and malignant non-Hodgkin's lymphoma. Br J Surg 77: 443–449

18. DeVita VT jr, Hubbard SM (1993) Hodgkin's disease. N Engl J Med 328: 560–565

19. Dimopoulos MA, Alexanian R (1994) Waldenstrom's macroglobulinemia. Blood 83: 1452–1459

20. Ebaugh FG, McIntyre OR (1979) Palpable spleens: ten-year follow-up. Ann Intern Med 90: 130–131

21. Ejeckam GC (1976) Diffuse cavernous hemangioma of the spleen. Can J Surg 19: 354–356

22. Falk S, Stutte HJ (1990) Primary malignant lymphomas of the spleen. A morphologic and immunohistochemical analysis of 17 cases. Cancer 66: 2612–2619

23. Fisher RI, Dahlberg S, Nathwani BN, Banks PM, Miller TP, Grogan TM (1995) A clinical analysis of two indolent lymphoma entities: mantle cell lymphoma and marginal zone lymphoma (including the mucosa-associated lymphoid tissue and monocytoid B-cell subcategories): a Southwest Oncology Group study. Blood 85: 1075–1082

24. Flandrin G, Sigaux F, Sebahoun G, Bouffette P (1984) Hairy cell leukemia: clinical presentation and follow-up of 211 patients. Semin Oncol 11 [Suppl 2]: 458–471

25. Goerg C, Schwerk WB, Goerg K (1991) Splenic lesions: sonographic patterns, follow-up, differential diagnosis. Eur J Radiol 13: 59–66

26. Golomb HM, Catovsky D, Golde DW (1978) Hairy cell leukemia: a clinical review based on 71 cases. Ann Intern Med 89: 677–683

27. Gomez GA, Sokal JE, Mittelman A, Aungst CW (1976) Splenectomy for palliation of chronic myelocytic leukemia. Am J Med 61: 14–22

28. Gratwohl A, Goldman J, Gluckman E, Zwaan F (1985) Effect of splenectomy before bone-marrow transplantation on survival in chronic granulocytic leukaemia. Lancet 2: 1290–1291

29. Gratwohl A, Hermans J, von Biezen A, Arcese W, de Witte T, Debusscher L, Ernst P, Ferrant A, Frassoni F, Gahrton G, et al (1992) No advantage for patients who receive splenic irradiation before bone marrow transplantation for chronic myeloid leukaemia: results of a prospective randomized study. Bone Marrow Transplant 10: 147–152

30. Greenberger JS, Chaffey JT, Rosenthal DS, Moloney WC (1977) Irradiation for control of hypersplenism and painful splenomegaly in myeloid metaplasia. Int J Radiat Oncol Biol Phys 2: 1083–1090

31. Guiney MJ, Liew KH, Quong GG, Cooper IA (1989) A study of splenic irradiation in chronic lymphocytic leukemia. Int J Radiat Oncol Biol Phys 16: 225–229

32. Hancock SL, Scidmore NS, Hopkins KL, Cox RS, Bergin CJ (1994) Computed tomography assessment of splenic size as a predictor of splenic weight and disease involvement in laparotomy staged Hodgkin's disease. Int J Radiat Oncol Biol Phys 28: 93–99

33. Hays DM, Fryer CJ, Pringle KC, Collins RD, Hutchinson RJ, O'Neill JA, Constine LS, Heller RM, Davis PC, Nachman J, et al (1992) An evaluation of abdominal staging procedures performed in pediatric patients with advanced Hodgkin's disease: a report from the Children's Cancer Study Group. J Pediatr Surg 27: 1175–1180

34. Hehlmann R, Heimpel H, Hasford J, Kolb HJ, Pralle H, Hossfeld DK, Queisser W, Loffler H, Heinze B, Georgii A, et al (1993) Randomized comparison of busulfan and hydroxyurea in chronic myelogenous leukemia: prolongation of survival by hydroxyurea. The German CML Study Group. Blood 82: 398–407

35. Hoppe RT (1990) Radiation therapy in the management of Hodgkin's disease. Semin Oncol 17: 704–715

36. Hoppe RT, Cox RS, Rosenberg SA, Kaplan HS (1982) Prognostic factors in pathologic stage III Hodgkin's disease. Cancer Treat Rev 66: 743–749

37. Italian Cooperative Study Group on Chronic Myeloid Leukemia (1984) Results of a prospective randomized trial of early splenectomy in chronic myeloid leukemia. Cancer 54: 333–338

38. Jaiyesimi IA, Kantarjian HM, Estey EH (1993) Advances in therapy for hairy cell leukemia. A review. Cancer 72: 5–16

39. Jockovich M, Mendenhall NP, Sombeck MD, Talbert JL, Copeland EM III, Bland KI (1994) Long-term complications of laparotomy in Hodgkin's disease. Ann Surg 219: 615–621

40. Kaldor JM, Day NE, Clarke EA (1990) Leukemia following Hodgkin's disease. N Engl J Med 322: 7–13

41. Kehoe J, Straus DJ (1988) Primary lymphoma of the spleen: clinical features and outcomes after splenectomy. Cancer 62: 1433–1438

42. Kim H, Dorfman RF (1974) Morphological studies of 84 untreated patients subjected to laparotomy for the staging of non-Hodgkin's lymphoma. Cancer 33: 657–674

43. King DJ, Dawson AA, Thompson WD (1987) Splenectomy in patients with malignant lymphoma presenting with massive splenomegaly. Eur J Haematol 38: 162–165

44. Koeffler HP, Cline MJ, Golde DW (1979) Splenic irradiation in myelofibrosis: effect on circulating myeloid progenitor cells. Br J Haematol 43: 69–77

45. Kraemer BB, Osborne BM, Butler JJ (1984) Primary splenic presentation of malignant lymphoma and related disorders: a study of 49 cases. Cancer 54: 1606–1619

46. Lehne G, Hannisdal E, Langholm R, Nome O (1994) A 10-year experience with splenectomy in patients with malignant non-Hodgkin's lymphoma at the Norwegian Radium Hospital. Cancer 74: 933–939

47. Lindgren PG, Hagberg H, Eriksson B, Glimelius B, Magnusson A, Sundstrom C (1985) Excision biopsy of the spleen by ultrasonic guidance. Br J Radiol 58: 853–857

48. Long JC, Aisenberg AC (1974) Malignant lymphoma diagnosed at splenectomy and idiopathic splenomegaly. A clinicopathologic comparison. Cancer 33: 1054–1061

49. MacRae HM, Yakimets WW, Reynolds T (1992) Perioperative complications of splenectomy for hematologic disease. Can J Surg 35: 432–436

50. Malmaeus J, Akre T, Adami HO, Hagberg H (1986) Early postoperative course following elective splenectomy in haematologic disease: a high complication rate in patients with myeloproliferative disorders. Br J Surg 73: 720–723
51. Manoharan A, Smart RC, Pitney WR (1982) Prognostic factors in myelofibrosis. Pathology 14: 455–461
52. Marble KR, Deckers PJ, Kern KA (1993) Changing role of splenectomy for hematologic disease. J Surg Oncol 52: 169–171
53. McGlave P, Bartsch G, Anasetti C, Ash R, Beatty P, Gajewski J, Kernan NA (1993) Unrelated donor marrow transplantation therapy for chronic myelogenous leukemia: initial experience of the National Marrow Donor Program. Blood 81: 543–550
54. Medical Research Council's Working Party for Threrapeutic Trials In Leukemia (1983) Randomized trial of splenectomy in Ph1-positive chronic granulocytic leukaemia, including an analysis of prognostic features. Br J Haematol 54: 415–430
55. Meloni G, De Fabritiis P, Alimena G, Malagnino F, Montefusco E, Sandrelli A, Pinto R, Vignetti M, Lo Coco F, Mandelli F (1989) Autologous bone marrow or peripheral blood stem cell transplantation for patients with chronic myelogenous leukaemia in chronic phase. Bone Marrow Transplant 4 [Suppl 4]: 92–94
56. Mendenhall NP, Cantor AB, Williams JL, Ternberg JL, Weiner MA, Kung, FH, Marcus RB jr, Ferree CR, Leventhal BG (1993) With modern imaging techniques, is staging laparotomy necessary in pediatric Hodgkin's disease? A Pediatric Oncology Group study. J Clin Oncol 11: 2218–2225
57. Mollejo M, Menarguez J, Lloret E, Sanchez A, Campo E, Algara P, Cristobal E, Sanchez E, Piris MA (1995) Splenic marginal zone lymphoma: a distinctive type of low-grade B-cell lymphoma. A clinicopathological study of 13 cases. Am J Surg Pathol 19: 1146–1157
58. Montemayor P, Caggiano V (1980) Primary hemangiosarcoma of the spleen associated with leukocytosis and abnormal spleen scan. Int Surg 65: 369–373
59. Morgenstern L, Rosenberg J, Geller SA (1985) Tumors of the spleen. World J Surg 9: 468–476
60. Mulder NH, Dolsma WV, Mulder PO, De Vries EG, Willemse PH, Sleijfer, DT, Hospers GA, Van der Graaf WT (1995) Long-term results of induction and intensification chemotherapy supported with autologous bone marrow reinfusion in patients with disseminated or T4 breast cancer. Anticancer Res 15: 1565–1568
61. Muskat PC, Johnson RA, Bowers GJ (1991) Staging laparotomy in Hodgkin's lymphoma: 1979 to 1988. Am J Surg 162: 603–606; discussion 606–607
62. Nagai M, Ikeda K, Nakamura H, Ohnishi H, Amino Y, Irino S, Sato A, Uda H (1991) Splenectomy for a case with Waldenstrom macroglobulinemia with giant splenomegaly (letter). Am J Hematol 37: 140
63. Narang S, Wolf BC, Neiman RS (1985) Malignant lymphoma presenting with prominent splenomegaly. A clinicopathologic study with special reference to intermediate cell lymphoma. Cancer 55: 1948–1957
64. Parker SL, Tong T, Bolden S, Wingo PA (1996) Cancer statistics, 1996. CA 46: 5–27
65. Parmentier C, Charbord P, Tibi M, Tubiana M (1977) Splenic irradiation in myelofibrosis. Clinical findings and ferrokinetics. Int J Radiat Oncol Biol Phys 2: 1075–1081
66. Pegourie-Bandelier B, Sotto JJ, Hollard D, Bolla M, Sarrazin R (1995) Therapy program for patients with advanced stages of chronic lymphocytic leukemia. Chlorambucil, splenectomy, and total lymph node irradiation. Cancer 75: 2853–2861
67. Phillips EH, Carroll BJ, Fallas MJ (1994) Laparoscopic splenectomy. Surg Endosc 8: 931–933
68. Rai KR, Sawitsky A, Cronkite EP (1975) Clinical staging of chronic lymphocytic leukemia. Blood 46: 219–234
69. Ramani P, Shah A (1993) Lymphangiomatosis. Histologic and immunohistochemical analysis of four cases. Am J Surg Pathol 17: 329–335
70. Ratain MJ, Vardiman JW, Barker CM, Golomb HM (1988) Prognostic variables in hairy cell leukemia after splenectomy as initial therapy. Cancer 62: 2420–2424

71. Richards MA, Webb JA, Jewell SE, Stansfeld AG, Lister TA, Wrigley PF (1988) Low field strength magnetic resonance imaging of the spleen: results from volunteers and patients with lymphoma. Br J Cancer 57: 408–411
72. Risdall R, Hoppe RT, Warnke R (1979) Non-Hodgkin's lymphoma: a study of the evolution of the disease based upon 92 autopsied cases. Cancer 44: 529–542
73. Robles AE, Andrews HG, Garberolgio C (1994) Laparoscopic splenectomy: present status and future outlook. Int Surg 79: 332–334
74. Roncadin M, Arcicasa M, Trovo MG, Franchin G, DePaoli A, Volpe R, Carbone A, Tirelli U, Grigoletto E (1987) Splenic irradiation in chronic lymphocytic leukemia: a 10-year experience at a single institution. Cancer 60: 2624–2628
75. Schmid C, Kirkham N, Diss T, Isaacson PG (1992) Splenic marginal zone cell lymphoma. Am J Surg Pathol 16: 455–466
76. Sessarego M, Fugazza G, Frassoni F, Defferrari R, Bruzzone R, Carella AM (1992) Cytogenetic analysis of hemopoietic peripheral blood cells collected by leukapheresis after intensive chemotherapy in advanced phase Philadelphia-positive chronic myelogenous leukemia. Leukemia 6: 715–719
77. Shanberge JN, Tanaka K, Gruhl MC (1971) Chronic consumption coagulopathy due to hemangiomatous transformation of spleen. Am J Clin Pathol 56: 723
78. Siler J, Hunter TB, Weiss J, Haber K (1980) Increased echogenicity of the spleen in benign and malignant disease. AJR: 1011–1014
79. Silverman ML, LiVolsi VA (1978) Splenic hamartoma. Am J Clin Pathol 70: 224–229
80. Simanski DA, Schiby G, Dreznik Z, Jacob ET (1986) Rapid progressive dissemination of hemangiosarcoma of the spleen following spontaneous rupture. World J Surg 10: 142–145
81. Skillings JR, Bramwell V, Nicholson RL, Prato FS, Wells G (1991) A prospective study of magnetic resonance imaging in lymphoma staging. Cancer 67: 1838–1843
82. Soderstrom N (1976) How to use cytodiagnostic spleen puncture. Acta Med Scand 199: 1–5
83. Sombeck MD, Mendenhall NP, Kaude JV, Torres GM, Million RR (1993) Correlation of lymphangiography, computed tomography, and laparotomy in the staging of Hodgkin's disease . Int J Radiat Oncol Biol Phys 25: 425–429
84. Spier CM, Kjeldsberg CR, Eyre HJ, Behm FG (1985) Malignant lymphoma with primary presentation in the spleen. A study of 20 patients. Arch Pathol Lab Med 109: 1076–1080
85. Straus DJ, Filippa DA, Lieberman PH, Koziner B, Thaler HT, Clarkson BD (1983) The non-Hodgkin's lymphomas: a retrospective clinical and pathologic analysis of 499 cases diagnosed between 1958 and 1969. Cancer 51: 101–109
86. Straus DJ, Gaynor JJ, Myers J (1990) Prognostic factors among 185 adults with newly diagnosed advanced Hodgkin's disease treated with alternating potentially non-cross-resistant chemotherapy and intermediate-dose radiation therapy. J Clin Oncol 8: 1173–1186
87. Strijk SP, Boetes C, Bogman MJ, De Pauw BE, Wobbes T (1987) The spleen in non-Hodgkin's lymphoma. Diagnostic value of computed tomography. Acta Radiol 28: 139–144
88. Suzuki T, Shibuya H, Yoshimatsu S, Suzuki S (1987) Ultrasonically guided staging splenic tissue core biopsy in patients with non-Hodgkin's lymphoma. Cancer 60: 879–882
89. Swerdlow AJ, Douglas AJ, Vaughan Hudson G, Vaughan Hudson B, MacLennan KA (1993) Risk of second primary cancer after Hodgkin's disease in patients in the British National Lymphoma Investigation: relationships to host factors, histology and stage of Hodgkin's disease, and splenectomy. Br J Cancer 68: 1006–1011
90. Klein B, Stein M, Kuten A, Steiner M, Barshalom D, Robinson E, Gal D (1987) Splenomegaly and solitary spleen metastasis in solid tumors. Cancer 60: 100–102
91. Szczylik C, Skorski T, Nicolaides NC, Manzella L, Malaguarnera L, Venturelli D, Gewirtz AM, Calabretta B (1991) Selective inhibition of leukemia cell proliferation by BCR-ABL antisense oligodeoxynucleotides. Science 253: 562–565

92. Tallman MS, Hakimian D, Variakojis D, Koslow D, Sisney GA, Rademaker AW, Rose E, Kaul K (1992) A single cycle of 2-chlorodeoxyadenosine results in complete remission in the majority of patients with hairy cell leukemia. Blood 80: 2203–2209

93. Tefferi A, Silverstein MN, Noel P (1995) Agnogenic myeloid metaplasia. Semin Oncol 22: 327–333

94. Tura S, Baccarani M, Corbelli G, The Italian Cooperative Study Group on Chronic Myeloid Leukaemia (1981) Staging of chronic myeloid leukaemia. Br J Haematol 47: 105–119

95. Tura S, Fiacchini M, Zinzani PL, Brusamolino E, Gobbi PG (1993) Splenectomy and the increasing risk of secondary acute leukemia in Hodgkin's disease. J Clin Oncol 11: 925–930

96. van Krieken JH, Feller AC, te Velde J (1989) The distribution of non-Hodgkin's lymphoma in the lymphoid compartments of the human spleen. Am J Surg Pathol 13: 757–765

97. Van Leuween FF, Somers R, Hart AAM (1987) Splenectomy in Hodgkin's disease and second leukemia. Lancet 2: 210–211

98. Van Norman AS, Nagorney DM, Martin JK, Phyliky RL, Ilstrup DM (1986) Splenectomy for hairy cell leukemia. A clinical review of 63 patients. Cancer 57: 644–648

99. Varki A, Lottenberg R, Griffith R, Reinhard E (1983) The syndrome of idiopathic myelofibrosis. A clinicopathologic review with emphasis on the prognostic variables predicting survival. Medicine 62: 353–371

100. Visani G, Finelli C, Castelli U, Petti MC, Ricci P, Vianelli N, Gianni L, Zuffa E, Aloe Spiriti MA, Latagliata R, Pileri S, Magrini U, Gugliotta L, Morra E, Bernasconi C, Mandelli F (1990) Myelofibrosis with myeloid metaplasia: clinical and haematological parameters predicting survival in a series of 133 patients. Br J Haematol 75: 4–9

101. Wagner H Jr, McKeough PG, Desforges J, Madoc-Jones H (1986) Splenic irradiation in the treatment of patients with chronic myelogenous leukemia or myelofibrosis with myeloid metaplasia. Results of daily and intermittent fractionation with and without concomitant hydroxyurea. Cancer 58: 1204–1207

102. Wetzler M, Kurzrock R, Lowe DG, Kantarjian H, Gutterman JU, Talpaz M (1991) Alteration in bone marrow adherent layer growth factor expression: a novel mechanism of chronic myelogenous leukemia progression. Blood 78: 2400–2406

103. Wolf DJ, Silver RT, Coleman M (1978) Splenectomy in chronic myeloid leukemia. Ann Intern Med 89: 684–689

104. Zeppa P, Vetrani A, Luciano L, Fulciniti F, Troncone G, Rotoli B, Palombini L (1994) Fine needle aspiration biopsy of the spleen. A useful procedure in the diagnosis of splenomegaly. Acta Cytol 38: 299–309

105. Zhang A, Zhang JN, Liu EK (1981) Clinical analysis of 414 cases of chronic granulocytic leukaemia. Chin J Intern Med 20: 194–197

106. Zhang B, Lewis SM (1989) The splenomegaly of myeloproliferative and lymphoproliferative disorders: splenic cellularity and vascularity. Eur J Haematol 43: 63–66

107. Ziemski JM, Rudowski WJ, Jaskowiak W, Rusiniak L, Scharf R (1987) Evaluation of early postsplenectomy complications. Surg Gynecol Obstet 165: 507–514

Splenectomy for Hematologic Disorders

S. I. SCHWARTZ

> "The spleen is not the site of formation of platelets but their place of death; the spleen also has a thrombolytic function which after its removal is assumed by the lymph nodes and liver.
> It must be accepted that the cause of severe [essential] thrombocytopenia is the overwhelming destruction of platelets in the spleen."
> *Paul Kaznelson*, Czech medical student; suggesting splenectomy for ITP (1916)

Introduction

In 1887, Sir Spencer Wells [1] operated on a patient with the preoperative diagnosis of a uterine fibroid, but instead he noted a "wandering spleen," which he removed. The patient later proved to have hereditary spherocytosis; thus, the first surgical cure of a hematologic disorder was inadvertent and became manifest postoperatively when the patient's anemia and chronic jaundice disappeared. Micheli is generally given credit for introducing the concept of splenectomy for hemolytic anemia in an article published in 1911 [2]. As a medical student in Prague, Kaznelson proposed to Schloffer, a professor of surgery, that splenectomy for idiopathic thrombocytopenic purpura be performed in a 36-year-old woman. The case and the successful elevation of the platelet count to above normal levels was reported 4 weeks after the procedure in 1916 [3].

Anemias

Hereditary Spherocytosis

Hereditary spherocytosis is transmitted as an autosomal dominant trait and is the most common congenital anemia for which splenectomy is performed. Elliptocytosis is a rare variant of this disorder, and all issues pertinent to hereditary spherocytosis pertain to elliptocytosis. In these disorders there is a fundamental abnormality in the red cell membrane that causes the cells to be less deformable and more susceptible to trapping and consequent disintegration within the spleen.

The clinical manifestations include anemia, reticulocytosis, jaundice, and splenomegaly. Periodic increases in the severity of the anemia and parallel rises in the jaundice may occur. Fatal crises are extremely rare. Pigmented gallstones are present in 30%–60% of patients. The diagnosis is readily established by peripheral blood smear, which demonstrates a predominance of spherocytic red cells with a mean diameter less than normal and a thickness greater than normal. The osmotic fragility test, which demonstrates increased fragility, is rarely performed.

Only splenectomy is curative and the success rate approximates 100%. Although the inherent membrane abnormality and the spherocytosis persist, hemolysis ceases after splenectomy, and the jaundice disappears. It is recommended that the operation be delayed until the fourth year of life. If cholelithiasis exists, the gallbladder should be removed at the time of splenectomy.

Thalassemia

Thalassemia (Mediterranean anemia) is transmitted as a dominant trait and is characterized by a defect in hemoglobin synthesis. The development of intracellular precipitation contributes to premature red cell destruction. The disease is classified into alpha, beta, and gamma types; in the United States most patients suffer from the beta type. The peripheral blood smear is characterized by many nucleated red blood cells (target cells) that have a washed-out appearance.

Thalassemia occurs in two major degrees of severity: homozygous thalassemia major, with severe clinical manifestations that may result in early death, and heterozygous thalassemia minor, that is often not detected until a blood smear is reviewed. Patients with thalassemia major usually require transfusions at regular intervals, but because most of these patients accommodate to low hemoglobin levels, transfusions should be directed toward maintaining the hemoglobin in the range of 10 g/dl. Splenectomy is reserved for a limited number of patients and is specifically indicated for symptomatic splenomegaly and recurrent pain caused by splenic infarction. Removal of the spleen has also been shown to reduce transfusion requirements. Although the complication rate associated with splenectomy in these patients is extremely high, generally related to infections, the benefit-to-risk ratio favors splenectomy for specific indications [4].

Sickle Cell Anemia

Sickle cell anemia is a hereditary hemolytic anemia seen predominantly in blacks and is characterized by sickle-shaped erythrocytes. The normal Hb-A is replaced by Hb-S that undergoes crystallization when oxygen tension is reduced. The crystallization elongates and distorts the cells, resulting in increased blood viscosity and circulatory stasis. In turn, this action results in ischemia, infarction, and tissue necrosis, with the spleen as a target organ. Early in the course of disease splenomegaly may occur, but eventually the spleen undergoes infarction and autosplenectomy results.

Sickle cell anemia occurs in 0.3%–1.3% of blacks, usually when the trait is inherited from both parents or when Hb-S is combined with Hb-C or thalassemia. The chronic anemia and associated jaundice is often highlighted by acute symptoms known as crises; this is related to the vascular occlusion. Abdominal pain simulates an acute surgical abdomen. Bone pain, hematuria, priapism, neurologic manifestations, and leg ulcers can be caused by small vessel thrombosis. Splenic abscesses occasionally follow infarction of the spleen. The diagnosis of sickle cell anemia is established by the characteristic peripheral blood smear and the electrophoretic definition of Hb-S.

Although splenectomy does not affect the sickling process, it may benefit patients in whom acute splenic sequestration of red cells is demonstrated and those who develop splenic abscesses [5].

Other Congenital Anemias

Splenectomy has improved the lot of patients with profound anemia associated with PK deficiency, but in some patients postoperative thrombosis involving the portal and/or hepatic veins, or the inferior vena cava, has developed if the hemolysis was unabated. Splenectomy is not indicated for anemia associated with glucose-6-phosphate deficiency and is contraindicated in patients with hereditary high red phosphatidylcholine anemia.

Idiopathic Autoimmune Hemolytic Anemia

In idiopathic autoimmune hemolytic anemia (IAHA) normal erythrocytes exposed to circulating antibodies that are hemaglutinins undergo hemolysis, with consequent anemia and jaundice. There is evidence that the spleen serves as a source of antibodies and that sequestration of the red blood cells occurs primarily in the spleen, but the entire reticuloendothelial system can be involved. Both "warm" and "cold" antibodies have been described.

IAHA occurs at all ages but generally after the age of 50 and more commonly in women. Mild jaundice is usually present, and the spleen is palpably enlarged in half the cases. In severe cases, hemoglobinuria and tubular necrosis have been reported. The diagnosis is made by demonstrating anemia and reticulocytosis accompanied by the detection of products of red cell destruction in the serum and urine. Characteristically, the direct Coombs' test is positive.

In some patients the disease runs a self-limiting course. If the anemia persists and intensifies, steroid therapy is often effective. In the presence of "warm" antibodies, splenectomy is indicated if steroids are ineffective or contraindicated. Splenectomy is effective in about 80% of cases, but late relapses have been reported [6].

Idiopathic Thrombocytopenic Purpura

Idiopathic thrombocytopenic purpura (ITP) is an acquired disorder caused by the destruction of platelets exposed to IgG antiplatelet factors. The spleen is the source of these factors and the major site for sequestration and destruction of the sensitized platelets. The term ITP is reserved for the clinical disorder characterized by a significant reduction in the number of circulating platelets in the presence of a normal or increased number of megakaryocytes in the bone marrow, and in the absence of any systemic disease or ingestion of drugs capable of inducing thrombocytopenia. Women are affected three times more frequently than men.

ITP occurs in some patients with HIV positivity and as part of the acquired immunodeficiency syndrome (AIDS). When ITP is accompanied by an autoimmune hemolytic anemia this is known as Evans's syndrome. ITP is also a component of systemic lupus erythematosus (SLE). The clinical manifestations of ITP include ecchymoses, purpura, bleeding gums, vaginal bleeding, gastrointestinal bleeding, and hematuria. The bleeding is rarely intense and is occasionally cyclic, occurring at the time of menses. Intracranial bleeding, which can be lethal, occurs in 1%–2% of cases and usually early in the course of the disease. The spleen is characteristically small or of normal size; the presence of an enlarged spleen should suggest a diagnosis other than ITP.

The platelet count is generally reduced to $50\,000/\mathrm{mm}^3$ or less, and at times no platelets are detected by count or in the peripheral smear. The bleeding time is often prolonged but the clotting time, the prothrombin time, and the activated partial thromboplastin times are normal. Platelet survival following the transfusion of ^{51}Cr-labeled platelets is short, and there is evidence of platelet sequestration in the spleen. The megakaryocytes in the bone marrow are characterized by degranulation of the cytoplasm, a varying degree of cytoplasmic vacuolization, and the disappearance of the usual pseudopodia-containing granule-free platelets.

In adults, initial therapy usually consists of steroids for 6–8 weeks, intravenous gamma globulin and, at times, plasmapheresis. If the patient does not respond with elevation of the platelet count to over $80\,000/\mathrm{mm}^3$, splenectomy is performed. If the patient does respond and the thrombocytopenia recurs when the steroids are tapered or discontinued, splenectomy is indicated. If there is evidence of intracranial bleeding, emergency splenectomy should be done [7]. The same criteria pertain for patients with SLE, HIV, and AIDS [8]. In children, the thrombocytopenia usually is acute and self-limiting; splenectomy is rarely required.

For patients with platelet counts approaching zero, platelet packs are held in reserve for intraoperative use but are not administered preoperatively. Intraoperative platelet therapy is administered only if diffuse bleeding persists after the spleen has been removed. Medical therapy achieves permanent cure in about 15% of patients with ITP. Between 75% and 85% of patients subjected to splenectomy are permanently cured of their thrombocytopenia [9–12].

Opinions differ regarding a correlation between an initial response to steroid therapy and the efficacy of splenectomy. There is a better correlation with the response to IgG; the platelet count reaches $100\,000/mm^3$ in most instances within the first week after splenectomy. Even in those patients in whom the platelet count remains reduced, petechiae and ecchymoses rarely recur. An integral part of the operative procedure is a deliberate search for accessory spleens, which have been noted in 15%–30% of patients with ITP. An inadequate elevation of the platelet count after splenectomy or recurrent thrombocytopenia may be caused by an accessory spleen that can be detected by technetium scan, and removal can effect a permanent cure [13].

Thrombotic Thrombocytopenic Purpura

Thrombotic thrombocytopenic purpura (TTP) is a widespread occlusion of arterioles and capillaries by hyaline membranes with minimal inflammation, accompanied by significant hematologic changes. The cause has not been defined, but immune mechanisms have been indicated. The clinical manifestations comprise a pentad and the five features are present in almost all patients. These include purpura, fever, hemolytic anemia, neurologic manifestation, and sign of renal disease, i.e., hematuria and/or renal failure. In about 5% of cases the symptoms and signs first appear during pregnancy. At times, it is difficult to distinguish between TTP and the toxemia of pregnancy, the manifestations of which disappear with interruption of the pregnancy.

In most instances there is no splenomegaly. The laboratory findings include anemia with reticulocytosis, leukocytosis, and profound thrombocytopenia, at times accompanied by hyperbilirubinemia, proteinuria, hematuria, urinary casts, or azotemia. The peripheral blood smear is characterized by pleomorphic, fragmented, and distorted red blood cells. The bone marrow reveals erythroid and myeloid hyperplasia and a normal or increased number of megakaryocytes.

The disorder has a rapid onset and progression; the fatal outcome is due to intracerebral hemorrhage or renal failure [14]. Repeated plasmapheresis usually reverses the process, but in occasional cases where no response was effected, splenectomy, coupled with high-dose steroids, has resulted in cure.

Secondary Hypersplenism

Congestive splenomegaly, secondary to cirrhosis or other disorders that result in postsinusoidal obstruction, and also to those associated with presinusoidal obstruction such as schistosomiasis, and hepatic fibrosis, often results in pancytopenia, thrombocytopenia, anemia, leukopenia, or any combination of these. The hematologic disorders are due to delayed passage and consequent cellular destruction within the spleen. Because there is no correlation between the degree of hypersplenism and the prognosis of patients with hepatic disease, splenectomy is not indicated in these patients. Splenectomy alone should not be performed in patients with portal hypertension because there is no persistent effect on this condition. In the unusual circumstance that a profound thrombocytopenia mandates splenectomy in these patients, it should be combined with a splenorenal shunt. Thrombocytopenia is generally improved by decompression of portal hypertension.

Myeloproliferative Disorders

The myeloproliferative disorders constitute a spectrum of panproliferative processes manifested by increased connective tissue proliferation within the bone marrow, liver, spleen, and lymph nodes, coupled with simultaneous proliferation of hematopoietic elements in the liver, spleen, and long bones. Myeloid metaplasia, therefore, is closely related to polycythemia vera, idiopathic thrombocytosis, and myelogenous leukemia. The largest spleens encountered occur in patients with myeloproliferative disorders, and the splenomegaly is occasionally associated with portal hypertension, due either to obstructive hepatic fibrosis or to increased blood flow through the markedly enlarged spleen.

Symptoms and signs usually become apparent in middle-aged and older patients. The marked splenomegaly is often accompanied by pain caused by splenic infarcts, and the degree of splenic enlargement is manifest by diffuse abdominal discomfort and early satiety. Other symptoms include spontaneous bleeding, bone pain, pruritus, hypermetabolism, and complications ascribed to hyperuricemia. The spleen is readily palpable, and hepatomegaly is present in three quarters of these patients.

The circulating red blood cells are characterized by fragmentation and immature forms, and by poikilocytosis with tear-drop and elongated shapes. A normochromic anemia is generally present. The white blood count is markedly elevated and immature myeloid cells are present in the peripheral smear. The platelet count is variable; thrombocytopenia is present in about one third of the patients while thrombocytosis, with counts greater than $1\,000\,000/mm^3$, is observed in one quarter. The leukocyte alkaline phosphatase is usually high, as is the serum uric acid level. The bones manifest increased density on radiographs, and marrow biopsies show bone replacement by fibrous tissue.

Although the management of patients with myeloproliferative disorders is based in most instances on periodic transfusions, alkylating agents such as busulfan, and male hormones in patients with anemia due to marrow failure, splenectomy may be indicated for symptomatic splenomegaly and significant increases in transfusion requirements or thrombocytopenia that precludes chemotherapy. In patients with portal hypertension and esophagogastric varices, splenectomy often results in reduction in size or disappearance of the engorged veins.

Splenectomy does not remove a significant compensatory hematopoietic organ, but the operation is associated with a high complication rate. Postoperative thrombocytosis and/or thrombosis of the splenic vein with extension into the superior mesenteric vein and portal vein occurs more commonly in these patients. The complication is characterized by intractable ascites, hepatic failure, and renal failure that is often not noted until a week after the operation. The incidence of this complication is reduced by correcting an existing thrombocytosis preoperatively and preparing the patient with a combination of antiplatelet aggregating drugs such as aspirin or dipyridamole and low-dose heparin or coumarin [15–17].

Lymphomas, Leukemias, and Hodgkin's Disease

Although chemotherapy and/or radiation therapy constitute the main approaches to these disorders, splenectomy is occasionally applicable for symptomatic splenomegaly and for thrombocytopenia or leukopenia of a degree that precludes continuing the medical regimen [18]. The cytopenia is improved in 75% of these patients, but there is no evidence of extended survival. Hairy cell leukemia, characterized by malignant cells with filamentous cytoplasmic projections, requires no treatment in the absence of symptomatic splenomegaly, and those who live 4 years have a favorable long-term prognosis. When hairy cell leukemia is accompanied by anemia, leukopenia, and thrombocytopenia, however, splenectomy is very effective. A complete response occurs in two thirds of the patients, and the 5-year survival is between 61% and 76% [19].

The indications for surgical staging of Hodgkin's disease have decreased significantly because of greater reliance on CT scans and the more liberal use of chemotherapy that eliminates the need to determine the presence of infradiaphragmatic involvement. Currently, the indications for surgical staging focus on stage-I patients, in whom the disease is apparently limited to one anatomic region, and stage-II patients, in whom the disease is detected in two regions above the diaphragm and the pathology demonstrates nodular sclerosis.

The staging procedure begins with a wedge biopsy of the liver before retractors are applied and cause confusing white blood cell migration. Splenectomy is then carried out, followed by removal of representative retroperitoneal, mesenteric, and hepatoduodenal nodes. An iliac marrow biopsy is usually included. Surgical staging upgraded the clinical stage in 27%–36% of cases and decreased it in 7%–15%, for a total alteration of 42% [20]. The current consensus is that surgical staging is not indicated for non-Hodgkin's lymphoma. In these patients the combination of CT scans, marrow biopsy, and laparoscopically directed nodal and liver biopsies offers a reasonable alternative to diagnostic celiotomy.

Other Disorders

Felty's Syndrome

Felty's syndrome consists of rheumatoid arthritis, splenomegaly, and neutropenia, at times accompanied by anemia and/or thrombocytopenia. Fluorescent staining demonstrates an antibody against neutrophil nuclei. When corticosteroids fail, splenectomy is often effective as a means of reversing a profound neutropenia and thereby facilitating the healing of a resistant infection. Splenectomy is indicated for patients with serious or recurrent infections, anemia requiring repeated transfusions, and marked thrombocytopenia. Although neutropenia may persist after splenectomy, the neutrophilic response to infection is improved. The arthritis is not affected by removal of the spleen.

Sarcoidosis

Splenomegaly is present is about 25% of patients with sarcoidosis, and hypersplenism is a consequence in about 20% of the patients with splenomegaly. This is usually characterized by thrombocytopenia with purpura, but anemia, neutropenia, and spontaneous splenic rupture also have been noted. Splenectomy is indicated for symptomatic splenomegaly and hypersplenism. Removal of the spleen is almost always followed by correction of the hematologic abnormality.

Gaucher's Disease

This familial disorder, in which there is abnormal storage or retention of glycolipid cerebrosides in the reticuloendothelial cells, is often accompanied by significant splenomegaly and enlargement of the lymph nodes. Many patients present with the signs of hypersplenism, which is corrected by splenectomy.

There is no evidence that splenectomy alters the course of the disease. Partial splenectomy has been performed in children with symptomatic splenomegaly and hypersplenism to reduce the incidence of overwhelming postsplenectomy infection [21].

Porphyria Erythropoietica

This recessively transmitted trait is characterized by an excessive deposition of porphyrins in the tissues. The patients present with bullous dermatitis. When the disease is complicated by splenomegaly and anemia, splenectomy results in improvement of the anemia and reduced deposition of porphyrins in the red blood cells, marrow, and urine.

Systemic Mast Cell Disease

Urticaria pigmentosa and mast cell infiltration of the skin, marrow, and gastrointestinal tract is improved by splenectomy, and survival is extended [22].

Special Considerations

All adult patients undergoing splenectomy for hematologic disorders should receive pneumococcus vaccine as prophylaxis, and children should also receive the vaccine against *Haemophilus influenzae*. Vaccination is best performed at least 10 days before splenectomy but should be performed postoperatively if preoperative vaccination was neglected. Children continue to receive daily penicillin until they reach the age of 18 years; antibiotics are not routinely used in adults postoperatively. Patients with diseases associated with a higher rate of overwhelming postoperative sepsis, such as thalassemia, autoimmune hemolytic anemia, and thrombocytopenia, should seek medical attention at the onset of any febrile illness.

Platelets are not administered preoperatively to patients with ITP, regardless of the level of thrombocytopenia, and are reserved for intraoperative use in patients with diffuse bleeding after removal of the spleen. Insertion of a nasogastric tube for decompression of the stomach facilitates handling of the short gastric veins. If ligation of these veins encroaches on the stomach, enfolding of the seromuscular layers will reduce the incidence of gastric fistulization. The nasogastric tube can be removed in the recovery room. Every procedure should include a careful search for accessory spleens, which should be removed. The splenic bed is not drained routinely; drainage is reserved for patients in whom there has been evidence of oozing from distended collateral veins. Laparoscopic removal of the spleen is most readily performed for the smaller spleens associated with ITP.

Bleeding that occurs either immediately after completion of the procedure or during the first postoperative day should not be ascribed to thrombocytopenia or a coagulation abnormality. Most often, the bleeding is the result of inadequate ligation of a vessel or vessels, and the short gastric vessels are usually implicated. Immediate reexploration of the abdomen is indicated. Atelectasis and subphrenic abscess formation are rare complications. In most instances, postoperative thrombocytosis, even to levels above $10^6/mm^3$, requires no treatment, and no correlation has been demonstrated between an elevated platelet count and deep venous thrombosis. In patients with hereditary hemolytic anemia and associated enzyme deficiency, postoperative thrombosis may lead to hepatic, portal, or caval thrombosis if the hemolytic rate is unabated.

References

1. Wells TS (1888) Remarks on splenectomy with a report of a successful case. Med Chir Trans 71: 255–263
2. Micheli F (1911) Effetti immediati della splenectomia in un caso di ittero emolitico splenomegalico acquisitio tipo Hayem-Widal (ittero splenomolitico). Clin Med Ital 50: 453–468
3. Kaznelson P (1916) Verschwinden der hämorrhagischen Diathesis bei einem Falle von "essentieller Thrombopenia" (Frank) nach Milzexstirpation. Splenogene thrombolytische Purpura. Wien Klin Wochenschr 29: 1451–1454
4. Pinna AD, Argiolu F, Marongiu L, Pinna DC (1988) Indications and results for splenectomy for beta thalassemia in two hundred and twenty-one pediatric patients. Surg Gynecol Obstet 167: 109–113
5. Emond AM, Morais P, et al (1984) Role of splenectomy in homozygous sickle cell disease in childhood. Lancet 1: 88–90
6. Bowdler AJ (1976) The role of the spleen and splenectomy in autoimmune hemolytic disease. Semin Hematol 13: 335–348
7. Wanachiwanawin W, Piankijagum A, et al (1989) Emergency splenectomy in adult idiopathic thrombocytopenic purpura: a report of seven cases. Arch Intern Med 149: 217–219
8. Tyler DS, Shaunak S, et al (1990) HIV-1-associated thrombocytopenia: the role of splenectomy. Ann Surg 211–217
9. Schwartz SI (1985) Splenectomy for thrombocytopenia. World J Surg 9: 416–421
10. Akwari OE, Itani KMF, et al (1987) Splenectomy for primary and recurrent immune thrombocytopenic purpura (ITP): current criteria for patient selection and results. Ann Surg 206: 529–539
11. Coon WW (1987) Splenectomy for idiopathic thrombocytopenic purpura. Surg Gynecol Obstet 164: 225–229
12. Chirletti P, Cardi M, Barillari P, et al (1992) Surgical treatment of immune thrombocytopenic purpura. World J Surg 16: 1001–1005
13. Rudowski WJ (1985) Accessory spleens: clinical significance with particular reference to the recurrence of idiopathic thrombocytopenic purpura. World J Surg 9: 422–430
14. Onundarson PT, Rowe JM, Heal JM, Francis CW (1992) Response to plasma exchange and splenectomy in thrombotic thrombocytopenic purpura: a 10-year experience at a single institution. Arch Intern Med 152: 791–796
15. Schwartz SI (1975) Myeloproliferative disorders. Ann Surg 182: 464–471

16. Gordon DH, Schaffner D, Bennett JM, Schwartz SI (1978) Postsplenectomy thrombocytosis: its association with mesenteric, portal and/or renal thrombosis in patients with myelo-proliferative disorders. Arch Surg 113: 713–715
17. Brenner B, Nagler A, et al (1988) Splenectomy in agnogenic myeloid metaplasia and postpolycythemic myeloid metaplasia. A study of 34 cases. Arch Intern Med 148: 2501–2505
18. Delpero JR, Houvenaeghel G, Gastaut JA, et al (1990) Splenectomy for hypersplenism in chronic lymphocytic leukaemia and malignant non-Hodgkin's lymphoma. Br J Surg 77: 443–449
19. Jacobs P, King HS, Dent DM, Van der Westhuizen N (1987) Splenectomy as primary treatment for hairy cell leukaemia. Br J Surg 74: 1169–1170
20. Schwartz SI, Cooper RA jr (1972) Surgery in the diagnosis and treatment of Hodgkin's disease. Adv Surg 6: 175–203
21. Morgenstern L, Verham R, Weinstein T, Phillips EH (1993) Subtotal splenectomy for Gaucher's disease: a follow-up study. Am Surg 59: 860–865
22. Friedman B, Darling G, Norton J, et al (1990) Splenectomy in the management of systemic mast cell disease. Surgery 107: 94–100

Infections of the Spleen

R. A. WILLIAMS and R. A. DUENSING

"Yet I cannot help thinking I have some right to discharge the overflowing of my spleen upon you, whose province is to remove those disorders that occasioned it."

Tobias Smollett, Eighteenth Century

Introduction

Hippocrates is credited with the first description of focal suppuration in the spleen [1]. An array of splenic infections have since been described, with differences in etiology, pathogenesis, and microbiology. A change in the clinical spectrum has evolved as the result of advances in diagnostic techniques, antibiotic development, and an increasing frequency of immunocompromised patients. Advances in imaging technology have enabled earlier diagnosis of this potentially fatal intra-abdominal process with a characteristically subtle early presentation. The development of antimicrobial therapy has changed the profile of the infecting micro-organism. In the first half of this century, prior to the discovery of antibiotics, the majority of reports identified *Salmonella typhi*, staphylococci, various streptococci, and aerobic gram-negative bacilli as the primary organisms in infectious splenic abscesses [2–5]. Since the development of antibiotics, the incidence of splenic abscesses caused by *Salmonella typhi* has markedly decreased, and there have been more cases of splenic infections due to anaerobes, fungal organisms, and mycobacteria.

Splenic infection and abscess occur in a variety of clinical circumstances which can be used to classify patients. While some variations may be found in the literature, splenic infections can generally be grouped as being the result of either disseminated infection, traumatic abscess, hemoglobinopathies, or contiguous spread from an adjacent diseased organ.

Historically, splenic infections are uncommon. A compromised immune system has the highest prevalence among predisposing factors that lead to their development [5]. Understanding the presentation, diagnosis, and available treatments is important, given the rising number of splenic infections as the result of an expanding population of immunocompromised patients with the application of more aggressive chemotherapy, and patients with acquired immunodeficiency syndrome (AIDS).

Splenic Abscess

Epidemiology and Incidence

While the incidence of splenic abscess has historically been infrequent, ranging between 0.2% and 0.7% in autopsy-based reviews, an increasing incidence has been noted and is thought to be partly the result of sophisticated imaging techniques more readily allowing diagnoses [6, 7]. Also, a growing population of immunocompromised patients has resulted from more widespread use of cancer chemotherapy and the emergence of the AIDS epidemic [7]. Before the advent of antibiotics, the mean age of patients with splenic abscess was 32 years, compared with 37.9 years in the antibiotic era up to 1980 [8]. Since then, there has been an increase in younger children with splenic infections, due largely to an expanding population of immundeficient children infected with HIV and more aggressive cancer chemotherapy [9–11].

Etiology

Many conditions may result in splenic infection and abscess (Table 1). Grouping these predisposing causes is useful, as it allows a systematic approach to determining the etiology in each case. Metastatic infection from another primary infection has been reported as the most common source of splenic abscess [5, 8, 12]. In this category, hematologic spread and seeding in the spleen from ulcerative endocarditis occurs with the highest frequency, with an insignificant difference between the relative incidence in the preantibiotic versus the antibiotic era [5, 8, 13]. Hemaglobinopathies, particularly sickle cell disease, may result in secondary infection through obstruction of vital splenic blood flow leading to infarction, thus creating an environment for superinfection. The pathogenesis of abscesses secondary to endocarditis may also develop as the result of embolization of vegetations and subsequent splenic infarction. Once considered a relatively rare cause of splenic infection, intra-abdominal trauma with interruption of the normal splenic anatomy or infarction may represent a more frequent cause, as conservative management of splenic injury becomes more accepted and replaces splenectomy [8, 14, 15]. While not all patients with splenic infarction develop an abscess, hematogenous seeding of an organism which overwhelms the normal splenic immunologic filtering function will most likely result in abscess formation.

Splenic infections due to direct extension of an intra-abdominal process are relatively less common but are nonetheless an important predisposing factor. Primary sources for contiguous spread include carcinoma of the stomach or descending colon, gastic ulceration, perihepatic abscess, pancreatitis, or retroperitoneal abscess [7, 8, 15]. Chun et al. [8] site one mechanism for splenic abscess to be the result of splenic artery erosion from an adjacent pathologic process (tumor) with subsequent thromboses and infarction. Other uncommon causes of splenic abscesses have been associated with invasive radiologic procedures of the portal and splenic vessels [8].

Table 1. Factors predisposing to splenic infection/abscess. (Adapted from [5])[a]

Predisposing condition	Percent of cases
Combined immunodeficiency	24
Chemotherapy	23
Metastatic infection	22
Endocarditis	14
Intravenous drug use	11
Unknown	11
Trauma	8
Iatrogenic	8
Steroids	7
Contiguous infection	6
Diabetes	6
Sickle cell anemia	5
Cancer	4
Cirrhosis	2
Collagen/vascular disease	2
Hemolytic anemia/polycythemia	2
AIDS	1
Pheochromocytoma	1
Pregnancy	1
Parasitic infection	0
Mononucleosis	0

[a] Based on review covering 1978–1986 and comprising 171 patients.

Considering all predisposing conditions, the contribution of immunosuppression due to chemotherapy and AIDS is the most significant [5]. Other factors also related to alteration of immune function include diabetes mellitus, transplant immunotherapy, steroid use, and alcoholism [6, 8, 15, 16]. However, their contribution to splenic infection and abscess is relatively insignificant.

Presentation

The signs and symptoms of a patient with splenic infection and abscess are often nonspecific and may only be suspected. Table 2 lists common clinical findings in patients with splenic abscesses from a compilation of two large studies which include a worldwide literature review from 1900 to 1986. Patients predominantly present initially with abdominal pain and fever [8]; fever occurs in the largest proportion of patients [15]. Abdominal pain, which may be the result of splenic capsular irritation, may be localized to the left upper quadrant, left hypochondrium, or left costovertebral angle [8, 15]. Pain radiating to the left shoulder is the result of splenic rupture or diaphragmatic irritation from upper pole lesions [8, 16, 17]. Left-sided pleuritic chest pain has also been associated with diaphragmatic irritation [8, 15]. Signs of peritonitis are more likely with focal lesions in the lower splenic pole due to

Table 2. Physical signs and symptoms in patients with splenic abscesses. (Adapted from [5, 8])

Findings	Percent of patients[a]
Fever	90
Abdominal pain	50
Nausea/vomiting	15
Left-sided chest symptoms	13
Left shoulder pain	6
Abdominal tenderness	46
Splenomegaly	41
Friction rub	5

[a] Percentage values based on population of 329 patients for abdominal pain, left chest pain, left shoulder pain, nausea and vomiting; 308 patients for fever; 295 patients for abdominal tenderness and splenomegaly; and 247 patients for friction rub.

peritoneal irritation [3]. Abdominal pain maybe absent, however, with constitutional symptoms [8] as the only clinical clues.

Physical examination may reveal splenomegaly in 40%–54%, left upper quadrant tenderness in 46%–59%, and rarely, friction rub [5, 8]. However, some have reported that at least one chest auscultatory abnormality, such as basilar lung dullness, is evident in approximately two thirds of patients [8].

There appears to be no appreciable difference between the presentation of bacterial and fungal abscesses [5]. Similarly, no difference has been noted between multiple and solitary lesions with regard to the presence of fever, abdominal pain or tenderness, splenomegaly, pulmonary involvement, blood cultures, and average age at onset [8].

Microbiology

Bacterial Infections

Prior to 1977, splenic infections due to streptococci and staphylococci were most common, together comprising 41.9%. While there has not been a significant decline in the overall comparative incidence, both staphylococci and streptococci have been surpassed in frequency by a significant rise in fungal and anaerobic organisms (Table 3). However, a splenic abscess associated with infective endocarditis is usually still due to streptococci or staphylococci [16].

Prior to the use of antibiotics, autopsy findings reported a 1.5%–1.8% incidence of splenic abscess in patients who died of typhoid fever; since 1940, they have rarely been described [18, 19]. However, there has been a relative increase in splenic involvement by *Salmonella* species other than *S. typhi* [5]. Gram-negative aerobic organisms, most commonly *Escherichia coli,* and anaerobic organisms have increased over the past decades due to the development and use of more specific antibiotic agents, improved critical care, and

Table 3. Comparison of organisms identified in splenic abscesses before and after 1978. (Adapted from [5, 8])

Organism	1900–1977 (%)[a]	1978–1986 (%)[b]
Staphylococci	20.2	15.7
Streptococci	21.7	13.2
Salmonella	10.9	10.7
Fungal species	0.8	25.8
Anaerobes	5.4	17.6
Sterile cultures	37.0	11.9

[a]1900–1977: total patients cultured=129.
[b]1978–1986: total patients cultured=159.

increased nosocomial infections [8, 20]. Of the anaerobic bacteria, *Bacteroides fragilis* and *Clostridium, Proprionibacterium,* and *Fusobacterium* species have been most commonly reported [16, 21–23].

Fungal Infections

Fungal splenic infections are rarely found in immunocompetent patients. In a review of 189 patients, Nelken et al. [5] discovered fungal splenic abscesses, due primarily to *Candida* species, in 26%. Only 5.2% of all fungal splenic abscesses were identified in immunocompetent patients. In a review of the world literature covering the period 1900–1977, only one case of a fungal abscess (*Candida pseudotropicalis*) was identified in a patient receiving cancer chemotherapy [8].

Amoebic/Protozoal Infections

Prior to 1930, there were several reports indicating that splenic abscesses due to *Plasmodium* species were common [2, 3, 24]. However, a large review of that period revealed only eight patients with splenic abscesses among a total of 107 000 cases of malaria [3, 8, 25]. In modern times, splenic abscesses secondary to parasites such as *Plasmodium* species and *Schistosoma* are rare, and no cases have been reported in over 15 years. As evidenced by the association of splenic abscess and splenomegaly with subcapsular infarction in patients in the tropics, the contribution of organisms such as *Plasmodium* and *Schistosoma* to abscess development may be related to splenic infarction and not direct infection. However, the exact pathogenesis remains to be determined. Parasitic splenic cysts have been reported and are usually the result of *Echinococcus*. In patients suspected of harboring an echinococcal cyst, caution is warranted if percutaneous aspiration is planned, due to the possibility of anaphylaxis should intra-abdominal spillage occur [26]. *Entamoeba histolytica* was identified in one patient reported in 1975 [8] and may be more frequent in underdeveloped countries where the organism is endemic.

Diagnosis

Laboratory Studies

While most laboratory findings are not helpful in the diagnosis of splenic infections, leukocytosis is usually present in patients with splenic abscesses. A review of 143 patients with splenic infections in whom the white blood count was obtained showed that 61.5% had leukocytosis, with an average of 16 500 ±8500 cells/mm^3 [12]. However, considerable variability may exist in absolute leukocyte number, as noted in another review which revealed a white cell count less than 10 000 cells/mm^3 in 30%, a range of 2400–41 000 cells/mm^3, and a mean of 15 631 cells/mm^3 [8].

Diagnostic Radiology

Plain film roentgenograms may provide information toward the diagnosis of a splenic abscess through nonspecific manifestations of the infectious process on adjacent structures. For example, chest X-rays may demonstrate abnormal findings such as left pleural effusion, left elevated hemidiaphragm, or basilar pulmonary infiltrates in the majority of patients [5]. Abdominal films may reveal a left upper quadrant soft tissue mass or air fluid levels, changes consistent with bowel obstruction, or splenic calcifications [5, 8]. Barium contrast studies may demonstrate evidence of mass effect; however, they are not specific enough to be used alone for the diagnosis of splenic abscess [6].

Splenic scintigraphy with gallium or technetium 99m has been reported to be 80%–90% accurate, but both are more reliable with larger lesions [5, 6, 8]. In addition, false-positive gallium scans may occur during sepsis in a hypermetabolic spleen [6, 27]. Since the development of less invasive imaging modalities, arteriography has essentially been replaced by ultrasonography and computed axial tomography (CAT) scans.

Transabdominal ultrasound to determine splenic abnormalities is useful and commonly performed as part of an abdominal sonographic examination in patients with nonspecific abdominal complaints or signs of sepsis. There is a lack of specificity, however, when the search is for splenic abscesses in particular, and suspicious lesions must be differentiated from hematoma, infarction, hemangioma, lymphoma, metastatic disease, and cystic structures [6, 28]. Additionally, there may be difficulty in obtaining proper images due to overlying bowel gas and maneuvering of the probe over ribs [29].

Computed axial tomography scans have proven superior in detecting splenic abscesses when compared with other imaging techniques, with specificity and sensitivity both ranging between 90% and 95% [5, 30, 31]. Features

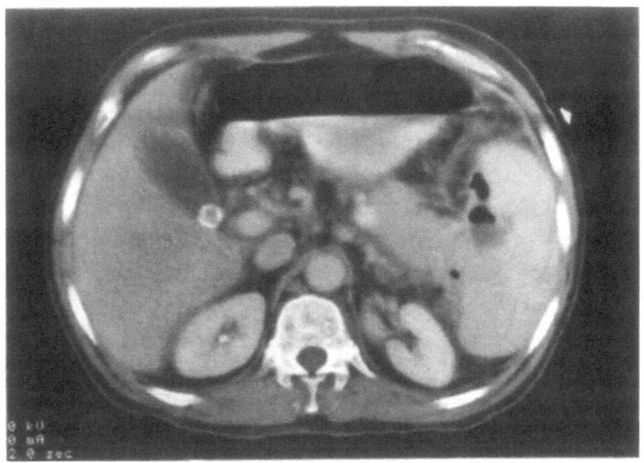

Fig. 1. CT scan of a hilar splenic abscess in a 48-year-old man. Note the presence of air within the abscess site

of splenic abscess on the CAT scan include single or multiple focal areas of homogeneous lucent densities, and there may be evidence of an air-fluid interface (Fig. 1). When intravenous contrast medium is used, a nonenhancing rim lesion is usually manifested. Features of CAT scanning that contribute to its improved sensitivity are multifactorial and include less reliance on technical aspects to perform the examination and better differentiation between tissue densities compared with ultrasonography [13]. Because splenic abscesses present predominantly in patients with nonspecific clinical features such as unexplained fever or sepsis, the use of abdominal CAT scanning early in the diagnostic algorithm may allow an earlier diagnosis. A CAT scan should be the diagnostic imaging examination of choice in patients with predisposing factors for splenic infection.

Treatment

The most widely accepted definitive management of splenic infections begins with antibiotic therapy, followed by splenectomy. In most instances the infecting organisms have not been identified at the time of diagnosis, and there is a variety of possibilities, necessitating wide-spectrum antimicrobial therapy. However, blood cultures which isolate particular microbial species should be used to guide early therapy in a patient with splenic infection.

Without identification of a particular organism, initial coverage for staphylococci, streptococci, gram-negative bacilli, and anaerobes would be appropriate. Previous studies have demonstrated the presence of similar infecting organisms in spleen and blood in 68.8%–74.4% of patients with positive blood cultures; an exception was polymicrobial infections, for which cultures were similar in only 9.1% of cases [8, 13]. In the absence of positive blood cultures, other clinical and radiological features may be helpful in choosing the most appropriate antimicrobial agent. Patients suspected of having splenic abscesses with recognized infectious endocarditis usually have similar pathogens seeding the spleen, most commonly *Streptococci* and *Staphylococcus aureus*. Occasionally, superinfections with organisms such as *Enterobacter*, *Klebsiella*, and *E. coli* have been identified; however, one report did question whether there may have been contamination in the isolation of these organisms [16]. Anaerobic infections should be considered in patients with an anaerobic process in another site, a prolonged intra-abdominal process, or if culture of a splenic suppuration fails to identify on organism [8]. Radiographic evidence of air, such as heterogeneous lucencies representing air-fluid levels on CAT scan or hypoechogenic lesions on ultrasonography, should elicit the suspicion of gas-producing organisms.

Immunocompromised patients have a greater frequency of fungal, mycobacterial, and bacterial infections compared with the immunocompetent host, and this should be considered in directing antimicrobial therapy. There is a large variety of possible infecting organisms and predisposing factors to splenic infections. Despite the diagnostic information provided by improved imaging techniques, the responsible organism(s) cannot be identified at initial diagnosis in the majority of patients, necessitating empiric antibiotic therapy.

Patients with fungal abscesses may be managed differently than those with suppurative bacterial splenic infections. Clinically stable patients suspected to have a fungal abscess may undergo definitive diagnosis via ultrasonographic- or CAT scan-guided percutaneous biopsy and culture. Sterile or nondiagnostic cultures in the presence of focal suppuration should be treated with prompt splenectomy and continued antibiotic therapy. However, there have been reports of successful management with antifungal therapy without splenectomy when cultures isolated specific fungal organisms. In one series, management of splenic fungal abscesses treated with antifungals alone was successful in 75% of patients and the mortality in this group was comparable to that for the group with fungal abscesses who also underwent splenectomy [5]. Patients managed in this manner should be closely observed to follow clinical improvement, and periodic CAT scan examinations should be performed to document regression of the abscess.

Following diagnosis of bacterial splenic abscess and initiation of antibiotic therapy, splenectomy is indicated and can be performed safely in the majority of patients. Splenectomy is considered the treatment of choice for patients with bacterial abscesses that are multiple, multilocular, large, perihilar, adjacent to, or involving other abdominal organs, or in the presence of splenomegaly. Technically, splenectomy can be performed safely in most patients and is usually the only procedure required; occasionally, external drainage may be needed for larger, complicated abscesses [13]. In patients with simultaneous small abscesses in other organs, prolonged antibiotics are usually needed for 2 or more weeks. Overall morbidity and mortality of patients with splenic abscess after splenectomy are less often related to procedural complications than to contributing factors related to patients' underlying health, as many patients are critically ill by the time a diagnosis is made.

Mortality after splenectomy has been reported to be 6.7%, due mainly to abscess in other organs, splenic rupture, or overwhelming sepsis [8, 13]. However, mortality of splenic suppuration without treatment approaches 100%, and treatment with antibiotics alone has only rarely been reported and is generally discouraged unless risk of death from operation and anesthesia supersedes [13].

An alternative to splenectomy has evolved since the development of more sophisticated imaging techniques. Percutaneous splenic abscess drainage guided by CAT scan or ultrasonography has been performed with some success. Whether this technique is more efficacious and safer than splenectomy remains unclear at this time. A review of 30 patients treated with percutaneous drainage and reported in the literature showed that 21 were cured, without need for further intervention [6]. However, patient selection for aspiration is limited and the procedure has proven most successful when the abscess is single, moderate to large in size, has a discrete wall and cavity, lacks internal septations, and contains a relatively liquefied medium without necrotic debris [5, 6]. Percutaneous drainage may be indicated in those patients considered to have significant underlying health risk factors which may result in death due to the stress of an invasive procedure and anesthesia. In addition, it may be appropriate in young patients when attempting to avoid potentially overwhelming infections associated with splenectomy. Antibiotic therapy should be incorporated, as in splenectomy, and periodic post-aspiration imaging studies should be performed to document abscess cavity resolution. If the patient fails to improve clinically or the abscess persists, splenectomy is indicated.

Viral Splenic Infections

Splenic infection and abscess due to a viral process are rare. Among viral causes, infectious mononucleosis is the most common. Splenomegaly in patients with Epstein-Barr virus and infectious mononucleosis is a recognized manifestation and is thought to be mainly the result of congestion and lymphoid cell infiltration into the white and red pulp. One of the most serious complications of splenomegaly is rupture, which is spontaneous or, more commonly, the result of blunt trauma, and has been reported to occur in 14% of patients with infectious mononucleosis [32]. Typically, patients present with acute-onset abdominal pain and a recent history of a viral syndrome. Without therapeutic intervention, patients with splenic rupture may develop hemorrhagic shock. If recognized immediately, splenic rupture can be managed effectively with splenectomy or, seldom, splenorrhaphy. If unrecognized, splenic rupture can be fatal, and it is the most frequent cause of death in patients with infectious mononucleosis [33]. Other reported causes of splenic rupture are less common and include viral hepatitis, malaria, endocarditis, and actinomycosis [34, 35].

Primary splenic abscesses due to viral infections, particularly in immuno-competent individuals, have been identified even less frequently than splenic rupture. Two cases of splenic abscesses associated with infectious mononu-cleosis have been reported in the literature between 1976 and 1992 [20, 36]. Both patients developed fever and abdominal pain and tenderness necessitat-ing splenectomy. In one patient a single 4 x 5 centimeter abscess cavity in an enlarged spleen was noted on a CAT scan. However, during laparotomy, the abscess ruptured and an inflammatory process began, involving the tail of the pancreas and the transverse colon. Athough this is only a single case sce-nario, these operative findings indicate that viral processes are insidious and may have relatively late clinical manifestations, emphasizing the importance of high clinical suspicion, early imaging studies, and prompt operative man-agement.

Splenic Infections in Patients with AIDS

Since the recognition of AIDS in 1981, the slope of its epidemic curve con-tinues to rise unremittingly, albeit with a varying trend. Over 610000 cases of AIDS have been reported worldwide, nearly one half of them in the United States [37]. The actual world AIDS population is currently estimated to be greater than 2.5 million, and the World Health Organization projects that 30–50 million people will be infected with HIV by the turn of the century [38]. The main impact of AIDS clinically has been the evolution of previously rare opportunistic infectious diseases and select malignancies. While surgeons have been operating on patients with AIDS since discovery of the syndrome, elective abdominal operations have been relatively uncommon [39, 40]. There are several HIV-associated sydromes which require operative intervention, and splenomegaly is an undoubtably well-recognized indication, particularly when associated with focal splenic loculation and signs of sepsis.

Presentation

As in all patients, infection of the spleen in immunocompromised patients, such as those with AIDS, is potentially fatal [41]. The importance of this fact is underscored with the understanding that unreliable parameters for clinical diagnosis and inconsistent febrile responses in immunocompromised patients may lead to a delay in diagnosis and therefore delay treatment [5, 42]. Due largely to the more widespread use of cancer chemotherapy and the epi-demic spread of AIDS, not only has the incidence of splenic abscesses in-creased, but there has also been a change in the demographics relating to age, presentation, microbiology, and treatment.

Historically, splenic infections occurred most commonly in the young-adult population, with a reported mean age of 37.9 years since the introduction of antibiotics [8]. A higher prevalence in the adult population is likely related to the predisposing clinical conditions that lead to infectious involvement of the spleen. However, with more aggressive chemotherapy of hematologic malignancies and the spread of HIV in the pediatric population over the past decade, a rise has been noted in the incidence of splenic abscesses in severely immunocompromised children [10, 11]. In a study of pediatric AIDS patients, two of 291 were diagnosed with splenic abscess after presentation of fever and abdominal pain [9]. Both children (aged 19 months and 9 years) had *Mycobacterium avium-intracellulare* growth in blood cultures and showed rapid therapeutic response to splenectomy. This study illustrates the role of splenectomy in the immunocompromised patient for diagnosis and treatment of the causative organism. In the two patients mentioned above, a trial of antiobiotics – which has been advocated by others [43, 44] – failed after 7 and 14 days, respectively, necessitating laparotomy, which led to a definitive diagnosis and eradication of the source of symptoms.

Diagnosis of splenic infection and abscess in patients with AIDS may be difficult based on clinical presentation alone, due to the nonspecific findings of HIV-associated intra-abdominal disease. The signs and symptoms may be similar to those in the immunocompetent patient, with unexplained fever and abdominal pain. However, it is recognized that inconsistencies exist with regard to pyrexic response and hematologic markers of infection seen in the peripheral blood smear of HIV-infected patients [9]. Additionally, patients may present with severe abdominal symptoms which may be due to a myriad of pathologic processes, including those for which operative intervention is not indicated. In two recent reports, only 4.5% of patients in a New York study and 35 patients at eight hospitals over 4 years in a Southern California review required abdominal procedures for AIDS-related disease; only a minority of these patients had splenic abscesses [39, 40].

Splenomegaly is an important physical finding in patients with HIV and is reported with a frequency of 72%, often with massive enlargement up to 3000 g [45]. Splenic infection will be associated in a significant proportion of these patients with splenomegaly, particularly in the setting of acute illness. It is important that the examining physician have a high level of suspicion in order to hasten the diagnosis and prevent an otherwise ultimately fatal outcome.

Etiology

AIDS and other causes of immunosuppression predispose patients to opportunistic infections believed to be the result of seeding reticuloendothelial cells in the spleen, leading to abscess and ineffective cellular immune cells [43, 46]. Studies indicate that candidiasis is the most common opportunistic pathogen associated with splenic abscess in immunocompetent and immunocompromised patients [9, 12]. Case reports specifically examining HIV/AIDS and splenic infection reveal a lower but increasing prevalence of several other fungal and mycobacterial infections.

Mycobacterium tuberculosis is recognized as an opportunistic infection in patients with HIV [47]. Splenic infection by tuberculosis is rare but is perhaps more common than previously suspected, given an increasing incidence in autopsy series [48–53]. Also, an increasing incidence of *M. tuberculosis* infection has been observed in HIV patients living in areas where tuberculosis is more prevalent [54].

Mycobacterium avium-intracellulare (MAI), the most commonly reported opportunistic infection in the liver of patients with AIDS [55–57], is a relatively rare cause of splenic abscess. Extrapulmonary dissemination of MAI is an AIDS-defining criterion in HIV-infected patients [58]. Reports indicate that 80% of patients with MAI splenic abscesses had a previous diagnosis of AIDS, and those who develop MAI infection are likely to have significant immunosuppression and therefore have a poor prognosis [57, 59]. It seems plausible that the prevalence may actually be higher, but that many cases are not identified due to the difficulty in distinguishing MAI from *M. tuberculosis* without positive culture, and that some patients die of other causes before specific infections are isolated. In a review of HIV-infected patients with abnormal CAT scans, *M. tuberculosis* was identified in 34 of 55 patients, MAI in two, and histoplasmosis and coccidioidomycosis in one and two of 55, respectively [60]. The study illustrates the large array of organisms that have been associated with splenic lesions in patients with HIV. However, the relative prevalence may be misleading. As noted in the study, patients with disseminated tuberculosis are more likely to be hospitalized and ill, and consquently to undergo a diagnostic abdominal CAT scan, which may reveal incidental intra-abdominal lesions [60] (Table 4).

Pneumocystis carinii is a well-known opportunistic organism in AIDS and has been reported as a pulmonary pathogen in up to 85% of patients [61]. Moreover, extrapulmonary manifestations are increasingly being identified, and some of these include splenic involvement [62, 63]. One of the most significant factors implicated in the increased incidence of *Pneumocystis* dissemination is the use of prophylactic pentamidine [64–66]. However, *P. carinii* involvement of the spleen is still considered infrequent, and diagnosis may be difficult due to the nonspecific physical findings and imaging characteristics, particularly on CAT scan. In one review of 55 patients reported to have extrapulmonary or disseminated *P. carinii*, 26 had splenic involvement, and only two of them had initially presented with splenomegaly [62]. Many times there is hepatic involvement, with clinical presentation of ascites, hypoalbuminemia, and edema accompanying splenomegaly and abdominal discomfort [62]. The splenomegaly represents splenic nodules due to involvement of *Pneumocystis* organisms after hematogenous and lymphatic spread. Figure 1 presents the typical multiple mass lesions seen on CAT scan.

An increase in splenic abscesses due to *Salmonella typhi* and other *Salmonella* species has been reported since the decline of the *S. typhi* type from 1940 to 1980 [8, 20]. There have been reported cases of *S. typhi, S. typhimur-*

Table 4. Relationship of imaging characteristics and disease process in 55 patients with low-attenuation confirmed splenic abscesses. (Adapted from [60])

Infection	Percentage of patients with largest lesion		
	<1 cm	2–4 cm	>5 cm
M. tuberculosis	60.0	0.02	0.0
M. avium-intracellulare	0.04	0.0	0.0
Histoplasmosis	0.0	0.02	0.0
Coccidioidomycosis	0.04	0.0	0.0
Candidiasis	0.04	0.0	0.0
P. carinii	0.0	0.04	0.02

ium, and other *Salmonella* species splenic abscesses in HIV-infected patients [45, 67, 68]. Splenomegaly and fever seem to be relatively constant clinical findings. The occurrence of splenic *Salmonella* infections in this patient population may reflect the fact that immunodeficient patients have a higher incidence of *Salmonella* bacteremia compared with immunocompetent populations [67–69].

Diagnosis

Diagnosis of splenic infection may be more difficult in immunocompromised patients than in the general population due to a lack of clinical indicators with sufficient specificity. Therefore, patients with febrile illness of an undetermined source who are believed to be immunocompromised should be evaluated promptly with a CAT scan of the abdomen. While ultrasonography is useful, it is comparatively less accurate than CAT scanning and may delay diagnosis [5, 10]. Other imaging modalities may have good diagnostic accuracy but are generally less readily available and/or more invasive. Diagnosis of splenic infection depends on a high degree of suspicion, and choosing the most appropriate diagnostic approach is important, given that the prognosis is likely to improve with early and aggressive treatment.

Characteristic patterns of splenic lesions on CAT scan have been associated with individual organisms. Lesions associated with disseminated candidiasis in HIV-infected and immunocompromised patients are typically multiple, small, and of low attenuation, occasionally involving the kidney, and there is an absence of lymphadenopathy or hepatosplenomegaly [60, 70]. Conversely, disseminated histoplasmosis may involve lymph nodes and hepatosplenomegaly, occasionally with low-attenuation splenic or hepatic lesions [60, 71]. Radin [60] describes lesions associated with coccidioidomycosis as multiple and small, lymph-node lesions with central low attenuation and mild splenomegaly. He also described the prominent features of two patients with disseminated cryptococcosis to be significant splenomegaly, lymphadenopathy, and mild hepatomegaly. The majority of patients with disseminated *M. tuberculosis* and MAI have lymphadenopathy. However, central low attenuation is more frequent in *M. tuberculosis*, whereas hepatomegaly and/or splenomegaly are more often seen in MAI [60, 72]. Patients with extrapulmonary *P. carinii* infection may demonstrate focal low-attenuation splenic lesions of varying size and number [60, 63, 73]. Splenic lesions accompanied by visceral or nodal calcifications have also been described, but the specificity of these findings when used alone is inadequate for the diagnosis of *P. carinii* [73].

Treatment

HIV-related intra-abdominal processes may present with splenomegaly alone, and some may be managed medically. While splenic abscess is a definite indication for splenectomy, several infections may not require invasive intervention. Fungal splenic abscesses have been successfully managed with antifungal therapy alone in immunocompromised patients [5, 43, 44]. In a series of documented fungal splenic abscesses, 12 of 16 immunocompromised patients treated with antifungal medication without surgery had resolution without a significant difference in mortality compared with patients treated with splenectomy and antifungals [5]. Those patients considered for nonoperative therapy should have a culture diagnosis of the splenic lesion, not only to determine the organism, but also to rule out other entities such as leukemic infiltrates and metastases. If nonoperative management is attempted, splenectomy should be reserved in case a reasonable period of appropriate antibiotic therapy is unsuccessful. When multiple organ involvement is noted at operation, splenectomy alone is usually satisfactory management, with the understanding that prolonged postoperative antibiotics may be required for these extrasplenic abscesses [44]. The fact that recovery occurs soon after splenectomy in the majority of cases of splenic infection, even where there is extrasplenic involvement, supports the claim that splenectomy is important and explains why it is considered the gold standard for treatment of fungal and bacterial splenic infections.

The best diagnostic and most effective therapeutic intervention for focal splenic lesions in patients with disseminated tuberculosis is splenectomy. However, antituberculous therapy alone has been successful in AIDS patients with *M. tuberculosis* splenic abscesses documented by needle aspiration [74]. MAI splenic abscesses are also most effectively managed by splenectomy. Conversely, one study has reported poor outcomes in patients with disseminated MAI presenting with splenomegaly and treated with splenectomy [45]. The authors recommend that all patients infected with HIV have blood or bone marrow cultures done prior to splenectomy, and that splenectomy be avoided in those cases where MAI is isolated. Similar experiences also led the authors to recommend the same approach for patients with splenomegaly and disseminated cytomegalovirus.

Patients with extrapulmonary *P. carinii* have not typically responded to medical management alone [65]. However, improved success has been reported with intravenous pentamidine or trimethoprim-sulfamethoxazole [62, 75–78].

For HIV patients with focal splenic suppuration, splenectomy is still the mainstay of management. Initial imaging techniques lack the specificity and sensitivity for definitive diagnosis of particular organisms. An operative approach hastens diagnosis and treatment, which will ultimately favorably affect morbidity and mortality.

References

1. Littre E (ed) (1849) Hippocrates: oeuvres completes d'Hippurates, vol 16. Libraire de l'Academie Nationale de Medicine, Paris, pp 155, 230
2. Billings A (1928) Abscess of the spleen. Ann Surg 88: 416
3. Etling AW (1915) Abscess of the spleen. Ann Surg 62: 182
4. Inlow WD (1927) Traumatic abscess of the spleen. Ann Surg 85: 368
5. Nelken N, Ignathius J, Skinner M, Christensen N (1987) Changing clinical spectrum of splenic abscess. Am J Surg 154: 27–34
6. Gleich S, Wolin DA, Herbsman H (1988) A review of percutaneous drainage in splenic abscess. Surg Gynecol Obstet 167: 211–216
7. Paris S, Weiss SM, Ayers WH jr, Clarke LE (1994) Splenic abscess. Am Surg 60: 358–361
8. Chun CH, Raff MJ, Contrareras L, Varghese R, Waterman N, Daffner R, Melo JC (1980) Splenic abscess. Medicine (Baltimore) 59: 50–65
9. Smith MD jr, Nio M, Camel JE, Sato JK, Atkinson JB (1993) Management of splenic abscess in immunocompromised children. J Pediatr Surg 28: 823–826
10. Alonso-Cohen MA, Galera MJ, Ruiz M, et al (1990) Splenic abscess. World J Surg 14: 513–516
11. Caslowitz PL, Labs JD, Fishman EK, et al (1989) The changing spectrum of splenic abscess. Clin Imaging 13: 71–74
12. Faught WE, Gilbertson JJ, Nelson EW (1989) Splenic abscess: presentation, treatment options, and results. Am J Surg 158: 612–614
13. Gadacz TR (1985) Splenic abscess. World J Surg 9: 410–415
14. Budd DC, Fouty WJ, Johnson RB, Lukash WM (1976) Occult rupture of the spleen. JAMA 236: 2884
15. Simson JNL (1980) Solitary abscess of the spleen. Br J Surg 67: 106–110
16. Johnson JD, Raff MJ, Barnwell PA, Chun CH (1983) Splenic abscess complicating infectious endocarditis. Arch Intern Med 143: 906–912
17. Lowenfels AB (1966) Kehr's sign – a neglected aid in rupture of the spleen. N Engl J Med 274: 1019
18. Cohen JI, Bartlett JA, Corey GR (1987) Extra-intestinal manifestations of *Salmonella* infections. Medicine (Baltimore) 66: 349–388
19. Ransohoff J, O'Rourke W (1940) Typhoid abscess of the spleen in hemolytic jaundice. JAMA 114: 2543
20. Chulay JD, Lankerani MR (1976) Splenic abscess. Am J Med 61: 513
21. Keidl CM, Chusid MJ (1989) Splenic abscesses in childhood. Pediatr Infect Dis J 8: 368–373
22. Gadacz T, Way LW, Dunphy JE (1974) Changing clinical spectrum of splenic abscess. Am J Surg 128:182–187
23. Wolff MJ, Bitran J, Northland RG, Levy IL (1991) Splenic abscesses due to *Mycobacterium tuberculosis* in patients with AIDS. Rev Infect Dis 13: 373–375

24. Spear WM (1903) Abscess of the spleen. JAMA 41: 304
25. Anderson ARS (1906) Splenic abscess in malarial fever. Lancet 2: 1159
26. Van Sonnenberg E, Ferrucci JT, Meuller PR, et al (1982) Percutaneous drainage of abscesses and fluid collections: technique, results and applications. Radiology 142: 1–10
27. Hertzanu Y, Mendelsogn DB, Goudie E, Butterworth A (1983) Splenic abscess: a review with the value of ultrasound. Clin Radiol 34: 661–667
28. Solbiati L, Bossi MC, Bellotti E, et al (1983) Focal lesions in the spleen: sonographic patterns and guided biopsy. AJR 140: 59–65
29. Synder SK, Hahn HH (1982) Diagnosis and treatment of intraabdominal abscess in critically ill patients. Surg Clin North Am 62: 229–239
30. Ferruchi JT, Van Sonnenberg E (1981) Intraabdominal abscess, radiological diagnosis and treatment. JAMA 246: 2728–2733
31. Koehler PR, Moss AA (1980) Diagnosis of intraabdominal and pelvic abscesses by computerized tomography. JAMA 244: 4 9–52
32. Bhattacharyya N, Ablin DS, Kosloske AM (1989) Stapled partial splenectomy for splenic abscess in a child. J Pediatr Surg 24: 316
33. Schwartz SI (1994) Spleen. In: Schwartz SI, Shires GT, Spenser FC (eds) Principles of surgery, chap 31, 6th edn. McGraw-Hill, New York
34. Wood LJ (1946) Pathologic aspects of acute epidemic hepatitis. Arch Pathol 41: 345
35. Sperling RL, Heredia R, Gillesby WJ, Chomet B (1967) Rupture of the spleen secondary to actinomycosis. Arch Surg 94: 344
36. O'Dell KB, Gordon RS (1992) Ruptured splenic abscess secondary to infectious mononucleosis. Ann Emerg Med 21: 1160–1162
37. Connall TP, Wilson SE, Williams RA (1995) Surgery in patients with acquired immune deficiency syndrome. In: Howard RJ, Simmons RL (eds) Surgical infectious disease, chap 53, 3rd edn. Appleton and Lange, Norwalk, Connecticut, pp 1371–1380
38. World Health Organization (1991) Update on AIDS. Wkly Epidemiol Rec 66: 353
39. LaRaja RD, Rothenberg RE, Odom JW, Meuller SC (1989) The incidence of intra-abdominal surgery in acquired immunodeficiency syndrome: a statistical review of 904 patients. Surgery 210: 428
40. Wilson SE, Robinson G, Williams R, et al (1989) Acquired immune deficiency syndrome (AIDS). Indications for abdominal surgery, pathology, and outcome. Ann Surg 210: 428
41. Pomerantz RA, Eckhauser FE, Thornton JW, et al (1986) Covert splenic abscess: a continuing challenge. Am Surg 52: 386–390
42. Wald BR, Ortega JA, Ross L, et al (1981) Candidal splenic abscesses complicating acute leukemia of childhood treated by splenectomy. Pediatrics 67: 296–299
43. Helton WS, Carrico CJ, Zaveruha PA, et al (1986) Diagnosis and treatment of splenic fungal abscesses in the immune-suppressed patient. Arch Surg 121: 580–586
44. Hatley RM, Donaldson JS, Raffensperger JG, et al (1989) Splenic microabscesses in the immune-compromised patient. J Pediatr Surg 24: 697–699
45. Mathew A, Raviglione MC, Niranjan U, Sabatini MT, Distenfeld A (1989) Splenectomy in patients with AIDS. Am J Hematol 32: 184–189
46. Stone HH, Kolb LD, Currie CA, Geheber CE, Cuzzell JZ (1979) *Candida* sepsis: pathogenesis and principles of treatment. Ann Surg 179: 697–710
47. Soriano E, Mallolas J, Gatell JM, et al (1988) Characteristics of tuberculosis in HIV-infected patients: a case-control study. AIDS 2: 429–432
48. Harries AD (1990) Tuberculosis and human immunodeficiency virus in developing countries. Lancet 335: 387–389
49. Weinberg JJ, Cohen P, Malhotra P (1988) Primary tuberculous liver abscess associated with the human immunodeficiency virus. Tubercle 69: 145–147
50. Moreno S, Pacho E, Lopez-Herce JA, Rodriquez-Creixems M, Martin-Scapa C, Bouza E (1988) *Mycobacterium tuberculosis* visceral abscesses in the acquired immunodeficiency syndrome (AIDS). Ann Intern Med 105: 437
51. Rumoid MJ, Orr TG (1933) Tuberculous abscess of the spleen. Ann Surg 98: 474–477
52. Alvarez S, McCabe WR (1984) Extrapulmonary tuberculosis revisited: a review of experience at Boston city and other hospitals. Medicine (Baltimore) 63: 25–55

53. Weir MR, Thornton GF (1985) Extrapulmonary tuberculosis: experience of a community hospital and review of the literature. Am J Med 79: 467–478
54. Gatell JM, Soriano E, Mallolas J, Mariscal D (1988) Tuberculosis and the new CDC case definition for AIDS (letter). Lancet 1: 832–833
55. Cappell MS (1991) Hepatobiliary manifestations of the acquired immune deficiency syndrome. Am J Gastroenterol 86: 1–15
56. Grumbach K, Collman BG, Gal AA, et al (1989) Hepatic and biliary tract abnormalities in patients with AIDS. J Ultrasound Med 8: 247–254
57. Schneiderman DJ, Arenson DM, Cello JP, Margaretten W, Weber TE (1987) Hepatic disease in patients with the acquired immune deficiency syndrome (AIDS). Hepatology 7: 925–930
58. Centers for Disease Control (1992) 1993 revised classification system for HIV infection and expanded surveillance case definition for AIDS among adolescents and adults. MMWR 41 (RR-17): 1–19
59. American Thoracic Society (1987) Mycobacterioses and the acquired immunodeficiency syndrome. Am Rev Respir Dis 136: 492–496
60. Radin R (1995) HIV infection: analysis in 259 consecutive patients with abnormal abdominal CT findings. Radiology 197: 712–722
61. Gal AA, Koss MN, Strigle S, et al (1989) *Pneumocystis carinii* infection in the acquired immune deficiency syndrome. Semin Diagn Pathol 6: 287–299
62. Rockley PF, Wilcox CM, Moynihan M, Hewen-Lowe K, Schwartz DA (1994) Splenic infection simulating lymphoma: an unusual presentation of disseminated *Pneumocystis carinii* infection. South Med J 87: 530–536
63. Lubat E, Megibow AJ, Balhazar EJ, Goldenberg AS, Birnbaum BA, Bosnik MA (1990) Extrapulmonary *Pneumocystis carinii* infection in AIDS: CT findings. Radiology 174: 157–160
64. Telzak EE, Cote RJ, Gold JWM, et al (1990) Extrapulmonary *Pneumocystis carinii* infections. Rev Infect Dis 12: 380–386
65. Berman SM, Shah B, Wyle F, et al (1990) Disseminated *Pneumocystis carinii* in a patient receiving aerosolized pentamidine prophylaxis. West J Med 153: 82–86
66. Spouge AR, Wilson SR, Gopinath N, et al (1990) Extrapulmonary *Pneumocystis carinii* in a patient with AIDS: sonographic findings. AJR 155: 76–78
67. Torres JT, Rodriguez Casas J, Balda E, Cebrian J (1992) Multifocal *Salmonella* splenic abscess in an HIV-infected patient. Trop Geogr Med 44: 66–68
68. Sperber SJ, Schleupner CJ (1987) Salmonellosis during infection with human immunodeficiency virus. Rev Infect Dis 9: 925–934
69. Jacobs JL, Gold JWM, Murray HW, Roberts RB, Armstrong D (1985) *Salmonella* infections in patients with acquired immunodeficiency syndrome. Ann Intern Med 102: 186–188
70. Shirkhoda A (1987) CT findings in hepato-splenic and renal candidiasis. J Comput Assist Tomogr 11: 795–798
71. Radin DR (1991) Disseminated histoplasmosis: abdominal CT findings in 16 patients. AJR 157: 955–958
72. Radin DR (1991) Intraabdominal *Mycobacterium tuberculosis* vs *Mycobacterium avium-intracellulare* infections in patients with AIDS: distinction based on CT findings. AJR 156: 487–491
73. Radin DR, Baker EL, Klatt EC, et al (1990) Visceral and nodal calcification in patients with AIDS-related *Pneumocystis carinii* infection. AJR 154: 27–31
74. Pedro-Botet J, Maristany MT, Miralles R, Lopez-Colomes, Rubies-Prat J (1991) Splenic tuberculosis in patients with AIDS. Rev Infect Dis 13: 1069–1071
75. Coulman CU, Greene I, Archibald RWR (1987) Cutaneous pneumocystosis. Ann Intern Med 106: 396–398
76. Carter TR, Cooper PH, Petri WA, et al (1988) *Pneumocystis carinii* infection of the small intestine in a patient with acquired immune deficiency syndrome. Am J Clin Pathol 89: 679–683

77. Sparling TG, Dong SR, Hegedus C, et al (1989) Aerosolized pentamidine and disseminated infection with *Pneumocystis carinii*. Ann Intern Med 111: 442
78. Problete RB, Rodriguez K, Foust RT, et al (1989) *Pneumocystis carinii* hepatitis in the acquired immunodeficiency syndrome (AIDS). Ann Intern Med 110: 737–738

Metabolic Disorders and the Spleen

W. R. Wilcox

> "I walk as I were girdles with my spleen;
> And look as if my belly carried twins –
> Wretch that I am! I fear me I shall burst."
> *Plautus*, Second Century B.C.

Introduction

The spleen is frequently enlarged in genetic disorders, particularly those characterized by hemolysis, storage, infiltration, portal hypertension, immune deficiency, or abnormal phagocytic function (Table 1). The topic of this chapter is metabolic disorders, or inborn errors of metabolism, that result in splenomegaly, especially those disorders with surgical implications for the spleen. Hemolytic disorders are discussed in another chapter in this volume. I will summarize the genetic and biochemical aspects of the diseases with storage or infiltration, as well as the indications for and results of surgical intervention, and any alternative therapies available. For a more complete discussion of each disorder, the reader is referred to Scriver et al. [45].

Storage Disorders

The lysosome is an acidic membranous compartment of the cell containing numerous hydrolases. In part, it is responsible for the degradation of glycoproteins, lipids, etc. that are normally turned over during cellular metabolism. Genetic defects in the degradative capacity of the lysosome lead to storage of incompletely degraded macromolecules within it. The storage ultimately causes cellular dysfunction. The manifestations of any specific biochemical defect depend on the distribution and turnover rate of the substrate in each cell type. Many people with lysosomal storage disorders have concomitant organomegaly. Splenomegaly in these diseases generally results from storage within an increased number of lymphoreticular cells in the spleen. The splenic pathology of these disorders has been reviewed by Elleder [16]. All the storage disorders listed in Table 1 are inherited in an autosomal recessive manner, except for mucopolysaccharidosis type II (Hunter), which is X-linked recessive.

Table 1. Genetic conditions with splenomegaly

Hematologic disorders
  Hemolytic
  - Disorders of erythrocyte membranes – spherocytosis, elliptocytosis, etc.
  - Hemoglobinopathies – sickle cell, hemoglobin C, SC, etc.
  - Disorders of erythrocyte metabolism – pyruvate kinase deficiency,
    glucose-6-phosphate-dehydrogenase, congenital erythropoietic porphyria

Extramedullary hematopoiesis
  - Thalassemia major
  - Osteopetrosis

Immune deficiencies
  - Chédiak-Higashi
  - Chronic granulomatous disease

Abnormal phagocytic function
  - Familial erythrophagocytic lymphohistiocytosis

Storage disorders
  - Gaucher's disease
  - Niemann-Pick diseases
  - GM_1 gangliosidosis
  - Mucolipidosis types II and III
  - Mucopolysaccharidosis types I, II, VII
  - Galactosialidosis
  - β-Mannosidosis
  - Fucosidosis
  - Sialidosis
  - Sialic acid storage disease
  - Farber disease
  - Multiple sulfatase deficiency
  - Wolman and cholesterol ester storage diseases
  - Tangier disease
  - Chylomicronemia

Disorders with portal hypertension
  - Cystic fibrosis
  - Wilson disease
  - $β_1$-Antitrypsin deficiency
  - Galactosemia
  - Cystinosis
  - Tyrosinemia
  - Fructose intolerance
  - Zellweger syndrome
  - Neonatal hemochromatosis
  - Glycogen storage disease type IV

Disorders with infiltration
  - Amyloidosis

Gaucher's Disease

Gaucher's disease is the most common disorder in the storage disease category and the one with the most surgical implications for the spleen. However, the recent introduction of enzyme replacement therapy has substantially altered the management of patients with Gaucher's disease, largely supplanting the need for surgical intervention.

The manifestations of β-glucosidase (or glucocerebrosidase) deficiency were first described in 1882 by Gaucher in his doctoral thesis. The defect in Gaucher's disease is a deficiency of lysosomal β-glucosidase (or glucocerebrosidase; see Fig. 1) leading to a storage of glucocerebrosides (*N*-acyl-sphingosyl-1-O-β-D-glucoside, components of the plasma membrane) within the lysosomes of macrophages (Gaucher cells). β-Glucosidase is membrane associated and requires the presence of the protein saposin C to efficiently hydrolyze its substrate [8]. Variant forms of Gaucher due to defects in saposin C have been described [42].

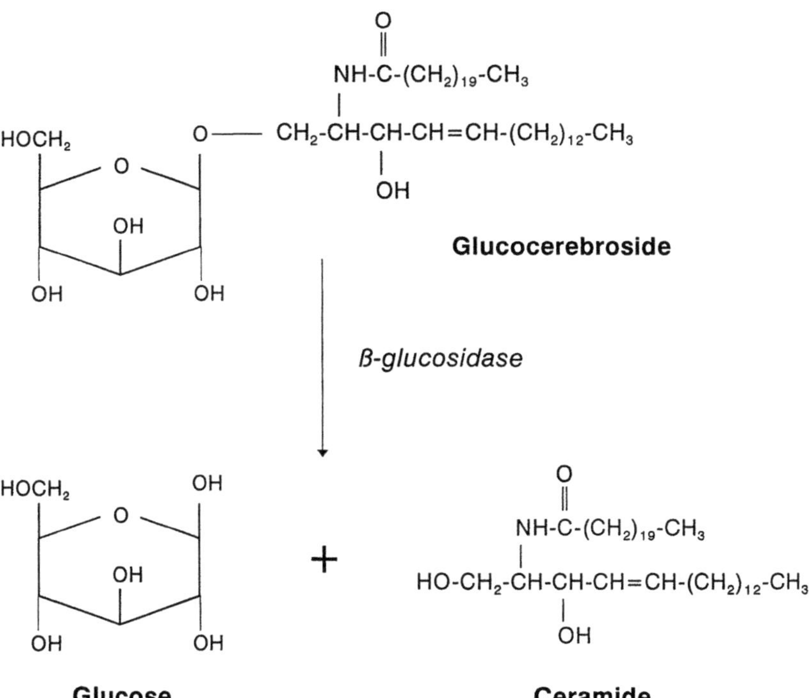

Fig. 1. Biochemical defect in Gaucher's disease. The hydrolysis of glucocerebroside to glucose and ceramide within the lysosome by acid β-glucosidase is impaired

Gaucher's disease is traditionally divided into three phenotypic groups (types I, II, and III) depending on the degree of central nervous system (CNS) involvement. Type I, or non-neuronopathic, is the most common form of Gaucher and lacks CNS involvement. The age at onset and severity of the disease are extremely variable; patients may present in childhood with significant involvement, or mild splenomegaly may be an incidental finding in old age. Splenomegaly is the most consistent feature of type-I Gaucher disease, but it can range from mild enlargement to quite massive, compromising pulmonary function. Splenic infarctions can occur and subcapsular infarcts may present as localized abdominal pain [8]. Pathological examination of the spleen reveals fibrosis, usually associated with infarcts and nodularity [16, 31]. The appearance of the spleen on ultrasonographic examination is abnormal, with hypoechoic areas corresponding to focal accumulations of Gaucher cells, and hyperechoic lesions reflecting Gaucher cells and fibrosis [22]. Magnetic resonance imaging of the spleen often reveals splenic infarcts and nodules [23]. The appearance of the spleen on imaging studies can raise concerns of malignant disease in a patient not yet diagnosed with Gaucher's disease. Hypersplenism is common, resulting in thrombocytopenia and usually mild anemia. Hepatomegaly is also common, but hepatic function is usually normal. In some patients, displacement of the bone marrow by Gaucher cells leads to thinning of bony trabeculae, infarctions, and pathological fractures. Erlenmeyer flask deformities of the distal femur are characteristic, and painful bone crises often involve the femur. The bone disease frequently progresses more rapidly during pubertal growth. Significant involvement of the lungs is a rare, but serious, complication resulting in compromised pulmonary function and pulmonary hypertension [8].

The other types of Gaucher's disease are less common than type I and involve the CNS. Type-II Gaucher's disease, or the acute neuronopathic type, can present at birth with hydrops fetalis, but more commonly, affected children develop hepatosplenomegaly, oculomotor abnormalities, and retroflexion of the head. There is progressive involvement of the CNS, eventually leading to death. Type-III Gaucher's disease, also known as the Norrbottnian or subacute neuronopathic form, is characterized by later-onset neurologic disease in addition to the features of type I [8].

The diagnosis of Gaucher can be suggested by a bone marrow aspirate demonstrating Gaucher cells, but similar cells can also be seen in other disorders such as chronic myelogenous leukemia [25]. An enzymatic assay of leukocytes or cultured fibroblasts is the preferred diagnostic method. The amount of residual enzyme activity in vitro does not correlate with the severity of the disease. Carriers cannot be detected reliably by enzyme assay because of overlap with noncarriers. Detection of causative DNA mutations is the only possible method for carrier screening, in selected populations [8]. However, even when carriers are detected it is difficult to provide genetic counseling because of the clinical variability of the disease (see below).

Gaucher's disease is panethnic in distribution, but there is a higher incidence of type I in Ashkenazi Jews and of type III in the Norrbottnian region of Sweden. In the Ashkenazim, the incidence of type I may be as high as 1:1000, but not all affected individuals come to medical attention because the disease can be quite mild [8].

Many mutations have been found in the β-glucosidase gene in Gaucher patients. Mutations in β-glucosidase are designated in the literature by either the amino acid or the nucleotide change (designated inside parentheses here). The N370S (1226G) mutation results in decreased catalytic activity and is the most frequent in the Ashkenazi Jewish population, carried by about 6%. The (84GG) insertion mutation, with no associated enzyme activity, is the second most common, carried by 0.6% of Ashkenazim. The L444P (1448C) mutation, with decreased enzyme activity and stability, is panethnic but more frequent in the Norrbottnian population of Northern Sweden. The combination of N370S (1226G), (84GG), (IVS2(+1)), and L444P (1448C) accounts for 95% of the mutant alleles in Jews, while in the general population, N370S and L444P account for 75% of the mutant alleles; all the other mutations are individually rare [8, 10].

Some general phenotype/genotype correlations are possible, but there is a great deal of variability among individuals with the same mutations in β-glucosidase. However, there is more phenotypic variability between unrelated affected individuals than within families, suggesting that there are other genetic factors involved in determining the phenotype. What is clear is that the N370S (1226G) mutation precludes neurologic disease, and that the L444P (1448C) is associated with more severe disease – homozygotes for L444P all have severe disease and usually have neurologic involvement. N370S/N370S homozygotes have a later onset of disease with milder manifestations. In fact, they may never come to medical attention. Among *symptomatic* patients, the mean age at onset is 30.8 years. N370S/L444P and N370S/(84GG) compound heterozygotes have more severe manifestations, with a mean age at onset of 13.5 and 7.4 years, respectively [47].

Prior to the advent of enzyme replacement therapy, splenectomy was frequently performed (although not for type II because of the aggressive CNS involvement) for indications including thrombocytopenia ($<40\,000/\mu l$), growth retardation, and cardiopulmonary compromise. It also helped to alleviate the associated anemia [8]. However, since the spleen is the major reservoir for storage of the glucocerebroside, eliminating it may increase the pace of storage elsewhere. In fact, there have been several reports of more rapid bone involvement following total splenectomy. Rose et al. [39] reported a 4.5-year-old who underwent total splenectomy. The preoperative skeletal radiographs were normal, but 3 months later there was extensive involvement of the femora and spine. Ashkenazi et al. [1] reported more rapid progression of bone disease in six of eight cases following total splenectomy. Similarly, Fleshner et al. [19] found that 11 of the 34 patients in their series who underwent a total splenectomy had accelerated bone disease, whereas none of the 13 patients with a partial splenectomy did, although the duration of follow-up was not as long. Cohen et al. [15] reported seven patients who underwent partial splenectomy with a 7- to 8-year follow up and six patients who underwent total splenectomy with a follow-up of 7–12 years. Three patients in the partial group had preoperative bone pain and two continued to have it afterwards. In contrast, no patients in the total group had bone pain preoperatively, but five did postoperatively. However, other authors have not found progression of bone disease after splenectomy to be a common occurrence [31, 50].

Aside from concerns about more rapid progression of disease at other sites, the only other notable complication of total splenectomy is thrombocytosis, predisposing patients to thromboembolic events. Treatment with aspirin and dipyridamole may be indicated in the perioperative period [19].

Because of the concerns about total splenectomy, partial splenectomy has been advocated as an alternative. The advantages of partial splenectomy are that it retains a reservoir for storage and preserves immune function. However, there are numerous problems that may occur with partial splenectomy, in addition to it being a more technically demanding procedure. Zimran et al. [53] reported postoperative bleeding requiring a total splenectomy in seven of the 31 patients in their series, but other authors have not described a similar incidence of bleeding [4, 15, 19, 33]. Regrowth of the splenic remnant has frequently been found when the duration of follow-up was long enough [4, 33, 53]. In the largest series, Zimran et al. [53] reported the results of partial splenectomy in 24 patients with a mean follow-up of 7.3 years: 21 of the 24 had significant, symptomatic regrowth of the spleen and either underwent a total splenectomy or were treated with enzyme replacement therapy.

Partial splenectomy in patients with aggressive disease may be contraindicated. Holcomb and Greene [24] reported a partial splenectomy in an 18-month-old with type-III Gaucher's disease. The splenic remnant regrew quickly, and 7.5 months later the child died of a splenic rupture opposite to the site of the operative division. Kyllerman et al. [29] reported a partial splenectomy in a 28-month-old with type III. The hypersplenism and splenomegaly returned within 3 months and the authors felt the rest of the disease may have been accelerated; the patient died at 32 months of age.

There have been two reports of splenic embolization for hypersplenism in Gaucher's disease. Thanopoulos et al. [49] reported partial splenic embolization in a single case with resolution of the hypersplenism and without apparent acceleration of the other findings 4 years later. Samama et al. [41] reported total embolization of the spleen in a 12-year-old. Eight months later the patient was doing well with resolution of the hypersplenism. However, since large organ size is often one of the indications for splenomegaly and the spleen is frequently fibrotic, embolization may not be appropriate in most circumstances.

As a variation on partial splenectomy, Miyano et al. [32] reported two cases of splenectomy followed by splenic autotransplantation of slices in an omental pouch. The hypersplenism resolved and there was slow enlargement of the transplanted splenic remnant over the course of 6.5 and 7 years.

The advent of enzyme replacement therapy (alglucerase injection, Ceredase, Genzyme Corporation, Cambridge Mass.) has changed the management of Gaucher. Before enzyme replacement therapy became available, the only therapeutic option besides splenectomy was bone marrow transplantation, with its attendant risks. Bone marrow transplantion can be curative for type I and can retard or prevent CNS deterioration in type III [38]. The enzyme currently available is purified from human placentas and then processed enzymatically to a high mannose form that can be recognized by receptors on the macrophage. A recombinant form of the enzyme should be available soon. When infused intravenously into the patient, the enzyme binds to the surface of the macrophage, is endocytosed and delivered to the lysosome, where it can degrade the stored glucocerebroside. The enzyme was originally administered as infusions of 60 units/kg every 2 weeks [5, 6, 9, 17]. However, because of the high cost of the enzyme (approximately US $3.50 per unit), alternative low-dose administration schedules (such as 30 units/kg per month divided into 3 weekly infusions) have been studied and found to be as effective as the high-dose regimen [18, 51, 52]. However, even with home-infusion low-dose therapy, the annual cost for a 70-kg adult is at least $94000 per year [51].

Enzyme replacement leads to a rapid rise in platelet counts in splenectomized patients and a slower increase if the spleen is present. Anemia improves gradually over months and organomegaly improves over 6 months. The bone disease improves more slowly. Approximately 10%–15% of patients develop antibodies, and some patients have had allergic reactions but not enough to stop therapy [5, 6, 8, 9, 17, 18, 51, 52]. After 1 year of therapy in one series, hepatomegaly had decreased by 20%–30% and splenic volume by 30%–50%, anemia had improved by 1.5 g Hb/dl, and platelet counts had doubled where thrombocytopenia had originally been present [36].

What, then, are the indications for splenectomy in the enzyme replacement era? The answer is not yet clear, but Zimran et al. [53] suggest the following: "(1) When enzyme replacement is not a suitable option (e.g., where the cost is prohibitive), (2) life-threatening thrombocytopenia or a critical need for surgery (such as coronary bypass) in a patient with a very low platelet count, (3) inferior vena cava syndrome, (4) unremitting abdominal pain resulting from recurrent splenic infarction, and (5) severe restrictive pulmonary disease with incipient respiratory failure."

Niemann-Pick Diseases

Niemann-Pick is similar to Gaucher in that both disorders are characterized by lysosomal lipid storage and splenomegaly. Unlike Gaucher, however, hypersplenism is not common. Niemann-Pick is currently classified into three types: A, B, and C. Types A and B are both due to deficiencies in lysosomal acid sphingomyelinase, while type C is due to an as yet unidentified abnormality in intracellular cholesterol and lipid trafficking. Although the sphinomyelinase-deficient forms of Niemann-Pick (A and B) and Niemann-Pick type C share the common feature of lysosomal lipid storage, they are otherwise distinct clinical entities [37, 44].

Sphingomyelinase Deficiency

Sphingomyelin is an important component of the plasma membrane, comprising 5%–20% of the total phospholipids. The biochemical defect in types A and B is shown in Fig. 2.

Individuals with type-A Niemann-Pick or the infantile form of sphingomyelinase deficiency present in early infancy with hepatosplenomegaly and poor feeding. By 6 months of age psychomotor retardation is evident and they begin to lose what skills they have. They usually die by 2–3 years of age. In contrast, type-B patients present in childhood and adolescence with hepatosplenomegaly; the CNS is spared. The major sites of storage are the spleen, lymph nodes, bone marrow, lungs, liver, and kidneys. Pulmonary involvement frequently appears in adolescence or adulthood and eventually is the cause of death. Although the spleen may be quite enlarged in this disease, there are seldom functional consequences [44]. Tassoni et al. [48] re-

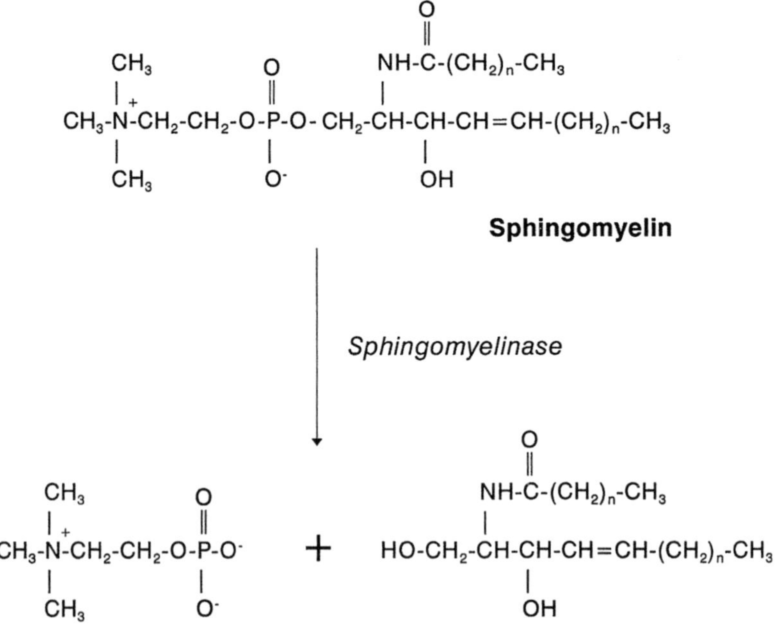

Fig. 2. Biochemical defect in Niemann-Pick disease types A and B. The hydrolysis of sphingomyelin to ceramide and phosphocholine within the lysosome by acid sphingomyelinase is diminished

ported a 33-year-old woman with Niemann-Pick type B, cirrhosis, portal hypertension, and thrombocytopenia secondary to hypersplenism. The thrombocytopenia resolved after splenectomy, and the spleen was found to have infarcts and calcifications.

The diagnosis of Niemann-Pick can be suggested by the finding of foam cells and sea-blue histiocytes on a bone marrow biopsy. A definitive diagnosis must be made with an enzymatic assay of fibroblasts or leukocytes. Heterozygote detection is possible only through DNA methods, since there is overlap of enzymatic activity between heterozygotes and noncarriers [44].

Similar to Gaucher's disease, sphingomyelinase-deficient Niemann-Pick has an elevated incidence in the Ashkenazi Jewish population; the incidence of type A is 1/40 000 while that of type B is 1/80 000. The carrier frequency is estimated to be about one in 60. Three mutations account for 92% of type-A alleles in the Ashkenazim [44].

There is no specific treatment for sphingomyelinase deficiency, only supportive care. Enzyme replacement therapy is a possibility, but is not currently available.

Niemann-Pick Type C

Niemann-Pick C is not due to sphingomyelinase deficiency, but rather to a defect in a gene on chromosome 18p [14]. In the classic form of type C, the child has a slow loss of cognitive abilities starting at the time of school entry. Ataxia, dysarthria, dysphagia and drooling, and dystonias develop later. Patients may also have seizures, cataplexy, and psychiatric disturbances. Vertical supranuclear ophthalmoplegia is a consistent and helpful diagnostic finding. Hepatosplenomegaly is frequent, but there are no functional consequences. Earlier-onset variants of type C are characterized by fetal ascites or neonatal jaundice and hepatic failure, and a later-onset form is notable for cognitive and psychiatric disturbances; the gaze palsy and other neurologic signs appear later [37].

Pathologically, the presence of foam cells and sea-blue histiocytes is similar to sphingomyelinase deficiency. Biopsies of the liver may be falsely negative. Biochemically, there is lysosomal storage of many different lipids and cholesterol. A definitive diagnosis is currently possible only by demonstrating a decreased ability of cultured fibroblasts to synthesize cholesterol esters after endocytic uptake of low-density lipoprotein and an abnormal cellular location of the unesterified cholesterol. Plasma lipids are normal.

Type C is panethnic in distribution and may be as common as types A and B. Carrier detection is not possible because of overlap with normal.

The only treatment for Niemann-Pick type C is symptomatic management. Liver (in man) and bone marrow transplants (in a mouse model) do not affect the progression of neurologic disease [37].

Tangier Disease

Tangier disease is a rare autosomal recessive disorder of cholesterol metabolism resulting in cholesterol ester storage, predominantly in the reticuloendothelial system. The basic defect is unknown. Patients present with a low plasma cholesterol, normal to increased triglycerides, very low levels of high-density lipoprotein and apolipoprotein A-I, hyperplastic orange tonsils, a peripheral neuropathy that may be relapsing, and corneal opacities that do not interfere with vision. There does not appear to be an increased risk of atherosclerosis. The liver may be enlarged and the intestinal mucosa, when examined, is notable for orange-brown lesions, but the function of both is usually normal [3]. Splenomegaly was described in 22 of the 37 reported patients reviewed by Assmann et al. [3], but hypersplenism was rare. Pathologically, the lesions in the tonsils, spleen, intestinal mucosa, etc. consist of foam cells or histiocytes full of lipid. Unlike the lysosomal storage disorders discussed above, this lipid is not contained within a separate membranous compartment of the cell [3, 16].

There have been two reports of splenectomy in Tangier disease. Labbé et al. [30] reported a 15-year-old patient with hypersplenism. The patient had persistent fevers after splenectomy and died 6 months later of a gastrointestinal hemorrhage (felt to be a peptic ulcer). The history of the inbred pedigree was significant for hypersplenism and death, also from a gastrointestinal hemorrhage, in an apparently affected uncle. Schaefer et al. [43] reported a 44-year-old man who underwent splenectomy for hypersplenism. The patient did well after surgery until the age of 63, when he was found to have very thickened small bowel mesentery and omentum due to infiltration by foam cells.

Other Storage Disorders

The other storage disorders with splenomegaly listed in Table 1 generally will not come to the attention of a surgeon. In the case of cholesterol ester storage disease and chylomicronemia, the splenomegaly is not massive and is reversible with dietary therapy [2, 13]. In the other disorders, the splenomegaly has little functional consequence compared with the involvement of the CNS and skeletal system.

Infiltrative Disorders

Amyloidosis

Amyloidosis is different from the other disorders discussed in this chapter because it is an infiltrative process rather than an intracellular storage disease. In amyloidosis, there is extracellular deposition of fibrillar protein with green birefringence on Congo-red staining. While localized forms of amyloid deposition do occur (in the thyroid in multiple endocrine neoplasia type II, in the skin in autosomal dominant and X-linked forms of cutaneous amyloidosis, and in the brain in Alzheimer's disease), amyloidosis is most commonly a systemic disorder. Systemic forms of amyloidosis can be divided into three basic types: immunoglobulin (AL), reactive (AA), and hereditary [7].

AL amyloidosis can be primary or associated with multiple myeloma. AL amyloid is composed of aggregated immunoglobulin light chains. Renal involvement progressing to the nephrotic syndrome is the most common finding. Amyloid infiltration of the liver can result in hepatomegaly, infiltration of the heart in cardiomyopathy and arrhythmias, infiltration of the bowel in diarrhea, and infiltration of the nervous system in carpal tunnel syndrome and peripheral and autonomic neuropathy. Involvement of the spleen by AL may cause factor-X deficiency and a bleeding diathesis, because AL amyloid can bind the factor in the spleen [20]. The general treatment for AL amyloidosis is with prednisone and alkylating agents [7].

AA or reactive amyloidosis is secondary to chronic inflammation from infection, rheumatologic disorders, inflammatory bowel disease, or familial Mediterranean fever (FMF). Nephrotic syndrome, hepatosplenomegaly, and gastrointestinal bleeding are manifestations of specific organ involvement. The amyloid is composed of the acute-phase reactant SAA, synthesized by the liver. AA amyloidosis is treated by controlling the underlying inflammatory process and, in FMF, with colchicine [7].

Amyloidosis can also be heritable in an autosomal dominant fashion. Many mutations in different genes have been identified as predisposing carriers to various clinical syndromes. One of the most common is familial amyloid polyneuropathy due to mutations in transthyretin (prealbumin), although kindreds with renal and cardiac involvement have also been described. Mutations in apolipoprotein A-I, gelsolin, fibrinogen, and lysozyme have all been reported with varying involvement of the peripheral nervous system, kidneys, cornea, and heart. Significant involvement of the spleen is not a finding in the hereditary forms of amyloidosis [7]. The most current information on individual hereditary amyloidoses can be obtained by accessing Online Mendelian Inheritance in Man at their worldwide web site (http://www3.ncbi.nlm.nih.gov/Omim/).

Involvement of the spleen in amyloidosis is frequent – 90% in AL and 96% in AA in one series [12], whereas splenic enlargement is less common – 4 [28]–15% [12] in AL and 20% in AA [12]. Patients may be functionally hyposplenic [11, 46]. The pattern of amyloid deposition in the spleen is somewhat different in AA and AL; both always involve the blood vessels, but 35% of AA involves the white pulp while in AL 52% had infiltration of the red pulp and 70% of the white [34]. Splenic infarctions can occur [27], and spontaneous rupture of the spleen is a rare complication that may be the presenting feature of systemic amyloidosis [27, 35]. Symptomatic factor-X deficiency in AL has been reversed by splenectomy in two reported cases [21, 40].

Future Directions

Over the past few decades, our understanding of the basic molecular, biochemical, and pathophysiological abnormalities in the metabolic disorders has increased exponentially. In contrast to these rapid advances, our ability to provide anything but symptomatic management has increased slowly. The recent introduction of enzyme therapy in Gaucher's disease represents a major advance in the field. While therapy for more mildly affected patients is currently prohibited by the cost of the drug and the inconvenience of frequent infusions, it has significantly altered the management and lives of patients with more severe disease. In the future, somatic cell gene therapy will provide an ultimate cure for patients afflicted with metabolic disorders. Because the diagnosis and management of these disorders is complex and requires the expertise of many different disciplines, the patient is best managed by a team consisting of internists or pediatricians, geneticists, surgeons, and other health-care professionals.

References

1. Ashkenazi A, Zaizov R, Matoth Y (1986) Effect of splenectomy on destructive bone changes in children with chronic (type I) Gaucher disease. Eur J Pediatr 145: 138–141
2. Assmann G, Seedorf U (1995) Acid lipase deficiency: Wolman disease and cholesterol ester storage disease. In: Scriver CR, Beaudet AL, Sly WS, Valle D (eds) The metabolic and molecular bases of inherited disease, 7th edn. McGraw-Hill, New York, pp 2563–2587
3. Assmann G, von Eckardstein A, Brewer HB (1995) Familial high density lipoprotein deficiency: Tangier disease. In: Scriver CR, Beaudet AL, Sly WS, Valle D (eds) The metabolic and molecular bases of inherited disease, 7th edn. McGraw-Hill, New York, pp 2053–2072
4. Bar-Maor JA (1993) Partial splenectomy in Gaucher's disease: follow-up report. J Pediatr Surg 28: 686–688
5. Barton NW, Furbish FS, Murray GJ, Garfield M, Brady RO (1990) Therapeutic response to intravenous infusions of glucocerebrosidase in a patient with Gaucher disease. Proc Natl Acad Sci U S A 87: 1913–1916
6. Barton NW, Brady RO, Dambrosia JM, Di Bisceglie AM, Doppelt SH, Hill SC, Mankin HJ, Murray GJ, Parker RI, Argoff CE, Grewal RP, Yu K-T et al (1991) Replacement therapy for inherited enzyme deficiency – macrophage-targeted glucocerebrosidase for Gaucher's disease. N Engl J Med 324: 1464–1470
7. Benson MD (1995) Amyloidosis. In: Scriver CR, Beaudet AL, Sly WS, Valle D (eds) The metabolic and molecular bases of inherited disease, 7th edn. McGraw-Hill, New York, pp 4157–4191
8. Beutler E, Grabowski GA (1995) Gaucher disease. In: Scriver CR, Beaudet AL, Sly WS, Valle D (eds) The metabolic and molecular bases of inherited disease, 7th edn. McGraw-Hill, New York, pp 2641–2670
9. Beutler E, Kay A, Saven A, Garver P, Thurston D, Dawson A, Rosenbloom B (1991) Enzyme replacement therapy for Gaucher disease. Blood 78: 1183–1189
10. Beutler E, Nguyen NJ, Henneberger MW, Smolec JM, McPherson RA, West C, Gelbart T (1993) Gaucher disease: gene frequencies in the Ashkenazi Jewish population. Am J Hum Genet 52: 85–88

11. Boyko WJ, Pratt R, Wass H (1982) Functional hyposplenism, a diagnostic clue in amyloidosis. Report of six cases. Am J Clin Pathol 77: 745–748
12. Briggs GW (1961) Amyloidosis. Ann Intern Med 55: 943–957
13. Brunzell JD (1995) Familial lipoprotein lipase deficiency and other causes of the chylomicronemia syndrome. In: Scriver CR, Beaudet AL, Sly WS, Valle D (eds) The metabolic and molecular bases of inherited disease, 7th edn. McGraw-Hill, New York, pp 1913–1932
14. Carstea ED, Parker CC, Fandino LB, Vanier MT, Overhauser J, Weissenbach J, Pentchev PG, Brady RO, Polymeropoulos MH (1994) Localizing the human Niemann-Pick C gene to 18q11-12. Am J Hum Genet 55: A182
15. Cohen IJ, Katz K, Freud E, Zer M, Zaizov R (1992) Long-term follow-up of partial splenectomy in Gaucher's disease. Am J Surg 164: 345–347
16. Elleder M (1994) The spleen and storage disorders. In: Cuschieri A, Forbes CD (eds) Disorders of the spleen. Blackwell Scientific, Oxford, pp 151–190
17. Fallet S, Grace ME, Sibille A, Mendelson DS, Shapiro RS, Hermann G, Grabowski GA (1992) Enzyme augmentation in moderate to life-threatening Gaucher disease. Pediatr Res 31: 496–502
18. Figueroa ML, Rosenbloom BE, Kay AC, Garver P, Thurston DW, Koziol JA, Gelbart T, Beutler E (1992) A less costly regimen of alglucerase to treat Gaucher's disease. N Engl J Med 327: 1632–1636
19. Fleshner PR, Aufses AH, Grabowski GA, Elias R (1991) A 27-year experience with splenectomy for Gaucher's disease. Am J Surg 161: 69–75
20. Furie B, Voo L, McAdam KPWJ, Furie BC (1981) Mechanism of factor X deficiency in systemic amyloidosis. N Engl J Med 304: 827–830
21. Greipp PR, Kyle RA, Bowie EJW (1979) Faxtor X deficiency in primary amyloidosis. Resolution after splenectomy. N Engl J Med 301:1050–1051
22. Hill SC, Reinig JW, Barranger JA, Fink J, Shawker TH (1986) Gaucher disease: sonographic appearance of the spleen. Radiology 160: 631–634
23. Hill SC, Damaska BM, Ling A, Patterson K, Di Bisceglie AM, Brady RO, Barton NW (1992) Gaucher disease: abdominal MR imaging findings in 46 patients. Radiology 184: 561–566
24. Holcomb GW, Green HL (1993) Fatal hemorrhage caused by disease progression after partial splenectomy for type II Gaucher's disease. J Pediatr Surg 28: 1572–1574
25. Kattlove HE, Williams JC, Gaynor E, Spivack M, Bradley RM, Brady RO (1969) Gaucher cells in chronic myelocytic leukemia: an acquired abnormality. Blood 33: 379–390
26. Kim E, Mattar AG (1976) Scan findings in a case of splenic infarction due to amyloidosis: case report. J Nucl Med 17: 902–903
27. Kozicky OJ, Brandt LJ, Lederman M, Milcu M (1987) Splenic amyloidosis: a case report of spontaneous splenic rupture with a review of the pertinent literature. Am J Gastroenterol 82: 582–587
28. Kyle RA, Greipp PR (1983) Amyloidosis (AL). Clinical and laboratory features in 229 cases. Mayo Clin Proc 58: 665–683
29. Kyllerman M, Conradi N, Mnsson J-E, Percy AK, Svennerholm L (1990) Rapidly progressive type III Gaucher disease: deterioration following partial splenectomy. Acta Paediatr Scand 79: 448–453
30. Labbé A, Dechelotte P, Meyer M, Dubray C, Jouanel P (1985) La maladie de Tangier. Une thésaurismose rare. Presse Med 14: 1189–1192
31. Lee RE (1982) The pathology of Gaucher disease. In: Desnick RJ, Gatt S, Grabowski GA (eds) Gaucher disease: a century of delineation and research. Liss, New York, pp 177–217
32. Miyano T, Yamataka A, Ohshiro K, Yamashiro Y (1994) Heterotopic splenic autotransplantation for splenomegaly secondary to Gaucher's disease – a case of siblings. J Pediatr Surg 29: 1572–1574
33. Morgenstern L, Verham R, Weinstein I, Phillips EH (1993) Subtotal splenectomy for Gaucher's disease: a follow-up study. Am Surg 59: 860–865
34. Ohyama T, Shimokama T, Yoshikawa Y, Watanabe T (1990) Splenic amyloidosis: correlations between chemical types of amyloid protein and morphological features. Mod Pathol 3: 419–422

35. Okazaki K, Moriyasu F, Shiomura T, Yamamoto T, Suzaki T, Kanematsu Y, Akasaka S, Kobashi Y (1986) Spontaneous rupture of the spleen and liver in amyloidosis – a case report and review of the literature. Gastroenterol Jpn 21: 518–524

36. Pastores GM, Sibille AR, Grabowski GA (1993) Enzyme therapy in Gaucher disease type 1: dosage efficacy and adverse effects in 33 patients treated for 6 to 24 months. Blood 82: 408–416

37. Pentchev PG, Vanier MT, Suzuki K, Patterson MC (1995) Niemann-Pick disease type C: a cellular cholesterol lipidosis. In: Scriver CR, Beaudet AL, Sly WS, Valle D (eds) The metabolic and molecular bases of inherited disease, 7th edn. McGraw-Hill, New York, pp 2625–2639

38. Ringdén O, Groth CG, Erikson A, Granqvist S, Mnsson J-E, Sparrelid E (1995) Ten years' experience of bone marrow transplantation for Gaucher disease. Transplantation 59: 864–870

39. Rose JS, Grabowski GA, Barnett SH, Desnick RJ (1982) Accelerated skeletal deterioration after splenectomy in Gaucher type 1 disease. Am J Radiol 139: 1202–1204

40. Rosenstein ED, Itzkowitz SH, Penziner AS, Cohen JI, Mornaghi RA (1983) Resolution of factor X deficiency in primary amyloidosis following splenectomy. Arch Intern Med 143: 597–599

41. Samama G, Brefort JL, Dolley M, Leporrier M (1989) Splénomégalie monstrueuse de la maladie de Gaucher. Traitement par embolisation puis splénectomie. Presse Med 18: 1078–1079

42. Sandhoff K, Harzer K, Fürst W (1995) Sphingolipid activator proteins. In: Scriver CR, Beaudet AL, Sly WS, Valle D (eds) The metabolic and molecular bases of inherited disease, 7th edn. McGraw-Hill, New York, pp 2427–2441

43. Schaefer EJ, Triche TJ, Zech LA, Stein LA, Kemeny MM, Brennan MF, Brewer HB (1983) Massive omental reticuloendothelial cell lipid uptake in Tangier disease after splenectomy. Am J Med 75: 521–526

44. Schuchman EH, Desnick RJ (1995) Niemann-Pick disease types A and B: acid sphingo-myelinase deficiencies. In: Scriver CR, Beaudet AL, Sly WS, Valle D (eds) The metabolic and molecular bases of inherited disease, 7th edn. McGraw-Hill, New York, pp 2601–2624

45. Scriver CR, Beaudet AL, Sly WS, Valle D (eds) (1995) The metabolic and molecular bases of inherited disease, 7th edn. McGraw-Hill, New York

46. Selby CD, Sprott VMA, Toghill PJ (1987) Impaired splenic function in systemic amyloidosis. Postgrad Med J 63: 357–360

47. Sibille A, Eng CM, Kim S-J, Pastores G, Grabowski GA (1993) Phenotype/genotype correlations in Gaucher disease type I: clinical and therapeutic implications. Am J Hum Genet 52: 1094–1101

48. Tassoni JP, Fawaz KA, Johnston DE (1991) Cirrhosis and portal hypertension in a patient with adult Niemann-Pick disease. Gastroenterology 100: 567–569

49. Thanopoulos BD, Frimas CA, Mantagos SP, Beratis NG (1987) Gaucher disease: treatment of hypersplenism with splenic embolization. Acta Paediatr Scand 76: 1003–1007

50. Zimran A, Kay A, Gelbart T, Garver P, Thurston D, Saven A, Beutler E (1992) Gaucher disease. Clinical, laboratory, radiologic, and genetic features of 53 patients. Medicine (Baltimore) 71: 337–353

51. Zimran A, Hollak CEM, Abrahamov A, van Oers MHJ, Kelly M, Beutler E (1993) Home treatment with intravenous enzyme replacement therapy for Gaucher disease: an international collaborative study of 33 patients. Blood 82: 1107–1109

52. Zimran A, Elstein D, Kannai R, Zevin S, Hadas-Halpern I, Levy-Lahad E, Cohen Y, Horowitz M, Abrahamov A (1994) Low-dose enzyme replacement therapy for Gaucher's disease: effects of age, sex, genotype, and clinical features on response to treatment. Am J Med 97: 3–13

53. Zimran A, Elstein D, Schiffmann R, Abrahamov A, Goldberg M, Bar-Maor JA, Brady RO, Guzzetta PC, Barton NW (1995) Outcome of partial splenectomy for type I Gaucher disease. J Pediatr 126: 596–597

Portal Hypertension and Disorders
of the Splenic Circulation

R. W. Busuttil and W. Arnaout

> "On the other hand, the spleen is merely a contingent necessity arising from the defectiveness of the liver and the stomach, like the wash-house to the kitchen …. Where there is more foul work than clean as in those in whom the whole composition of the body is vitiated, since their liver is vitiated, and who make use of an impure ailment, there the spleen is larger, the wash-house exceeds the kitchen."
>
> *William Harvey,* Seventeenth Century

The spleen plays an important role in conditions that affect the portal and splanchnic circulation. Without early diagnosis and treatment, both arterial and venous disorders of the splenic circulation result in various conditions that may produce a catastrophic outcome. These disorders are usually classified in terms of the underlying etiology as problems of venous outflow obstruction and portal hypertension or as anomalies of the arterial system. This chapter will focus on the role of the spleen in relation to these disorders and will review the current diagnostic and therapeutic options.

Anatomic Considerations

Splenic anatomy is discussed by Morgenstern (this volume). The relationship of the spleen to the splanchnic circulation is very intricate, as the spleen serves as the junction between the mesenteric venous circulation and the esophagogastric venous plexus. In this position, it becomes an important collateral channel in patients with portal hypertension, where elevated portal venous pressure causes alteration and possibly reversal of flow within the portal vein. In addition, the splenic ligaments, which are normally avascular, become highly vascularized with large varices that ultimately drain blood into the systemic circulation.

The splenic circulation is intimately related to the pancreas. Henschen [1] described the relationship of the splenic artery to the pancreas, finding it to be suprapancreatic in 90%, retropancreatic in 8%, and prepancreatic in 2% of specimens. The common splenic vein usually follows the splenic artery, running in the retropancreatic space and receiving multiple collaterals from the pancreas. Both the splenic artery and vein may be involved by inflammatory and neoplastic diseases of the pancreas and the retroperitoneum.

Portal Hypertension

Definitions

Portal hypertension is defined as an increase in portal vein pressure above the normal range of 5–10 mmHg. The condition results from a relative or absolute obstruction of splanchnic blood flow or, less commonly, from an increased portal venous flow [2]. In patients with portal hypertension, direct portal vein pressure ranges from 15 to 40 mmHg, while the hepatic vein wedge pressure measures 10–30 mmHg [3]. Sherlock [4] classified portal hypertension according to the underlying etiology as extrahepatic presinusoidal, intrahepatic presinusoidal, sinusoidal, and intra- and extrahepatic postsinusoidal. While cirrhosis of various causes remains the most common cause of portal hypertension, presinusoidal extrahepatic portal hypertension (EPH), as seen in cases of splenic outflow obstruction, is an extremely important form which comprises 5%–10% of all causes of portal hypertension. If the correct diagnosis is made early, these patients are easily managed, and life-threatening variceal bleeding can be avoided. The following discussion will focus upon this form of portal hypertension and the role of the spleen and its vasculature in the etiology and management of this disease.

Pathophysiology of Splenic Outflow Obstruction

Disorders of the spleen and its circulation are usually included with the extrahepatic presinusoidal causes of portal hypertension resulting either from outflow obstruction of the splenic vein or massive increase in portal flow. Consequently, pressures in the splenic vein and possibly the extrahepatic portions of the portal vein will be elevated, while hepatic sinusoidal pressure and hepatic parenchymal function will be normal.

Presinusoidal EPH secondary to isolated outflow obstruction of the splenic vein is found in approximately 5% of all patients with EPH [5], while infectious disorders, hypercoagulable states, and tumors constitute the remaining causes. Splenic artery aneurysm (SAA) and arteriovenous fistula have been reported to cause EPH. Outflow obstruction results either from splenic vein thrombosis or extrinsic compression of the splenic vein. Regardless of the underlying etiology, the associated pathophysiologic changes are similar, and the clinical picture depends on the rate of development and degree of obstruction. Acute splenic vein outflow obstruction causes rapid engorgement of the spleen and capsular swelling, with pain as a predominant symptom. Collateral venous channels to decompress the spleen are not present in this early stage, so that spontaneous variceal bleeding is most unlikely. However, splenic vascular congestion and stasis lead to entrapment and excessive consumption of blood products, which result in splenomegaly, consumptive coagulopathy, and thrombocytopenia.

Chronic venous outflow obstruction of the spleen, in contrast, presents a different clinical picture. As the splenic pressure increases gradually, a number of splenoportal collaterals develop, returning blood from the spleen into the portal vein. Splenic blood, unable to drain through the splenic vein, flows through the short gastric vessels in a retrograde fashion into the submucosal plexus in the gastric fundus and cardia to drain into the coronary vein. The coronary vein may drain directly into the portal vein (24%), into the confluence of the superior mesenteric vein and splenic vein (59%), or into the splenic vein itself (17%) [6, 7]. In the latter group of patients, a thrombosed splenic vein impairs drainage of the coronary vein, subsequently leading to the development of submucosal gastric varices. Retrograde flow through collaterals along the splenic ligaments as well as the gastroepiploic arcade and superior and inferior mesenteric veins serves to decompress the spleen and allow the return of blood into the portal circulation.

Sinistral Portal Hypertension and Splenic Vein Thrombosis

Sinistral portal hypertension is a rare form also referred to as left-sided portal hypertension, segmental, sectorial, regional, compartmental, or splenoportal hypertension [7–13]. Unlike patients with other forms of portal hypertension, these patients typically have elevated pressures to the left of the portal vein, isolated gastric varices, splenomegaly, and normal liver function [14]. Isolated splenic vein thrombosis is the most common cause of sinistral portal hypertension. Splenic vein occlusion due to extrinsic compresssion without partial or complete thrombosis of the splenic vein is a rare cause that has been described in patients with inflammatory retroperitoneal processes, where dense adhesions or fibrosis around the splenic vein cause complete occlusion of the lumen.

Incidence

Isolated splenic vein thrombosis (SVT) was first described at autopsy by Frick in 1922 [15]. The clinical syndrome and its radiographic diagnosis were reported by Greenwald and Wash in 1939 [16]. Sutton et al. [11] reviewed the English literature in 1970 and were able to find 54 cases during the period between 1900 and 1968. Since then, two separate reviews have been published: in 1985 by Moossa and Gadd [17], reporting 144 cases, and in 1986 by Madsen et al. [9], who collected 63 references describing a total of 209 patients between 1969 and 1984. More recently, Loftus et al. [18] reported the Mayo Clinic 20-year experience with 43 patients, six of whom were diagnosed at autopsy.

The true incidence of splenic vein occlusion and subsequent left-sided portal hypertension is unknown. Most cases have been described in association with disorders of the pancreas, both benign and malignant, as a result of the close anatomic relationship of the splenic vasculature and the pancreas. Newer noninvasive radiologic techniques, including duplex ultrasonography, computed tomography (CT), and magnetic resonance imaging (MRI) have resulted in more frequent diagnosis of this entity, even for asymptomatic patients in whom the condition would otherwise be unrecognized.

SVT affects patients of all ages (median age, 45 years; range, 10 months to 85 years). There is a definite male predominance, with a ratio of 1:1.5–2 [9, 11, 17], most likely due to an increased incidence of pancreatic disorders among middle-aged men.

Clinical Manifestations

Upper gastrointestinal (GI) bleeding is the most common symptom. Of the cases reviewed by Madsen et al. [9], 115 patients (72%) cases presented with massive hematemesis or melena (99 patients) or occult bleeding resulting in hypochromic microcytic anemia (16 patients). Splenomegaly was present in 32%–71% of patients, but was often missed on examination, especially when patients presented with massive bleeding. Recurrent abdominal pain was present in 26% of patients reviewed by Moossa and Gadd [17], usually secondary to repeated episodes of pancreatitis or pancreatic pseudocysts. Less common symptoms included chronic anemia and weight loss. Rare presentations, such as bleeding from colonic varices [19] or splenic rupture [20], have also been reported.

Etiology

Most cases of splenic vein occlusion have occurred in association with diseases of the pancreas. Madsen et al. [9] identified the cause of splenic vein occlusion to be pancreatitis, both acute and chronic, in 65% of cases (33% had a pseudocyst), benign and malignant pancreatic neoplasms in 18%, and miscellaneous causes in 17%. In a similar review, Moossa and Gadd [17] described 144 patients with sinistral hypertension and found the cause to be pancreatitis (characterized as chronic, acute, traumatic, hereditary, or associated with a pseudocyst in 56% the cases), while pancreatic malignancies, both islet and non-islet cell types, were the second most common cause of SVT.

While the exact prevalance of splenic vein occlusion in chronic pancreatitis is unknown, it was reported as 2.2% when not systematically sought [21] and 24–45% when clinically investigated using splenoportography [22, 23]. Splenic vein abnormalities were found in 70% of patients with chronic pancreatitsis who underwent splenoportography [24]. In a prospective study

[19], 266 patients with pancreatitis were followed over a period of 1–28 years (mean, 9.9 years); SVT was found in 22 patients (8.3%), including five patients with a single episode of acute pancreatitis and 15 patients with a history of pancreatic pseudocyst, while the cause was unknown in the remaining two patients. Gastric varices were seen in only one patient, after a median follow-up of 36 months.

In the first review of the English literature, Sutton found pancreatic cancer to be the most common cause of SVT, noted in 13 of 54 cases (35%), while pancreatitis was found in six patients and pancreatic pseudocyst in three. More recent reports, however, indicate that pancreatitis, both acute and chronic, was responsible for most cases of SVT (56%–65%) [9, 17], while 33% of patients had pancreatic pseudocysts. The increased incidence of SVT in patients with pancreatitis is most likely the result of greater awareness of the association and early diagnosis with noninvasive imaging. SVT may occur during any phase of pancreatic inflammation, and several studies have demonstrated altered splenic vein flow during the different phases of pancreatitis. Leger [22] found that 24% of a group of patients with chronic pancreatitis had complete occlusion of the splenic vein demonstrated by angiography, and 54% had abnormal flow. Similar prospective studies using splenoportography in patients with chronic pancreatitis revealed splenic vein flow abnormalities in 89% of patients, while advanced SVT was seen in 45% of patients [23, 24].

Less common pancreatic causes of SVT include pancreatic abscesses [25, 26], islet cells neoplasms [27], retroperitoneal tumors such as lymphomas and sarcomas [28], retroperitoneal fibrosis [29], SAA [30], renal cell carcinoma [31], abdominal trauma [12, 32, 33], umbilical vein catheterization in neonates [34], and hypercoagulable states such as myeloproliferative disorders, thrombocytosis, and protein S deficiency [35, 36, 20]. SVT also has been described in the postoperative period following distal splenorenal shunt [37] and orthotopic liver transplantation [38]. Wandering spleen syndrome may produce SVT by torsion of a redundant splenic pedicle [39].

Diagnosis

Isolated SVT is an uncommon condition which requires a high index of suspicion for early diagnosis. If undiagnosed, patients may develop gastric and occasionally esophageal varices that are complicated by massive, potentially fatal upper GI bleeding.

In the early report of SVT by Greenwald and Wasch [16] in 1939, barium upper GI studies were used for diagnosis of varices. Gastric varices appear as thick, tortuous mucosal folds, filling defects, or distorted mucosal configurations over the greater curvature of the stomach extending into the cardia [40]. The finding of gastric varices in patients with splenomegaly and normal liver function was considered diagnostic. More recently, direct visualization of the splenoportal system and its collaterals by splenoportography became popular (Fig. 1).

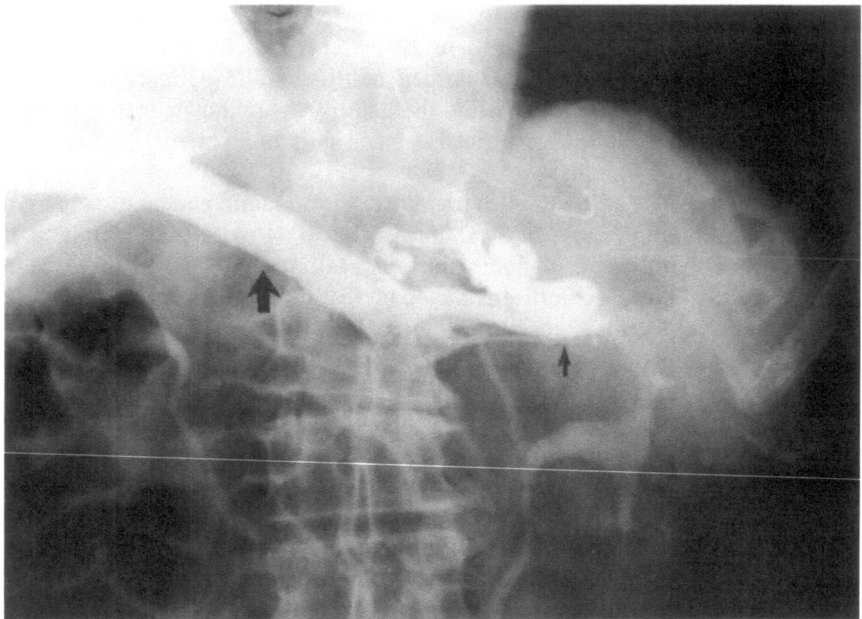

Fig. 1. Transhepatic portogram. Injection of catheter which traverses the portal vein and resides in the thrombosed splenic vein shows filling of portal vein (*large arrow*) through perihilar venous collaterals (*small arrow*)

Splenoportography was more accurate than upper GI contrast study for diagnosis of SVT, yet more invasive and associated with more complications. In a series [41] of 28 patients with gastric varices demonstrated by portography, standard upper GI radiography accurately diagnosed those varices in four patients, was suspicious in another two patients, and missed the diagnosis in 22 patients. Portographic changes in the splenic vein during chronic pancreatitis were described by Rignault et al. [23] in 1968. These changes fell into a spectrum ranging from slight alteration in the shape, course and filling of the splenoportal trunk (grade I) to complete obstruction of the splenic vein with propagation into the portal vein (grade V). Indirect splenoportography through the venous phase of selective celiac and superior mesenteric arteriograms subsequently became the gold standard for diagnosis of SVT (Fig. 2); however, unless there is complete nonvisualization of the splenic vein, the radiologic confirmation is rarely definitive.

Upper GI endoscopy is now considered to be the main diagnostic tool for suspected upper GI pathology. Demonstration of gastric varices in the absence of esophageal varices is highly suggestive of an underlying SVT. Unfortunately, gastric varices may be difficult to visualize, particularly in the fundus of the stomach, may be misinterpreted as prominent mucosal folds, or may be subserosal rather than submucosal, with loss of the typical bluish discoloration. In 30 patients with SVT reported by Loftus et al. [18], endoscopy showed gastric

Fig. 2. a Arterial phase of celiac angiogram shows filling of splenic and hepatic arteries. b Venous phase shows filling of gastric varices (*arrow*) and absent splenic vein

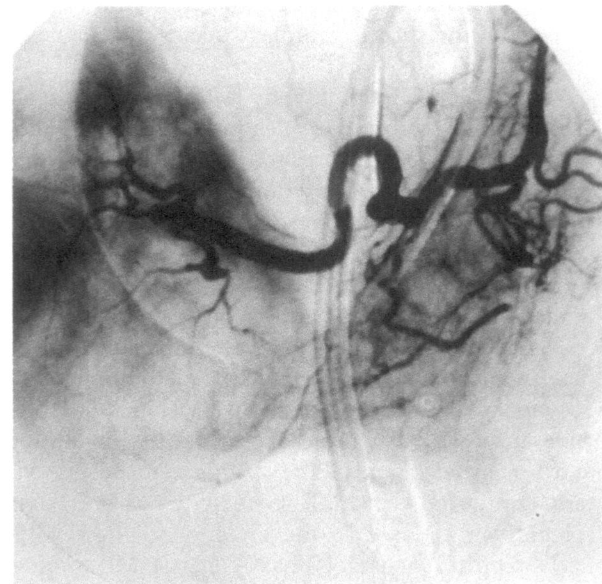

a

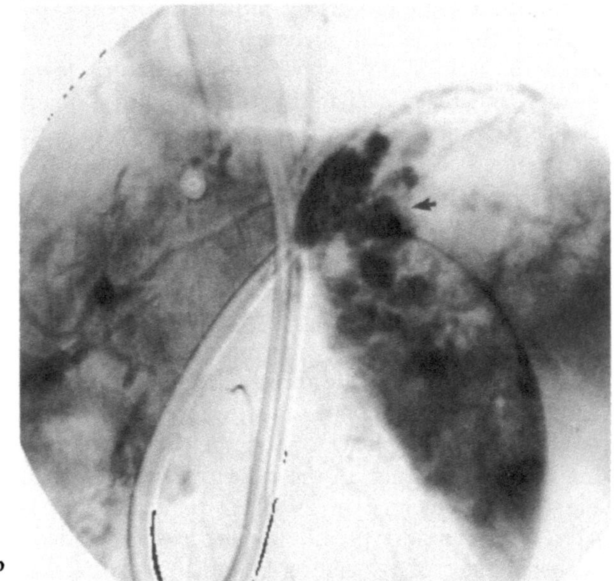

b

varices to be present in 80%, absent in 13.2%, and equivocal in 6.6% of patients. In another series [17] of 45 patients with SVT, gastric or esophageal varices were correctly diagnosed or suspected in 27 patients (60%) and missed in 18 patients (40%). This discrepancy is a result of multiple factors, including the technical skills and experience of the endoscopist as well as the site and size of the varices. The rate of bleeding and the presence of associated gastric pathology also influence the accuracy of endoscopic diagnosis.

Over the last two decades, newer noninvasive techniques to evaluate the patency of the splenic vein have become available. These include sonography, CT, and MRI.

Duplex Doppler sonography (DDS) is highly sensitive for detection of flow abnormalities within the splenoportal vessels. Sonography demonstrates lack of flow and presence of echoic material within the vessel lumen in patients with SVT [42]. The limitations of DDS are primarily technical and largely operator dependent.

CT with contrast enhacement has also been useful in evaluating splenic vein patency. The presence of an enlarged vein with a center of lower attenuation that does not show contrast enhancement is highly suggestive of SVT. Older thrombi may have an enhancing rim around the central lucency that is more likely to be due to proliferation of the vasa vasorum [43–45]. Secondary CT findings of main SVT include splenomegaly, an abnormally wide and tortuous splenic artery, varices in the region of the of the spleen, and nonvisualization of the splenic vein despite visualization of the mesenteric and portal veins. MR technology has been used to assess patency of the splenic vein as well as the direction of flow within the portal circulation. Early reports on use of phase-contrast MR angiography and gradient echo MRI appear to be promising, although current experience is limited [46, 47].

Given the consistent visualization of the abdominal vasculature by sonography, its lack of any hazard, painless nature, low cost, lack of radiation exposure, and ready availability, this modality remains the principal diagnostic choice. CT and MRI are reserved for cases in which sonography fails to visualize the bed of the splenic vein or is inconclusive.

Treatment

SVT is commonly associated with bleeding from gastric varices, which may be mild, presenting with intermittent hematochezia and iron-deficiency anemia, or massive and life-threatening. Most of the earlier reports of patients with SVT were of the latter type, where upper GI bleeding was the first manifestation of SVT. Splenectomy is the procedure of choice for control of bleeding in these patients. In the collective review by Sutton et al. [11], GI bleeding was documented in 29 of 52 patients, with splenectomy performed in 42%. Other authors [9, 17, 18] also recommended splenectomy for SVT and reported rates of rebleeding below 10% with follow-up of 1 year. While simultaneous oversewing of bleeding gastric varices was also advised by some authors, the theoretical benefit does not justify the increased risk of septic complications. Additional procedures have been undertaken at the time of splenectomy to treat the underlying causes of SVT, such as drainage of pancreatic pseudocysts or abscesses or resection of neoplasms.

The natural history of SVT due to chronic pancreatitis has been studied by Bradley [21], who followed 11 patients with chronic pancreatitis and angiographically demonstrated SVT for an average of 6.5 years (28–132 months). Three of seven patients with significant gastric varices eventually required surgical correction. Elective splenectomy was recommended, as the long-term risk of GI bleeding exceeds the risk of splenectomy.

In a retrospective study of 37 patients with SVT, Loftus et al. [18] compared patients with (n=27) and without (n=12) splenectomy and showed no advantage in survival (78% vs. 64%, p=1.0) or new or recurrent bleeding (16% vs. 24%, p=0.2) at 3.5 years of follow-up. Both groups had similar incidence of splenomegaly, abdominal pain, and gastric varices. A history of prior GI bleeding and blood transfusion was more common in patients who underwent splenectomy (p<0.05). The author concluded that in the absence of prior bleeding episodes, anemia, or severe hemorrhage, nonoperative management of patients with sinistral portal hypertension is justified.

Treatment of asymptomatic gastric varices, however, remains controversial. SVT was noted incidentally at autopsy and in 20%–40% of patients with chronic pancreatitis [23, 49]. Spontaneous resolution of SVT without further bleeding has been reported [14], particularly when associated with pancreatitis. It appears that in carefully selected patients there may be a role for nonoperative management of isolated SVT with asymptomatic gastric varices. Endoscopic sclerotherapy alone or with variceal banding has been attempted with variable results. More recently, Yoshida et al. [49] reported their experience in control of gastric varices using an endoscopic ligation technique with a detachable snare. Nine patients were treated electively without significant complications, and no patients experienced reappearance of varices or rebleeding within 4–12 months of observation. However, prospective randomized studies are not yet available. An algorithm for treatment of patients with SVT and sinistral portal hypertension is shown in Fig. 3.

Splenic Artery Aneurysms

Incidence

The splenic artery is the third most common intra-abdominal artery to become aneurysmal [50], following the infrarenal aorta and iliac arteries. The true incidence of SAA is unknown, as most patients are asymptomatic, and the diagnosis is generally made incidentally. These aneurysms are found in approximately 0.5%–1% of autopsy series, but the figure may reach 10% in patients over the age of 60 [51]. Based on arteriographic evidence, the incidence ranges between 0.78% and 7.1% [50–54]. Roughly four times as common in women of childbearing age as in men [54–57], SAA rarely occur in children. An increased incidence of SAA in association with portal hypertension has been reported [54, 58, 59]: the aneurysms were demonstrated in 7%–20% of patients with portal hypertension in whom arteriography was performed [54, 58]. SAA has also been reported in patients with potal hypertension and cirrhosis undergoing liver transplantation. Aylon et al. [60] reported a 10% incidence of SAA among

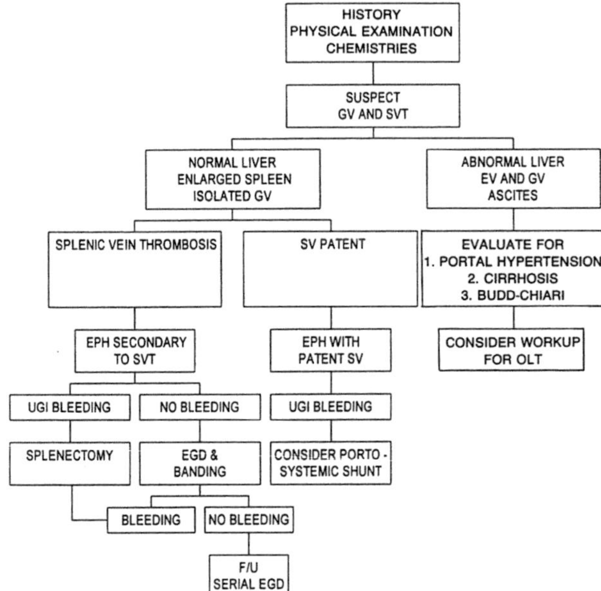

Fig. 3. Algorithm for evaluation and treatment of splenic vein thrombosis (*SVT*). *EGD*, esophagogastroduodenoscopy; *EPH*, extrahepatic portal hypertension; *EV*, esophageal varices; *GV*, gastric varices; *OLT*, orthotopic liver transplantation; *SV*, splenic vein; *UGI*, upper gastrointestinal tract

71 consecutive patients undergoing orthotopic liver transplantation, while in other series the incidence was significantly lower [61, 62].

Pathology

Seventy-five percent of splenic artery aneurysms are solitary, and the majority are between 1.5 and 3.5 cm, although sizes from 3 mm to 15 cm have been reported [63]. The records of 100 patients with documented SAA were reviewed by Trastek et al. [64]. Aneurysms were solitary in 71 patients, with diameters of 0.6–30 cm (mean, 2.1 cm). Nearly all of the solitary aneurysms were saccular, and most were within 2 cm of the bifurcation of the vessels. The main splenic artery was involved in 81% of the cases; of these, 79% of the aneurysms occurred in the distal third of the artery, 18% in the middle third, and 3% in the proximal third. The solitary aneurysms were calcified in 50 patients (70%). Multiple aneurysms occurred in 29 patients and ranged in size from 2 to 12 cm. These multiple aneurysms were located in the distal third of the splenic artery in 23 patients (79%). Points of arterial bifurcation, especially within the splenic hilum, appear to have a greater propensity for aneurysmal degeneration.

Pathogenesis

SAA are associated with various conditions, including atherosclerosis, trauma, pregnancy, portal hypertension, and liver transplantation [60, 62, 65–67].

Because the aneurysm wall is often calcified, atherosclerosis has generally been cited as the principal cause. However, the fact that many cases of SAA occur in young pregnant women without evidence of atherosclerosis suggests that this explanation is inadequate.

Physiologic changes during pregnancy which may figure in the pathogenesis of aneurysms include hormonally induced alterations of elastic tissue and medial ground substance, intimal hyperplasia, and fragmentation of the elastic lamina of the arterial wall [50, 68]. Stanley and Fry (54) reported that 88% of their female patients with SAA had been pregnant two or more times, and 39% were grand multiparas. The predilection for aneurysm formation in the splenic artery may also reflect excessive splenic arteriovenous shunting during pregnancy [51] or preexisting structural abnormalities inherent to this vessel. Another hypothesis is that increased cardiac output and blood volume during pregnancy may cause portal congestion and a propensity for aneurysmal dilatation [54, 67, 68].

In patients with chronic liver disease and portal hypertension, there is a need for increased portal inflow pressure in order to maintain portal perfusion. This state is achieved by an increase in splanchnic arterial flow through the splenic and superior mesenteric arteries [69–72]. Aneurysmal changes are thus thought to result from the combined effects of this state along with a high resistance to splenic artery outflow, splanchnic vasodilatation from hyperglucagonemia [73], and altered steroid metabolism [74].

Penetrating trauma may also be the cause of SAA. A famous example of this mechanism is the case of President James A. Garfield, who died from unrecognized rupture of a SAA 2 months after sustaining an abdominal gunshot wound in an assasination attempt. Finally, in rare instances, SAA may be congenital, mycotic, or associated with collagen vascular diseases, particularly periarteritis nodosa.

Clinical Manifestations

Splenic artery aneurysms may be asymptomatic, and a few patients (5%) present without any symptoms prior to rupture of the aneurysms [75]. There are no reliable symptoms or physical signs that indicate the presence of an SAA. Some patients report vague epigastric and left subcostal pain, and bruits may be audible [64]. A palpable mass in the left upper quadrant may be an SAA, but often the aneurysm is confused with an enlarged spleen in patients with portal hypertension. Sudden abdominal pain in the left upper quadrant associated with cardiovascular collapse usually signals rupture of the aneurysm.

Splenic artery aneurysms may either rupture freely into the peritoneum (75% of cases) or patients may present with so-called "double-rupture" syndrome of bleeding into the lesser sac (Fig. 4) followed by free rupture of the hematoma into the abdominal cavity [76]. SAA also may rupture into the GI tract, causing GI bleeding, but this occurs very rarely in pregnant women

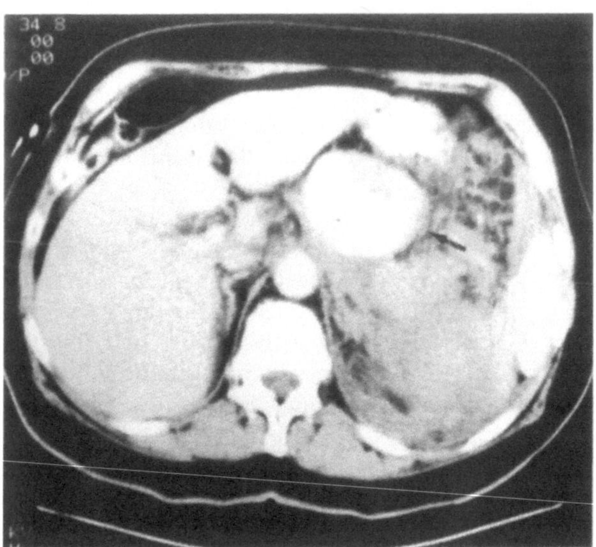

Fig. 4. Computed tomography (CT) scan of abdomen with intravenous contrast showing a ruptured splenic artery aneurysm (*arrow*) with a large hematoma in the lesser sac

[77]. SAA rupture into the common bile duct causing hemobilia, pancreatitis, and common bile duct obstruction has been reported [78], as has hemosuccus pancreaticus secondary to rupture of the aneurysm into the main pancreatic duct [79]; the latter represents an occult source of intermittent GI hemorrhage. An unusual case of SAA was complicated by arteriovenous fistula formation, in which high flow through the fistula led to the development of a mesenteric steal syndrome and acute lower GI hemorrhage secondary to nontransmural small-bowel ischemia [80].

More than 90 cases of pregnancy-related SAA ruptures have been reported. In a review of the first 61 cases, MacFarlane and Thorbjarnarson [81] found that 12% of the aneurysms ruptured in the first and second trimester, 69% in the third trimester, 13% during labor, and 6% in the puerperium. The maternal mortality rate from rupture during pregnancy is 71%, and fetal mortality is as high as 95% [50, 53, 82, 83].

Diagnosis

The diagnosis of splenic artery aneurysm is often suggested by the presence of a curvilinear calcification in the left upper quadrant on an abdominal film. Such calcification is nonspecific and can represent a tortuous splenic artery, calcified mesenteric lymph nodes, or calcified cysts of the spleen, kidney, or adrenal gland. As in the case of SVT, Doppler ultrasonography is a noninvasive test with minimal risk to the patient which, in addition to identifying SAA, provides a quantitative estimate of the volume of blood flow through the splenic artery and aneurysm [67, 69]. CT scanning, particularly with contrast enhancement, may also show an SAA. Angiography is the method used most commonly to confirm the diagnosis of SAA and localize the lesion. New technologies, such as MR angiography and spiral CT angiography, may provide more accurate assessments of SAA and deserve further investigation.

Treatment

The diagnosis of SAA alone is not an indication for operation, although splenectomy has usually been performed for emergency treatment. Trastek et al. [64] noted that one of 19 patients with an average aneurysm size of 1.4 cm had an increase in the size of aneurysm after a mean observation period of 19 years. This evidence suggests that treatment of asymptomatic aneurysms smaller than 2 cm in diameter is not necessary, especially given the operative mortality rate of greater than 0.5% [64, 84]. Symptomatic aneurysms are at increased risk of spontaneous rupture, especially if the diameter exceeds 2 cm. Elective resection should therefore be considered in good-risk patients.

An aneurysm detected in a woman who anticipates pregnancy should also be resected, as should one found before the third trimester of pregnancy, since maternal and fetal mortality from rupture during pregnancy is so high [50, 53, 83]. If the aneurysm is small, the physician may choose to allow the pregnancy to continue, hospitalize the patient, and plan for elective cesarean section and treatment of the aneurysm at the same time. For larger aneurysms, planned resection during the second trimester is preferred [85].

In a scheme for management of SAA proposed by Mattar and Lumsden [86], the decision to treat is based mainly on presence of risk factors for rupture (symptoms, expanding aneurysms, women anticipating pregnancy, pregnant women, patients undergoing liver transplantation). In the absence of risk factors, the decision depends upon the size of the aneurysm. Definite indications for treatment include lesions of diameter greater than 3 cm and lesions in patients of older than 60 years, provided that there are no prohibitive factors.

The choice of procedure is determined by the location of the aneurysm. Although splenectomy is often necessary, reasonable attempts at splenic preservation are warranted. Hashizume et al. [87] has reported laparoscopic ligation of an SAA. Laparoscopic approaches would be most feasible when the splenic artery is markedly tortuous and protrudes from the pancreas (see chap. by Phillips, this volume); young, pregnant women would be reasonable candidates for this treatment.

If the aneurysm is located near the celiac axis, aneurysmectomy or proximal and distal ligation with obliteration of all feeding vessels may be performed. The extensive blood supply from the stomach via the short gastric vessels will prevent infarction of the retained spleen. Aneurysm exclusion by ligation of all contributing vessels is preferred to excision in some cases, especially if excision will require excessive dissection within the body of the pancreas. Lesions proximal to the splenic hilum can be managed with proximal and distal ligation and, if possible, resection of the involved segment; however, lesions in close proximity to the splenic hilum and multiple lesions generally require splenectomy.

Transarterial embolization under local anesthesia provides an alternative nonoperative approach to the treatment of SAA in high-risk patients. Small metallic coils or particulate matter are introduced through a catheter to induce thrombosis of the aneursym [72, 88, 89].

Splenic artery aneurysms in liver transplant candidates present a unique problem and require special consideration, as spontaneous rupture of SAA has been reported in liver transplant recipients [60, 61]. It is suggested that the drop in portal pressure following transplantation may be associated with an increase in splenic arterial flow, which may lead to rupture of a preexisting aneurysm. Screening for SAA using ultrasonography should be performed during the transplant evaluation, and ligation of the splenic artery is recommended in all patients with demonstrated aneurysms who undergo transplantation.

Splenic Arteriovenous Fistula

Arteriovenous fistula (AVF) arising in the splenic circulation is an extremely rare condition with great potential for life-threatening complications. Similar to sinistral portal hypertension and SAA, early diagnosis and treatment are critical. The first case of splenic AVF was described by Weigert in 1886 [90], and several small series were reported subsequently. In the most comprehensive review, Brothers et al. [91] found 87 previously reported cases and added four additional ones. SAA represented the most common etiology (44%), with calcifications demonstrated in 30% of these aneurysms. Less frequent causes of splenic AVF included congenital (20%), postsplenectomy (13%), traumatic (10%), and miscellaneous (13%). There is a distinct female predominance, with a female to male ratio of 2:1.

Clinical presentation of splenic AVF was variable, ranging from incidental discovery of the fistula in an asymptomatic patient to an episode of massive intra-abdominal bleeding. GI bleeding was more common in patients with congenital lesions (60%). Other signs and symptoms included splenomegaly, audible bruit, anemia, nonspecific abdominal pain, abnormal liver chemistries, and ascites.

Portal hypertension is invariably present as a result of massively increased portal flow, and portal pressure exceeding 50 mmHg is not unusual. The exact mechanism by which liver function becomes impaired is unclear. Prolonged exposure of the portal venous system to arterial pressures and flow leads to progressive hypertrophy of the fibrous tissues in the portal triad, muscular hypertrophy of the portal vein radicals, and thickening of the vein wall. Subsequently, sinusoidal dilatation occurs, resulting in hepatoportal sclerosis. The increased risk of GI bleeding in congenital fistulas may simply reflect the long-standing portal hypertension and later development of porto-systemic collaterals. Congestive heart failure, sometimes seen with AVF in other locations, is uncommon, as the liver offers substantial vascular resistance and prevents the rapid venous return necessary for high-output failure.

Splenic AVF is treated with excision; the exact approach depends on the site of the fistula and the underlying cause. Splenectomy has been performed for lesions near the hilum, while four-quadrant ligation and excision is preferred for the more proximal lesions. Other operative approaches include distal pancreatectomy and central portosystemic shunt. The morbidity of operative interventions has been reported to be as high as 26% because of massive bleeding [92].

Recently, there has been an increased interest in nonoperative treatment of splenic AVF by percutaneous embolization. Four such patients were included in the review by Brothers et al. [91]; however, the complication rate was high, and at present the experience is insufficient to recommend this approach.

Summary

We have discussed the effects of portal hypertension upon the spleen and its circulation and have considered a group of vascular lesions which may affect the organ. Although heterogeneous, these vascular conditions have common features. They are relatively rare, often asymptomatic, may complicate other diseases, and have the potential to produce life-threatening GI or intra-abdominal bleeding, sometimes as their first manifestation. A variety of noninvasive and invasive radiologic studies are used for diagnosis, and multiple tests may be needed in some patients. Finally, treatment options are often complex, requiring subtle decisions regarding operative and nonoperative management, splenic preservation, and use of adjunctive radiologic techniques.

References

1. Henschen C (1923) Die chururgische anatomie der milzgefaze. Schweiz Med Wochenschr 58:164–167
2. Mahl TC, Groszmann RJ (1990) Pathophysiology of portal hypertension and variceal bleeding. Surg Clin N Am 70 (2):251–266
3. Brown SL, Busuttil RW (1983) Portal hypertension: In: Moore WS (ed) Vascular surgery – a comprehensive review. Grune and Stratton, New York, pp 777–819
4. Sherlock S (1974) Classification and functional aspects of portal hypertension. Am J Surg 127:121–128
5. Belli L, Puttini M, Marni A (1980) Extrahepatic portal obstruction: clinical experience and surgical treatment in 105 patients. J Cardiovasc Surg 21:439–448
6. Thavanathan J, Heughan C, Cummings T (1992) Splenic vein thrombosis as a cause of variceal bleeding. CJS 35 (6):649–652

7. Little AG, Moossa AR (1981) Gastrointestinal hemorrhage from left sided portal hypertension: an unappreciated complication of pancreatitis. Am J Surg 141:153–158
8. Turrill FL, Mikkelsen WP (1969) "Sinistral" (left-sided) extrahepatic portal hypertension. Arch Surg 99:365–369
9. Madsen MS, Petersen TH, Sommer H (1986) Segmental portal hypertension. Ann Surg 204 (1):72–77
10. Easter DW, Cuschieri A (1994) The spleen and disorders of its circulation: In: Cuschieri A, Forbes CD (ed) Disorders of the spleen. Blackwell Scientific, Oxford, pp 139–150
11. Sutton JP, Yarborough DY, Richards JT (1970) Isolated splenic vein occlusion. Arch Surg 100:623–626
12. Salam A, Warren D, Tyras DH (1973) Splenic vein thrombosis: a diagnosable and curable form of portal hypertension. Surgery 74:961–972
13. Itzchak Y, Glickman M (1977) Splenic vein thrombosis in patients with a normal size spleen. Invest Radiol 12:158–163
14. Glynn MJ (1986) Isolated splenic vein thrombosis. Arch Surg 121:723–725
15. Frick A (1922) Chronic splenomegaly with attacks of gastrorhagia due to recurrent thrombosis of the splenic vein. JAMA 78:424–425
16. Greenwald HM, Wasch MG (1939) The roentgenologic demonstration of esophageal varices as a diagnostic aid in chronic thrombosis of the splenic vein. J Pediatr 14:57–65
17. Moossa AR, Gadd MA (1985) Isolated splenic vein thrombosis. World J Surg 9:384–390
18. Loftus JP, Nagorney DM, Ilstrup D, Kunselman AR (1993) Sinistral portal hypertension: splenectomy or expectant management. Ann Surg 217 (1):35–40
19. Bernades P, Baetz A, Levy P, Belghiti J et al (1992) Splenic and portal vein obstruction in chronic pancreatitis. Dig Dis Sci 37 (3):340–346
20. Williams N, Gerrand C, London NJ, Chapman C, Bell PRF (1992) Splenic rupture following splenic vein thrombosis in a man with protein S deficiency. Postgrad Med J 68:928–929
21. Bradley EL III (1987) The natural history of splenic vein thrombosis due to chronic pancreatitis: indications for surgrey. Int J Pancreatol 2:87–92
22. Leger L (1951) Phlebographie portale par injection splenique intra-parenchmateuse. Mem Acad Chir 77:712
23. Rignault D, Mine J, Moine D (1968) Splenoportographic changes in chronic pancreatitis. Surgery 63 (4):571–575
24. Rosch J, Herfort K (1962) Contribution of splenoportography to the diagnosis of diseases of the pancreas. Acta Med Scand 171:251–272
25. Keith RG, Mustard RA, Saibil EA (1982) Gastric variceal bleeding due to occlusion of splenic vein in pancreatic disease. CJS 25 (3):301–304
26. Johnston FR, Myers RT (1973) Etiologic factors and consequences of splenic vein obstrution. Ann Surg 177:736–739
27. Metz DC, Benjamin SB (1991) Islet cell carcinoma of the pancreas presenting as bleeding from isolated gastric varices. Dig Dis Sci 36 (2):241–244
28. Yale CE, Crummy AB (1971) Splenic vein thrombosis and bleeding esophageal varices. JAMA 217:317–320
29. Lavender S, Lloyd-Davis RW, Lea-Thomas M (1970) Retroperitoneal fibrosis causing localized portal hypertension. Br Med Jr 3:627–628
30. Molnar WM, Rieber FA, McCormack KR (1958) Splenic vein thrombosis: three cases. Radiology 70:684–691
31. Koehler RE (1981) Splenic vein obstruction due to metastatic hypernephroma. Gastrointestinal Radiol 6:365–370
32. Bevin AG, Pickett LK (1967) Thrombosis of the splenic vein. J Pediatr Surg 2:320–324
33. Hassan A, Ahmed M (1982) Isolated splenic vein occlusion. JAMA 32:79–80
34. Vos LJM, Potocky V, Broker FL et al (1974) Splenic vein thrombosis with esophageal varices: a late complication of umbilical vein catheterization. Ann Surg 180:152–156

35. Shaldon S, Sherlock S (1962) Portal hypertension in myeloproliferative syndrome and the reticulosis. Am J Med 32:758–764
36. Hershfield NB, Morrow I (1968) Gastric bleeding due to splenic vein thrombosis. Can Med Assoc J 98:649–652
37. Law DK, Moore EE (1979) Compartmentalized gastrosplenic and mesenteric venous hypertension after distal splenorenal shunt occlusion: response to mesocaval shunt and splenectomy. Surgery 85 (5):579–582
38. Ranjan D, Purser R, Jonas M, Yrizzary J et al (1991) Isolated splenic vein thrombosis as a cause of massive upper gastrointestinal bleeding following orthotopic liver transplantation. Transplantation 52 (4):725–727
39. Angeras U, Almskog B, Lukes P, Lundstam S, Weiss L (1984) Acute gastric hemorrhage secondary to wandering spleen. Dig Dis Sci 29 (12):1159–1163
40. Marshall JP, Smith PD, Hoyumpa AM (1977) Gastric varices: problem in diagnosis. Dig Dis 22 (11):947–955
41. Gabrielsson N (1971) Diagnosis of gastric varices by conventional roentgenography as compared with splenoportal phlebography. Acta Radiol Diag 11:506–514
42. Rahmouni A, Mathieu D, Golli M, Douek P et al (1992) Value of CT and sonography in the conservative management of acute splenoportal and superior mesenteric venous thrombosis. Gastrointest Radiol 17:135–140
43. Schreiner V, Wilbur A, Sekosan M (1995) Intrasplenic venous thrombosis: CT findings. J Comput Assist Tomogr 19:225–227
44. Vogelzang RI, Gore RM, Anschuetz SL, Blei AT (1988) Thrombosis of the splanchnic veins: CT diagnosis. Am J Roentgenol 150:93–96
45. Belli AM, Jennings CM, Nakielny RA (1990) Splenic and portal venous thrombosis: a vascular complication of pancreatic disease demonstrated on computed tomography. Clin Radiol 41:13–16
46. Martinoli C, Cittadini G, Pastorino C, Rollandi G et.al (1992) Gradient echo MRI of portal vein thrombosis. J Comput Assist Tomogr 16:226–234
47. Nghiem HV, Freeny PC, Winter TC, Mack LA, Yuan C (1994) Phase-contrast MR angiography of the portal venous system: preoperative findings in liver transplant recipients. Am J Roentgenol 163:445–450
48. Evans GR, Yellin AE, Weaver FA, Stain SC (1990) Sinistral (left-sided) portal hypertension. Am Surg 56:758–763
49. Yoshida T, Hayashi N, Suzumi N, Miyazaki S et al (1994) Endoscopic ligation of gastric varices using a detachable snare. Endoscopy 26:502–505
50. Trastek VF, Pairolero PC, Bernatz PE (1985) Splenic artery aneurysms. World J Surg 9:378–383
51. Moore SW, Lewis RJ (1961) Splenic artery aneurysms. Ann Surg 153:1033–1046
52. Williams J (1988) Splenic artery aneurysms rupture: an uncommon obstetrical catastrophy. J Family Pract 26:73–75
53. DeVries J, Shattenkerk M, Malt R (1982) Complications of splenic artery aneurysm other than intraperitoneal rupture. Surgery 91:200–204
54. Stanley JC, Fry WJ (1974) Pathogenesis and clinical significance of splenic artery aneurysms. Surgery 76:898–909
55. Lie M, Ertresvag K, Skjennad A (1990) Rupture of a splenic artery aneurysm into the pancreatic duct. Acta Chir Scand 156:411–413
56. Busuttil RW, Brin BJ (1980) The diagnosis and management of visceral artery aneurysms. Surgery 88:619–624
57. Stanley JC, Thompson NW, Fry WJ (1970) Splanchnic artery aneurysms. Arch Surg 101:689–697
58. Boijsen E, Efsing HO (1969) Aneurysm of the splenic artery. Acta Radiolog 8:29–41
59. Feist JH, Gajaraj A (1977) Extra and intrasplenic artery aneurysm in portal hypertension. Radiology 125:331–334
60. Ayalon A, Wiesner RH, Perkins JD et al (1988) Splenic artery aneurysms in liver transplant patients. Transplantation 45:386–389

61. Brems JJ, Hiatt JR, Klein AS et al (1988) Splenic artery aneurysm rupture following orthotopic liver transplantation. Transplantation 45:1136–1137
62. Bronsther O, Merhav H, Van Thiel D, Starzl TE (1991) Splenic artery aneurysms occurring in liver transplant recipients. Transplantation 52:723–724
63. Sherlock S, Learmonth JR (1952) Aneurysm of the splenic artery with an account of an example complicating Gaucher's disease. Br J Surg 30:151–160
64. Trastek V, Pairolero P, Hollier L, Joyce J et al (1982) Splenic artery aneurysms. Surgery 91 (6):694–699
65. Tam TN, Lai KH, Tsai YT et al (1988) Huge splenic artery aneurysm after portocaval shunt. J Clin Gastroenterol 10:565–568
66. Furuta Y, Kashii A, Asaoka Y et al (1987) Splenic arteriovenous fistula formation due to angiodysplasia in a splenic aneurysm of a patient with liver cirrhosis – a report of a case. Gastroenterol Jap 22:374–378
67. Nishida O, Moriyasu F, Nakamura T et al (1986) Hemodynamics of splenic artery aneurysm. Gastroenterology 90:1042–1046
68. Barrett JM, Van Hooydonk JE, Boehm FH (1982) Pregnancy-related rupture of arterial aneurysms. Obstet Gynecol Surv 37:557–566
69. Sato S, Ohnishi K, Sugita S, Okuda K (1987) Splenic artery and superior mesenteric artery blood flow: nonsurgical Doppler US measurement in healthy subjects and patients with chronic liver disease. Radiology 164:347–352
70. Barrett J, Caldwell B (1981) Association of portal hypertension and ruptured splenic artery aneurysm in pregnancy. Obstet Gynecol 57:255–257
71. Graham JM, McCollum CH, DeBakey ME (1980) Aneurysms of the splanchnic arteries. Am J Surg 140:797–801
72. Probst P, Castaneda-Zuniga W, Gomes AS, Yonehiro EG et al (1978) Nonsurgical treatment of splenic artery aneurysms. Radiology 128:619–623
73. Lee SS, Moreau R, Hadengue A, Cerini R et al (1988) Glucagon selectively increases splanchnic blood flow in patients with well-compensated cirrhosis. Hepatology 8:1501–1505
74. Van Thiel DH, Gavaler JJ, Cobb CF et al (1980) Is feminization in diabetic men due in part to portal hypertension? A rat model. Gastroenterology 78:81–91
75. Czekelius P, Deicher L, Gesenhues T et al (1990) Rupture of an aneurysm of the splenic artery and pregnancy: a case report. Eur J Obst Gyn Reproduct Biol 38:229–232
76. Owens J, Coffey R (1953) Aneurysm of the splenic artery, including a report of six additional cases. Int Abst Surg 97:313–335
77. Lambert CJ, Williamson JW (1990) Splenic artery aneurysm: a rare cause of upper gastrointestinal bleeding. Am Surg 56:543–545
78. Harper P, Gammeli R, Kaye M (1984) Recurrent hemorrhage into the pancreatic duct from a splenic artery aneurysm. Gastroenterology 87:417–420
79. Wagner W, Cossman D, Treiman R, Foran R et al (1994) Hemosuccus pancreaticus from intraductal rupture of a primary splenic artery aneurysm. J Vasc Surg 19:158–164
80. Sendra F, Safran D, McGee G (1995) A rare complication of splenic artery aneurysm – Mesenteric steal syndrome. Arch Surg 130:669–672
81. MacFarlane JR, Thorbjarnarson B (1966) Rupture of splenic artery aneurysm during pregnancy. Am J Obstet Gynecol 95:1025–1037
82. Mehrotra D, diBenedetto R, Theriot E, Moreland J, Mehta P (1983) Spontaneous rupture of splenic artery aneurysm: sixth instance of both maternal and fetal survival. Obstet Gynecol 62:665–666
83. Bishop NL (1984) Splenic artery aneurysm rupture into the colon diagnosed by angiography. Br J Rad 57:1149–1150
84. Stanley JC, Messina LM, Zelenok GB (1991) Splanchnic and renal artery aneurysms. In: Moore WS (ed) Vascular surgery – a comprehensive review, 3rd edn. Saunders, Philadelphia, pp 335–349
85. Holdsworth RJ, Gunn A (1992) Ruptured splenic artery aneurysm in pregnancy: a review. Br J Obstet Gynecol 99:595–597

86. Mattar SG, Lumsden AB (1995) The management of splenic artery aneurysms: experience with 23 cases. Am J Surg 169:580–584
87. Hashizume M, Ohta M, Ueno K, Okadome K, Sugimachi K (1993) Laparoscopic ligation of splenic artery aneurysm. Surgery 113:352–354
88. Tihansky DP, Lluncor E (1986) Transcatheter embolization of multiple mycotic splenic artery aneurysms: a case report. Angiology 37:530–534
89. McDermott VG, Shlansky-Goldberg R, Cope C (1994) Endovascular management of splenic artery aneurysms and pseudoaneurysms. Cardiovasc Intervent Radiol 17:179–184
90. Weigert VC (1886) In die Milzvene geborstenes Aneurysma einer Milzarterie. Arch Pathol Anat 104:26–30
91. Brothers TE, Stanley JC, Zelenock GB (1995) Splenic arteriovenous fistula. Int Surg 80:189–194
92. Stone HH, Jordan WD, Acker JJ, Martin JD Jr (1965) Portal arteriovenous fistulas. Review and case report. Am J Surg 109:191–196

Section III: Splenic Surgery

Open Splenectomy

J. R. Hiatt, A. Allins, and L. R. Kong

"Extirpation of the spleen has been successful in cases of abdominal wounds with protrusion of the viscus. It has also been performed with fair results in many cases of hypertrophied spleen and of wandering spleen. The operation is not justifiable in cases of leukaemic enlargement of the organ, it having proved invariably fatal in such instances."

Sir Frederick Treves, 1883

Andriano Zaccarello performed the first splenectomy on a Neapolitan woman with massive splenomegaly in 1549 [1]. The colorful history of this operation is described in the first chapter of this volume.

Indications

Most of the early reported splenectomies in the United States were for trauma, including descriptions of the removal of spleens which had prolapsed through open wounds. An improved understanding of splenic physiology clarified and expanded the role of splenectomy in hematological diseases and resulted in a rapid increase in the number of splenectomies after the 1940s. In the 1950s, splenomegaly was the most common indication for splenectomy, but was replaced by staging operations for Hodgkin's disease in the 1970s. More recently, improved radiologic staging and the use of chemotherapy for Hodgkin's disease, combined with better and earlier medical management of infiltrative diseases causing splenomegaly, have limited the use of splenectomy for these indications. Today, the majority of splenectomies are performed for traumatic, cytopenic, or anemic disorders [2].

The role of splenectomy in treatment of various splenic disorders is considered in the other chapters of this volume, while this chapter discusses the general problem of splenomegaly. With increasing application of laparoscopic splenectomy (see the chap. by Phillips, this volume) and earlier treatment of hematologic diseases causing hypersplenism, massive splenomegaly will become a less frequent indication for open splenectomy.

Splenomegaly and Hypersplenism

By definition, splenomegaly is present when splenic weight exceeds 500 g. The condition is further subdivided into three types: mild (200–500 g), moderate (500–1000 g), and massive (greater than 1000 g) [3, 4]. Splenomegaly is one of the components of the clinical syndrome of hypersplenism, which also includes the following: anemia, leukopenia, thrombocytopenia, or a combination of these; compensatory bone marrow hyperplasia; and improvement after splenectomy [5]. In recent series, the frequency of splenomegaly was reported to range between 5.7% and 11.3% in all splenectomies performed for conditions unrelated to trauma [6, 7].

A number of pathologic conditions cause enlargement of the spleen. These may be classified in six broad categories, including infections, diseases of disordered immunoregulation, diseases of disordered splenic blood flow, diseases of abnormal red cell function, infiltrative diseases, and miscellaneous disorders or diseases of unknown cause [8]. In one series of 306 consecutive splenectomies, massive splenomegaly occurred most commonly in patients with myelofibrosis, hairy cell leukemia, chronic myelogenous leukemia, and chronic lymphocytic leukemia [6].

Preoperative Management

For patients with splenomegaly of uncertain cause, typical laboratory evaluations include serologic evaluation for rheumatoid factor, antinuclear antibodies, Coomb's test, cultures, and analysis for human immunodeficiency virus (HIV), hepatitis, and other infections. Radiologic studies may include plain films, computed tomography (CT) scans of the chest and abdomen, and gastrointestinal contrast studies. If not precluded by bleeding disorders, the investigation should also include biopsies of liver, bone marrow, and enlarged lymph nodes, as well as skin tests [9]. Biliary imaging studies are recommended in cases of splenomegaly complicated by hemolysis [10].

Blood products should be available for patients with cytopenias, but cross-matching may be difficult because of prior transfusions or circulating antibodies. In cases of idiopathic thrombocytopenic purpura (ITP) and thrombotic thrombocytopenic purpura (TTP), platelets should be withheld for as long as possible, preferably until the time of the surgical incision, because of their rapid destruction when administered. Due to the tendency for venous thrombotic complications in patients with myeloproliferative disorders, these patients usually benefit from low-dose heparin prophylaxis in the preoperative period. Pneumococcal, meningococcal, and *Haemophilus influenzae* vaccines should be given preoperatively for elective procedures and in the early postoperative period following emergency splenectomy [11, 12].

Use of intraoperative monitoring depends upon the medical condition of the patient and any associated diseases which may be present. Nasogastric tube decompression of the stomach facilitates exposure of the upper abdomen and the short gastric vessels. Preoperative antibiotics are administered before induction of anesthesia. Sequential compression stockings, placed preoperatively, are used at the discretion of the surgical team.

To minimize the perioperative risk of severe bleeding after elective splenectomy for hypersplenism, a comprehensive protocol has been proposed [13]. Malnutrition should be corrected by encouraging a diet rich in calories, protein, and vitamins. Patients with prolonged prothrombin time may require administration of vitamin K. Fever, common to the disorders underlying hypersplenism, should be controlled with acetaminophen or cooling blankets, thus avoiding aspirin and its antiplatelet effects. Patients with anemia should be transfused to a hemoglobin level of 10 g/dl before surgery, and all patients should have at least 4 U of cross-matched blood available at the time of the operation. Thrombocytopenia, also common in this patient population, should be corrected with platelet transfusions. Because of the short life span of transfused platelets, it is generally not advisable to give platelet transfusions in the days prior to operation, unless bleeding due to the low platelet count is a problem. A total of 6–10 U of platelets may be needed for transfusion in the immediate preoperative period to raise the platelet count above 100 000 per mm^3. In patients with uncompromised bone marrow and megakaryocyte function, administration of desmopressin (DDAVP) at a dose of 0.3 µg/kg IV over 15–30 min may be indicated. Hyperuricemia should be corrected well in advance of surgery to prevent postoperative gout and renal urate deposition. The preferred drug is allopurinol (administered in doses of 100 mg two to three times a day), which may be combined with uricosuric agents such as colchicine or probenecid. Acetazolimide may be given to increase uric acid excretion. Patients who have received corticosteroid therapy for temporary control of hemolysis or thrombocytopenia require perioperative supplementation with hydrocortisone or an equivalent glucocorticoid prior to operation.

Operative Procedure

Incision is chosen depending upon the surgeon's preference and the disease process (Fig. 1). Midline incisions are used when general abdominal exploration is needed, such as in cases of splenectomy for trauma or staging laparotomy for Hodgkin's disease. Most elective splenectomies are performed via a left subcostal incision, made two fingerbreadths below the costal margin. For cases of massive splenomegaly, options include a midline incision, extension of the left subcostal incision across the midline and into the right subcostal region (chevron incision), or very rarely a thoracoabdominal incision [3, 7]. As for all aspects of the splenectomy operation in patients with thrombocytopenia, meticulous hemostasis of the wound is very important.

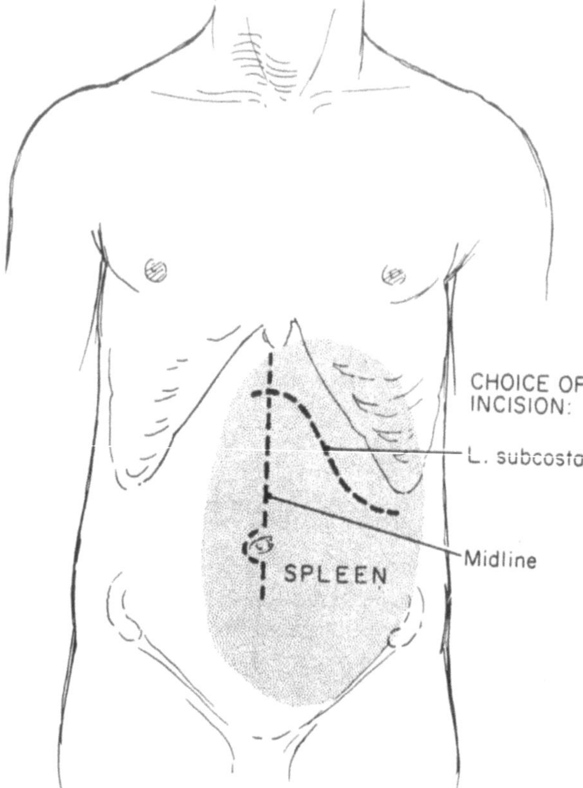

Fig. 1. Incisions for splenectomy. (Reprinted from [24]: Hiatt JR, Gomes AS, Machleder HI (1990) Massive splenomegaly: superior results with a combined endovascular and operative approach. Arch Surg 125: 1363–1367. Copyright 1990, American Medical Association)

The surgical approach to patients with massive splenomegaly is complicated by a number of factors, especially the problems of intraoperative hemostasis and perioperative hemorrhage. Manipulation of the enlarged and hypervascular organ is often made more difficult by previous abdominal procedures, infection, and radiation to the spleen (sometimes employed to control the proliferative process earlier in the disease). These result in multiple adhesions between the splenic capsule, the diaphragm, and the surrounding organs, increasing the danger of inadvertent injury to the capsule, and major bleeding from the parenchyma. Hemostasis is made more difficult by the typical thrombocytopenia, which is a consequence of platelet sequestration within the enlarged spleen, the underlying hematologic disease, and the drugs used to treat it.

For patients with massive splenomegaly, the splenic artery may be ligated along the superior edge of the pancreas once the lesser sac is assessed through the gastrohepatic or gastrocolic ligaments. This should be done prior to mobilization of the spleen. Care must be taken in these maneuvers, as the artery is quite large and thin-walled in patients with large spleens. Occlusion of the major arterial inflow allows for safer mobilization and hilar

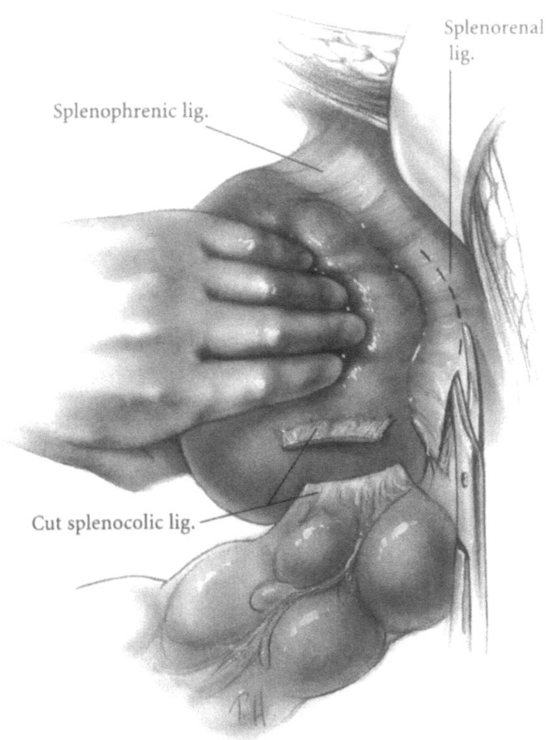

dissection of the enlarged organ, allowing it to shrink somewhat after arterial ligation, and provides an autotransfusion of blood and platelets.

Anatomic relationships which are important to the safe conduct of the operation are discussed in the chapter by Morgenstern and Skandalakis (this volume). The surgeon stands to the patient's right side and places traction on the convex surface of the spleen, exposing the various ligamentous attachments (Fig. 2). The splenocolic, splenorenal, inferior gastrosplenic, and splenophrenic ligaments are divided by electrocautery (Fig. 3). The few short gastric vessels leading from the proximal greater curvature of the stomach to the spleen are now exposed and may be divided (Fig. 4). These vessels should be ligated individually, as they may retract. Attempts at controlling bleeding from retracted short gastric vessels risks injury to the stomach, which may lead to a postoperative gastric fistula.

After division of the short gastric vessels, only the hilar dissection remains. It must be recognized that the tail of the pancreas often abuts the splenic hilum and is at risk of injury and subsequent fistula, especially in the face of splenic hemorrhage or hilar trauma. When hemorrhage is present, an atraumatic vascular clamp may be placed across the splenic pedicle and pancreatic tail to allow safer dissection in a less bloody field. The splenic artery and vein should be controlled and ligated individually. Generally, the splenic

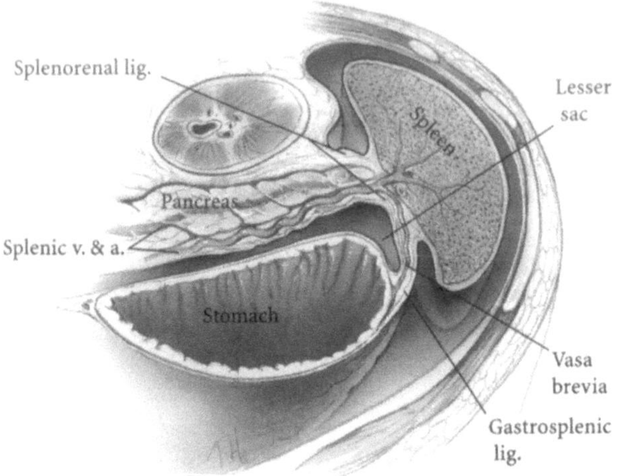

Fig. 3. Cross-section showing anatomic relationships and ligaments

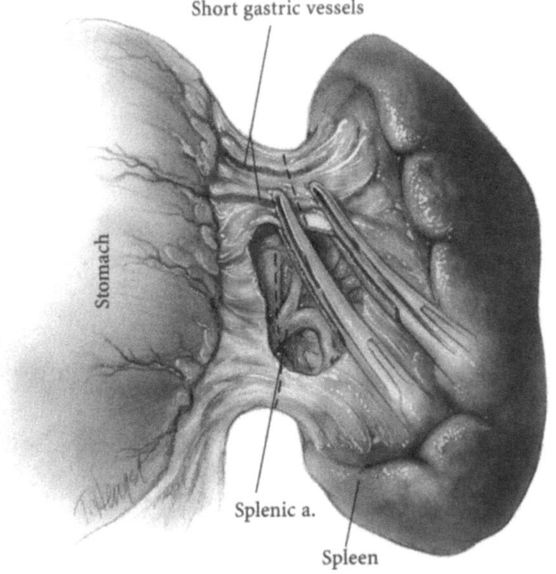

Fig. 4. Individual ligation and division of short gastric vessels

artery is ligated first, using proximal double and distal single ligation. In cases of massive splenomegaly (Fig. 5), the splenic vein may require control with a vascular clamp and closure with continuous vascular suture. A notched spleen usually has multiple arteries that should be singly ligated close to the hilum.

Mobilization of the spleen is begun by dividing the splenocolic ligament, followed by the retroperitoneal attachments. The organ is then brought medially, providing exposure to distal pancreas and splenic hilum. Care must be taken during the hilar dissection to avoid injury to the tail of the pancreas.

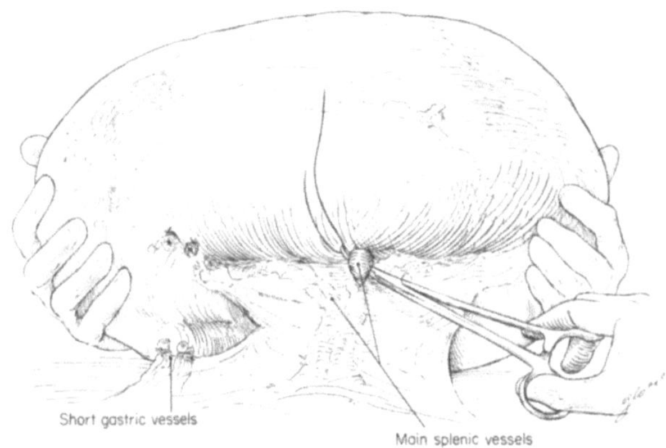

Fig. 5. Division of hilar vessels in massively enlarged spleen. (Reprinted from [24]: Hiatt JR, Gomes AS, Machleder HI (1990). Massive splenomegaly: superior results with a combined endovascular and operative approach. Arch Surg 125:1363–1367. Copyright 1990, American Medical Association)

The most frequent sources of hemorrhage at this point are splenic capsule, hilum, missed branches of short gastric vessels, and the splenic vein. Bleeding may be exacerbated by dense vascular adhesions from previous infarcts, neoplastic infiltration, or radiation.

Once the spleen is removed, hemostasis is achieved by inspecting the inferior surface of diaphragm, short gastric veins, and the hilar region. A rolled laparotomy pad is placed into the most dependent part of the now empty left upper quadrant space and slowly brought anteriorly. In this fashion, it is possible to inspect in turn the ligamentous attachments, short gastric vessels, and hilum and to control any bleeding points. Application of cellulose gauze and/or collagen powder followed by packing may be required in some cases.

Routine use of open drainage is currently discouraged, as it was shown to increase the incidence of subphrenic infection from 0.4%–12% to 6.5%–48% in undrained patients [14]. Indications for drainage of the splenic bed currently include continued oozing in the left upper quadrant, injury to the distal pancreas or greater curvature of the stomach, and resections complicated by presence of significant adhesions [7]. Under these circumstances, the use of closed drainage systems is preferred since, as demonstrated in one randomized prospective trial, these do not appear to increase the frequency of subphrenic infections [15].

When splenectomy is performed for hematologic disease, a search for accessory spleens must be conducted. These are found most commonly in the splenic hilum, ligamentous attachments, greater omentum, mesentery, ovaries, testicles, and presacral space [16].

Adjunctive Radiologic Techniques

The techniques of complete and partial splenic embolization have been in successful use for a number of years [17–23] and led to development of protocols for preoperative embolization of the spleen, aimed at facilitating the

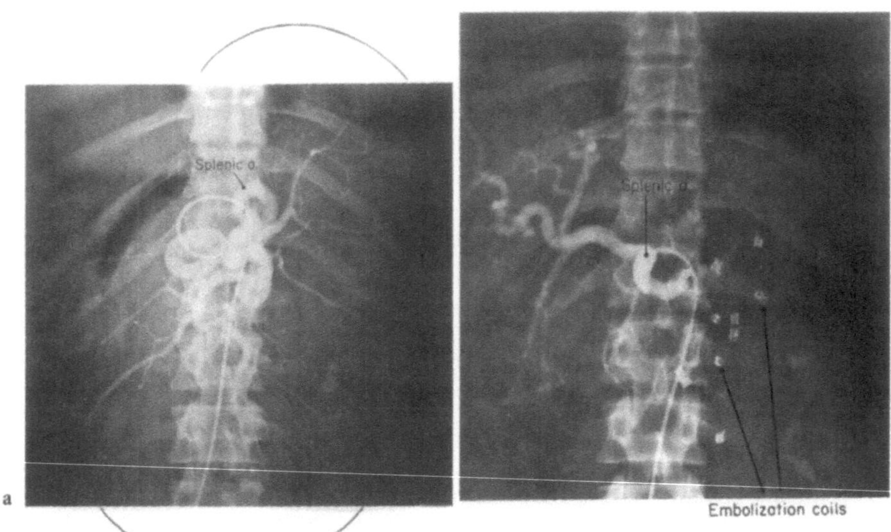

Fig. 6. Celiac arteriogram for angioembolization. **a** Splenic artery injection shows tortuous and elongated splenic artery supplying a massive spleen. **b** Postembolization arteriogram shows splenic artery occluded several centimeters beyond its origin with coils. With occlusion of the splenic artery, there is now filling of the hepatic artery on celiac injection. (Reprinted from [24]: Hiatt JR, Gomes AS, Machleder HI (1990). Massive splenomegaly: superior results with a combined endovascular and operative approach. Arch Surg 125:1363–1367. Copyright 1990, American Medical Association)

technical conduct of the operative procedures and reducing complications of postoperative bleeding. The splenic artery is assessed via a femoral approach, using a 5- or 6.5-F angiocatheter. Preliminary celiac and splenic arteriograms are obtained to visualize the size and the course of the splenic artery and the location of its major branches. The catheter is then advanced to the middle or distal portion of the splenic artery, and embolization is performed at this point with angiocoils, gelatin sponges, collagen (Avitene) globules, or detachable angioballoons (Fig. 6) [24].

Several reports using this approach in an attempt to minimize blood loss at the time of splenectomy in adult [24, 25] and pediatric [26] patients described a remarkable decrease in intraoperative blood loss and postoperative bleeding complications compared with prior reports (Table 1). Critics of preoperative embolization argue that the procedure adds additional risks of bleeding at the groin access site, ischemic injury to the pancreas, severe pain caused by iatrogenically induced splenic infarction, possibility of delay in the operation, and additional costs [24]. A recent report comparing splenectomies in patients with massive and normal-sized spleens, neither using preoperative embolization, showed no significant differences in morbidity, mortality, or transfusion requirements [27].

Table 1. Splenectomy for hypersplenism and splenomegaly

Reference	Preoperative Angio-embolization used	Total	Average Blood loss (ml)	Major complications (%)	Postoperative abdominal hemorrhage (%)	30-day mortality (%)
[13]	No	16	ND	19	13	13
[30]	No	34	ND	56	26	15
[31]	No	49	ND	43	10	2
[32]	No	47	ND	30	2	0
[25]	Yes	4	148	0	0	0
[3]	No	36	6241[a]	31	6	11
[47]	No	51	>1000	20	4	8
[24]	Yes	10	528	20	0	0
[7]	No	46	2686[b]	39	13	20
[26]	Yes	11	302	ND	0	0
[41]	No	156	ND	2	0.6	ND
[35]	No	47	ND	30	4	2
[4]	No	35	ND	37	3	3
[27]	No	20	690	20	ND	0

ND, no data.
[a] In patients with complications.
[b] Median blood loss, 1300 ml.

Complications

Splenectomy is associated with a number of complications related to the immunologic and hematologic functions of the organ. These can be subdivided into four broad categories, including hemorrhage, thrombosis, infectious complications, and technical problems. Splenic size was described to be the most important factor associated with bleeding by some investigators [28] and with the overall complication rate by others [3, 29, 30, 31, 32]. However, a statistical relationship between splenic size and complications was not corroborated by other authors [4, 27, 47].

Hemorrhage

Hemorrhage is a potentially grave complication of surgery for hypersplenism. In 1866, Bryant [33] reported the first documented case of splenectomy for leukemia in a young patient with massive splenomegaly. The patient died 2 h after the operation from intra-abdominal bleeding. In recent series, postoperative bleeding after splenectomy for massive splenomegaly occurs in 4%–16% of cases [3, 6, 7, 34, 35]. Exsanguination due to spontaneous rupture of an enlarged spleen is a special and almost uniformly fatal extreme of this complication [3, 7, 35].

Thrombosis

In recently reported series, the incidence of thrombosis and thromboembolic events after splenectomy for massive splenomegaly and hypersplenism was found to be 2% [6, 7, 35]. The frequency of postsplenectomy thrombosis is highest (5.4%) in patients with myeloproliferative disorders such as myelogenous leukemia, agnogenic myeloid metaplasia, and polycythemia vera. Thrombus formation is most likely a multifactorial event only partially explained by thrombocytosis, which occurs in 40%–50% of all splenectomized patients. Given that platelet function and kinetics are already abnormal in patients with myeloproliferative disorders, the combined effects of rising postsplenectomy platelet count, addition of young platelets to the circulating pool, and removal of regulatory humoral factors produced by the spleen may account for the increase in thromboembolic complications [14].

Thrombosis of the mesenteric venous system following splenectomy for hematologic disease is a rare, but lethal complication of this procedure. At autopsy, the thrombus appears to extend from the remnant of the splenic vein, implicating intimal injury and stasis in the venous remnant as etiologic factors. The presentation of mesenteric venous thrombosis frequently includes abdominal pain, bloody diarrhea, abdominal distention, oliguria, obtundation, and hepatic insufficiency. The condition is fatal in 70% of patients [14, 36].

No data are available at present to support routine use of anticoagulant or antiplatelet agents (heparin, aspirin, dextran, or dipyridamole) for prophylaxis of thromboembolic events in patients with postsplenectomy thrombocytosis (platelet count >400 000). Some authors [36] recommend preoperative therapeutic doses of alkylating agents such as busulfan and/or platelet phoresis to reduce the preoperative thrombocyte count to below 200 000 in patients at risk for mesenteric thrombosis. Once a thrombotic complication is diagnosed, treatment is supportive with intravenous heparin infusion, followed by oral administration of coumadin. Thrombolytic therapy may be of value in cases of mesenteric venous thrombosis [37].

Infection

Given the immunologic importance of the spleen, postoperative infectious complications are of primary concern in any condition requiring splenectomy. Infectious risk is compounded by immunosuppressive medications or chemotherapy, which are administered to most of the patients who undergo splenectomy for nontraumatic conditions. Infections after splenectomy can be separated into those occurring in the immediate postoperative period (within 30 days of surgery) and those of more latent onset.

Respiratory complications and subphrenic abscesses account for more than half of infections occurring immediately after operation [38]. The frequency of subphrenic abscess formation was originally attributed to the use of open drains placed within the splenic fossa [39, 40]. However, with the use of the modern closed drainage systems, the frequency of this complication was noted to be similar in patients with and without drains [15, 28]. Left subphrenic fluid collections, which occur in the early postoperative course, are now thought to result from technical errors such as inadequate hemostasis or injury to the nearby structures, especially pancreas and stomach. The incidence of this complication in most current series was noted to range between 1.2% and 5% [6, 7, 28, 29, 34, 35, 41]. When subphrenic abscess is due to unrecognized hollow visceral injury and treatment is delayed, mortality approaches 60%–90% [42].

Urinary tract infections account for 2%–6.5% of septic complications after surgery [6, 7, 35]. These are thought to be associated with bladder catheterization in the perioperative period and are usually due to *Escherichia coli, Staphylococcus aureus*, enterococci, *Klebsiella, Enterobacter, Pseudomonas*, and *Serratia* species [38].

Overwhelming postsplenectomy infection (OPSI) is one of the most dreaded sequelae of splenectomy and is discussed in greater detail by Stiehm and Trunkey (this volume). In a series of 306 splenectomies, half of all deaths were attributed to sepsis [6]. With aggressive use of antibiotics as well as immunosuppressive and chemotherapeutic regimens, new species of organisms have recently been reported to contribute to mortality from sepsis. *Enterobacter* species, *Candida albicans* [29], and herpes zoster viremia [14] have joined the classical pathogens responsible for OPSI, including *Streptococcus pneumoniae, Haemophilus influenzae, Neisseria meningitidis*, β-hemolytic *Streptococcus, Pseudomonas*, and *E. coli* [38]. Of note is the fact that in one series of 142 splenectomies performed for hematologic diseases in adults, the frequency of septic complications was not affected statistically by administration of preoperative antibiotics or steroids [28].

Technical Problems

Wound

Wound complications, including infections, hematomas, incisional hernias, and abdominal wall dehiscence, comprise 2%–7% of postoperative complications in some recent reviews [6, 7, 29, 34]. Use of agents known to impair wound healing (radiation therapy, chemotherapy, and steroids) in treatment of splenic diseases certainly contributes to the frequency of these complications.

Splenosis

As noted above, a diligent search for accessory spleens must be made at the time of splenectomy for hematologic conditions. Splenosis occurs in 15%–

30% [10] of such patients, with some authors observing an even higher incidence in more selected populations (40% incidence in patients with hereditary spherocytosis) [6]. Failure to remove accessory spleens at operation will result in failure of therapy [43–46]. Presence of Howell-Jolly bodies on the peripheral blood smear does not exclude the possibility that an accessory spleen was missed at exploration, and radiolabeled isotope scan (indium-111 or ^{99}Tc) in search of occult accessory spleens may be indicated in patients who continue to be symptomatic following splenectomy. Reexploration and removal of accessory spleens generally leads to improvement of symptoms, while attempts at medical therapy may be associated with a severe relapse [46].

Intestinal Complications

Small bowel obstruction is a rare complication of splenectomy, seen in 0.3%–2% of cases [6, 29, 34, 35]. Injuries to the surrounding organs are equally rare, but potentially far more serious.

Pancreatic injury may occur if the tail of the gland is not properly visualized when the splenic vessels are ligated and divided in the hilum. Even in the hands of experienced surgeons, pancreatitis and pancreatic fistula occur with a frequency of 2%–7% [6, 29, 35]. This technical error may be precipitated by dissection of dense adhesions around the enlarged spleen or by hasty and uncontrolled use of hemostats to control bleeding from splenic vessels. Careful dissection in the area of pancreatic tail, meticulous identification of the major splenic vessels, and ligation in continuity of large arteries and veins help to avoid this problem. If hemorrhage occurs, the splenic vessels should be compressed manually with the pancreatic tail rather than attempting to gain control with blind placement of hemostats.

Gastric fistula is avoided by use of perioperative nasogastric decompression of the stomach and good surgical technique, including care in application of clamps to the short gastric vessels and repair of any serosal tears which may occur. Gastric injury is now of largely historical significance; although common in the 1960s [14], this complication was not encountered in any of the most recent series of open splenectomies performed for malignancy or hematologic disorders [3, 6, 7, 28, 29, 34, 35].

References

1. Ellis H (1988) The spleen. In: Landes C (ed) Clio chirurgica. Silvergirl, Austin, p 1
2. Coon WW (1991) The spleen and splenectomy. Surg Gynecol Obstet 173:407–414
3. Johnson HA, Deterling RA (1989) Massive splenomegaly. Surg Gynecol Obstet 168:131–137
4. Lehne G, Hannisdal E, Langholm R, Nome O (1994) A 10-year experience with splenectomy in patients with malignant non-Hodgkin's lymphoma at Norwegian Radium Hospital. Cancer 74:933–939

5. Ellis LD, Dameshek HL (1975) The dilemma of hypersplenism. Surg Clin N Am 55:277–285

6. Musser G, Lazar G, Hocking W, Busuttil RW (1984) Splenectomy for hematologic disease – the UCLA experience with 306 patients. Ann Surg 200:40–45

7. Danforth DN, Fraker DL (1991) Splenectomy for the massively enlarged spleen. Am Surgeon 57:108–113

8. Haynes BF (1994) Enlargement of lymph nodes and spleen. In: Isselbacher KJ, Braunwald E, Wilson JD, Martin JB, Fauci AS, Kasper DL (eds) Harrison's principles of internal medicine, 13th edn. McGraw-Hill, New York, p 232

9. Cronin CC, Brady MP, Murphy C, Kenny E, Whelton MJ, Hardiman C (1994) Splenectomy in patients with undiagnosed splenomegaly. Postgrad Med J 70:288–291

10. Schwartz SI (1981) Splenectomy for hematologic disease. Surg Clin N Am 61:117–125

11. Rutherford EJ, Livengood J, Higginbotham M, Miles WS, Koestner J, Edwards KM, Sharp KW, Morris JA (1995) Efficacy and safety of pneumococcal revaccination after splenectomy for trauma. J Trauma 39:448–452

12. Lane PA (1995) The spleen in children. Curr Opin Pediatr 7:36–41

13. Morgenstern L (1971) Splenectomy for massive splenomegaly due to myeloid metaplasia. Am J Surg 122:288–293

14. Ellison EC, Fabri PJ (1983) Complications of splenectomy – etiology, prevention, and management. Surg Clin N Am 63:1311–1330

15. Patchen HL, Hofstetter SR, Spencer FC (1981) Evolving concepts of splenic surgery: splenorrhaphy versus splenectomy and post splenectomy drainage. Ann Surg 194:262–267

16. Schwartz SI, Adams JT, Bauman AW (1971) Splenectomy for hematologic disorders. Curr Prob Surg 5:1–57

17. Miyazaki M, Itoh H, Kaiho T, Ohtawa S, Ambiru S, Hayashi S, Nakajima N, Oh H, Asai T, Iseki T (1994) Partial splenic embolization for the treatment of chronic idiopathic thrombocytopenic purpura. Am J Roentgenol 163:123–126

18. Nakamura H, Ohishi A, Asano K, Hirose H, Hayakawa M, Iwai F, Kageyama T, Katsu M (1994) Partial splenic embolization for Felty's syndrome: a 10-year followup. J Rheumatol 21:1964–1966

19. Sangro B, Bilbao I, Herrero I, Corella C, Longo J, Beloqui O, Ruiz J, Zozaya JM, Quiroga J, Prieto J (1993) Partial splenic embolization for the treatment of hypersplenism in cirrhosis. Hepatology 18:309–314

20. Israel DM, Hassal E, Gordon Culham JA, Phillips RR (1994) Partial splenic embolization in children with hypersplenism. J Pediatr 124:95–100

21. Spigos DG, Tan WS, Mozes MF, Pringle K, Iossifides I (1980) Splenic embolization. Cardiovasc Intervent Radiol 3:282–288

22. Hocking WG, Machleder HI, Golde DW (1980) Splenic artery embolization prior to splenectomy in end-stage polycythemia vera. Am J Hematol 8:123–127

23. Sprayregen S (1986) Vascular interventional radiology of the spleen. Contemp Surg 29:26–32

24. Hiatt JR, Gomes AS, Machleder HI (1990) Massive splenomegaly – superior results with a combined endovascular and operative approach. Arch Surg 125:1363–1367

25. Fujitani RM, Johs SM, Cobb SR, Mehringer CM, White RA, Klein SR (1988) Preoperative splenic artery occlusion as an adjunct for high risk splenectomy. Am Surgeon 54:602–608

26. Hickman MP, Lucas D, Novak Z, Rao B, Gold RE, Parvey L, Tonkin IL, Hansen DE (1992) Preoperative embolization of the spleen in children with hypersplenism. J Vasc Intervent Radiol 3:647–652

27. Farid H, O'Connell TX (1996) Surgical management of massive splenomegaly. Am Surg (in press)

28. MacRae HM, Yakimets WW, Reynolds T (1992) Perioperative complications of splenectomy for hematologic disease. Can J Surg 35:432–436

29. Horowitz J, Smith JL, Weber TK, Rodrigues-Bigas MA, Petrelli N (1996) Postoperative complications after splenectomy for hematologic malignancies. Ann Surg 223:290–296

30. Goldstone J (1978) Splenectomy for massive splenomegaly. Am J Surg 135:385–388
31. Wobbes T, van der Sluis RF, Lubbers EC (1984) Removal of the massive spleen: a surgical risk? Am J Surg 147:800–802
32. Bickerstaff KI, Morris PJ (1987) Splenectomy for massive splenomegaly. Br J Surg 74:346–349
33. Bryant T (1866) Case of excision of the spleen from an enlargement of the organ attended with leukocythemia. Guys Hosp Rep 12:444–455
34. Jacobs P, Wood L, Dent DM (1992) Splenectomy in the chronic myeloproliferative syndromes. S Afr Med J 81:499–503
35. Letoquart J-P, La Gamma A, Kunin N, Grosbois B, Mambrini A, Leblay R (1993) Splenectomy for splenomegaly exceeding 1000 grams: analysis of 47 patients. Br J Surg 80:334–335
36. Gordon DH, Schaffner D, Bennet JM, Schwartz SI (1978) Postsplenectomy thrombocytosis – its association with mesenteric, portal, and/or renal vein thrombosis in patients with myeloproliferative disorders. Arch Surg 113:713–715
37. Bell WR, Meek AG (1979) Guidelines for the use of thrombolytic agents. New Engl J Med 301:1266–1270
38. Francke EL, Neu HC (1981) Postsplenectomy infection. Surg Clin N Am 64:135–155
39. Cerise EJ, Pierce WA, Diamond DC (1970) Abdominal drains: their role as a source of abdominal infection following splenectomy. Ann Surg 171:764–769
40. Cohn LH (1965) Local infection after splenectomy. Arch Surg 90:230–235
41. Marble KR, Deckers PJ, Kern KA (1993) Changing role of splenectomy for hematologic disease. J Surg Onc 52:169–171
42. Wang SM, Wilson SE (1977) Subphrenic abscess: the new epidemiology. Arch Surg 112:934–936
43. Krsnik I, Perez-Rus G, Calero MA, Perera F, Garcia-Suarez J, Ricard MP (1994) Peripheral thrombocytopenia, accessory spleen and Hodgkin's disease: an unusual combination. Acta Haematol 91:35–36
44. Kao NI, Musto PK, Richmond GW (1994) Refractory thrombocytopenia in a patient with systemic lupus erythematosus and prior immune thrombocytopenia, not responsive to accessory splenectomy. South Med J 87:941–943
45. Mintz SJ, Petersen SR, Cheson B, Cordell L, Richards RC (1981) Splenectomy for immune thrombocytopenic purpura. Arch Surg 116:645–650
46. Facon T, Caulier MT, Fenaux P, Plantier I, Marchandise X, Ribet M, Jouet JP, Baueters F (1992) Accessory spleen in recurrent chronic immune thrombocytopenic purpura. Am J Hematol 41:184–189
47. Coon WW (1989) Splenectomy for massive splenomegaly. Surg Gynecol Obstet 160:291–294

Laparoscopic Splenectomy

E. H. Phillips, J. E. Korman, and R. Friedman

> "If a fleshy tumour is found ... the patient will get worse and he will die .... If the liver passage falls to the right, the patient will live. If the gallbladder is long, the king will live long. If the *processus pyrimidalis* is shaped normally, he who makes the sacrifice [of the sheep] will be in good health and live long."
>
> *From a Babylonian cuneiform* of the eighteenth century B.C., describing hepatoscopy in animals

The technique of laparoscopic splenectomy (LS) was first described in 1992 [2, 6] and has become a well-accepted procedure. Approximately 600 cases have been reported, with the largest individual series comprising 70 cases, including a partial splenectomy. Initially, there was concern that the procedure would result in excessive blood loss, splenosis, and inaccurate pathologic examination of the specimen. For the most part, these fears have been proven unwarranted. While splenomegaly remains a technical challenge, LS has become the preferred surgical technique for idiopathic thrombocytopenic purpura (ITP) and other diseases with normal splenic size.

An important element of the technique to optimize exposure of the spleen is the proper positioning of the patient on the operating table. While the procedure was originally described with the patient in supine or lithotomy positions [2, 6], it was found that the lateral position [5] offered improved exposure of the splenic hilum. Many still prefer the lateral approach for LS, but we use a double-access position. The patient is placed on a bean bag in a semilateral angle (45°), which allows for operating in both the supine and lateral positions. The supine position is preferred for initiating pneumoperitoneum, inserting trocars, exploring for accessory spleens, and ligating the splenic artery in the lesser sac, while the lateral position offers excellent exposure of the hilum to facilitate dissection and vessel ligation [19].

To minimize the risk of excessive intraoperative blood loss, Poulin initially advocated the use of routine preoperative splenic artery embolization [23]. We perform routine operative ligation of the splenic artery in the lesser sac and reserve angioembolization for cases of splenomegaly, acquired immunodeficiency syndrome (AIDS), and obesity. At present, preoperative embolization is used infrequently by most surgeons.

The sequence of splenic hilar dissection remains controversial. We advocate division of the splenocolic and splenorenal ligaments prior to hilar dissection [20], while others recommend that the hilar vessels be dissected and divided first, leaving the lateral attachments to provide countertraction and elevation of the spleen [5].The method of vessel ligation has also evolved. Initially, clips and sutures were used, but most surgeons now rely on endovascular cutting devices.

Increasing operative experience and technical refinements have produced good results relative to open splenectomy (OS) in terms of outcome, patient discomfort, length of hospitalization, and costs. It is anticipated that the procedure may have greatest benefit in patients at greatest risk of complications of laparotomy, including those with hypersplenism who are treated with steroids and other immunosuppressive regimens. Wound problems, infections, and pulmonary complications, which are particularly troublesome with conventional splenectomy techniques, may be avoided with LS.

Indications

The indications for LS do not differ from those for OS. The diseases for which we have performed LS are the following:
- ITP
- Hereditary spherocytosis
- Autoimmune hemolytic anemia
- Staging for Hodgkin's disease
- Lymphoma
- Thrombocytopenic thrombotic purpura
- AIDS-related thrombocytopenia
- Leukemia
- Splenic abscess
- Gaucher's disease
- Myelofibrosis
- Splenic infarct

The size of the spleen is the single most important factor in determining whether or not the laparoscopic technique is appropriate. When the spleen is enlarged, the patient's body habitus influences the approach and the decision for preoperative arterial embolization to decrease the splenic size. Moreover, certain diseases such as AIDS, lymphoma, abscess, and infarction are associated with an inflammatory response with friable hilar vessels which may be obscured by enlarged lymph nodes.

The disease most commonly treated by LS is ITP; the laparoscopic approach is ideal for two reasons. First, exposure and dissection of the normal-sized spleen is simpler, and second, the specimen does not have to be delivered intact for pathologic analysis. Instead, it can be morcellated and extracted through a port site, in contrast to patients with Hodgkin's lymphoma, from whom the spleen must be removed intact for histologic examination. In our approach to laparoscopic staging for lymphomas, the splenectomy, liver and upper abdominal lymph node specimens are dissected laparoscopically, and a Pfannenstiel incision is performed to dissect the aortic, iliac, and femoral nodes and to remove the upper abdominal specimens.

In patients with borderline-sized spleens, body habitus and the volume of the spleen either allow or hinder adequate exposure. The laparoscopic approach is more difficult in obese patients. The massive omentum obscures the vasculature and makes dissection of the peritoneal attachments more challenging. Trocar locations and dissection sequences also have to be modified for the enlarged spleen, which may rotate and obscure the hilar vessels, leaving insufficient space in which to elevate the organ. Nevertheless, the avoidance of a large incision and pulmonary complications in these patients justifies the extra effort required to complete the procedure laparoscopically.

Patient Preparation

In preparation for splenectomy, patients should be immunized against pneumococcus, *Haemophilus influenzae B*, and meningococcus 2 weeks prior to operation, if possible. Preoperative splenic artery embolization, used only in selected patients with splenomegaly or AIDS or in obese patients, should be performed on the day of operation, since patients may experience considerable pain after infarction of the spleen. Embolization with coils is preferred to embolization with cellulose or microspheres, as the latter can embolize to unintended targets such as the pancreas [23]. A cephalosporin antibiotic is administered preoperatively to reduce the risk of wound infection.

Operative Technique

Patient Positioning

Positioning is a crucial consideration (Fig. 1). Three positions have been described, each with its advantages. The *anterior position* (patient supine) facilitates exploration of the abdomen for accessory spleens, which are present in 15%–30% of the population [27]. The *lateral position* (patient right side down) has been called the "hanged spleen" technique [5]. In this position, the viscera fall away from the hilum when the spleen is elevated, providing better exposure of the vasculature. The "double-access" position (patient right side down 45°, with a bean bag under the left flank) combines the advantages of the anterior and lateral positions. This technique allows for the creation of the pneumoperitoneum and abdominal exploration to be performed with the patient supine, while splenectomy is done in the lateral position.

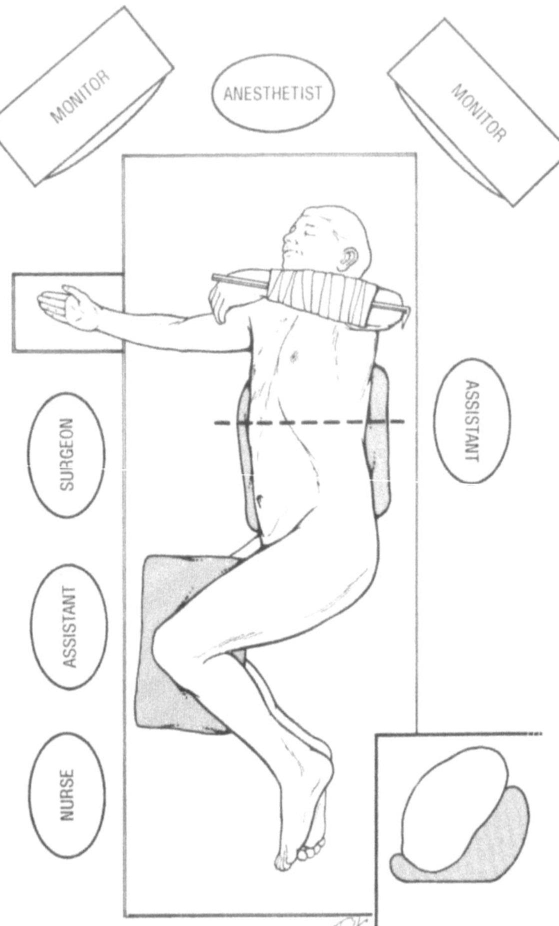

Fig. 1. a Double-access positioning of the patient and team. Patient in 45° right lateral decubitus, assisted by bean bag (*dotted line, inset*)

Trocar Placement

Six trocars are used. The camera port is placed first, except in some patients with prior abdominal surgery. Regardless of whether the pneumoperitoneum is created with a Veress needle or by open technique, the exact location of the first port varies with the body habitus of the patient. In average-sized patients, the subumbilical region is preferred, but in large and/or tall patients, this port should be placed above and to the left of the umbilicus. A 10/11-mm or 5-mm port is placed in the subxiphoid area to accommodate instruments the surgeon uses with the left hand, and a 10/11-mm trocar is placed midway between the umbilicus and the subxiphoid trocar for instruments he or she uses with the right hand. The most lateral trocar (10/11 mm) is then placed in the left axillary line, halfway between the costal margin and the iliac crest. A 12-mm trocar used to accommodate the endovascular cutter is

Fig. 1. b Lateral position

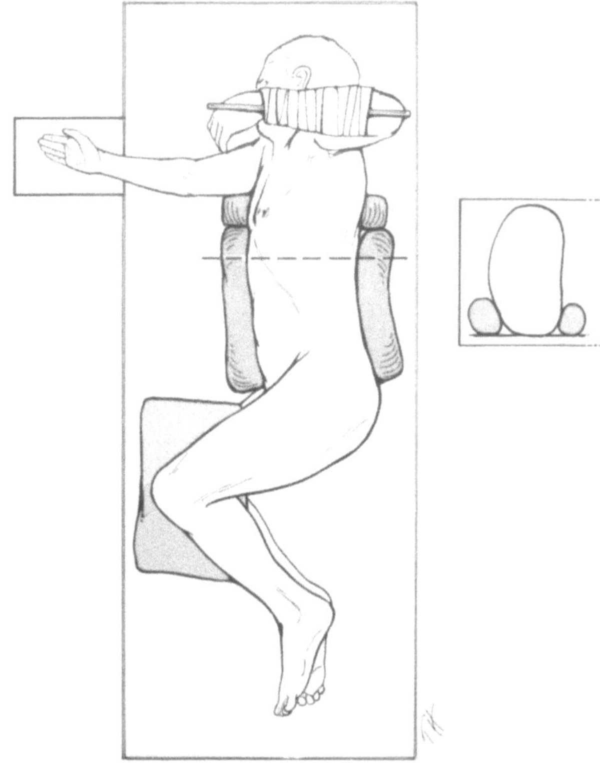

placed just lateral to the left rectus sheath, slightly above the level of the umbilicus between the optic and the most lateral trocar (Fig. 2). Infiltration
with local anesthesia prior to insertion of each trocar helps to reduce postoperative pain and to confirm the precise location of each trocar site.

General Inspection

The procedure is initiated by tilting the table to the left, so that the patient
is supine. This allows an easier search for accessory spleens, which may be
found in the splenic hilum, the splenic ligaments, the omentum, the small-
bowel mesentery, and the pelvic viscera (Fig. 3). All of these areas must be
carefully inspected. We have identified an accessory spleen on the abdominal
peritoneum in the right upper quadrant.

Ligation of the Splenic Artery

In most cases, the next step consists in ligation of the splenic artery in the
lesser sac. Though this may seem unnecessary and time-consuming in an un-

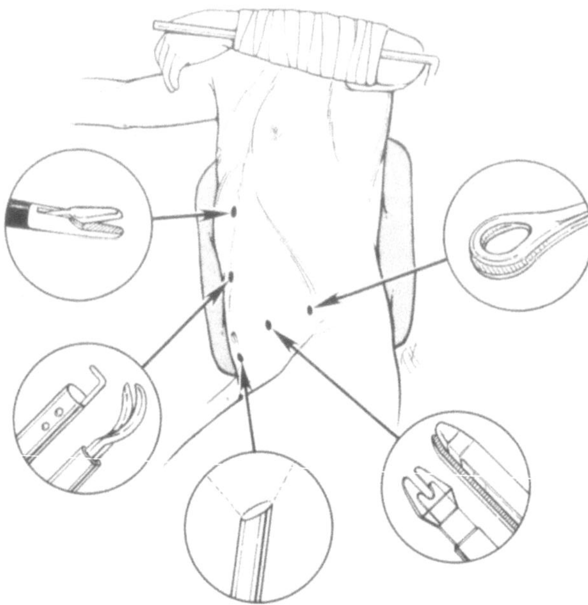

Fig. 2. Trocar sites and instrumentation

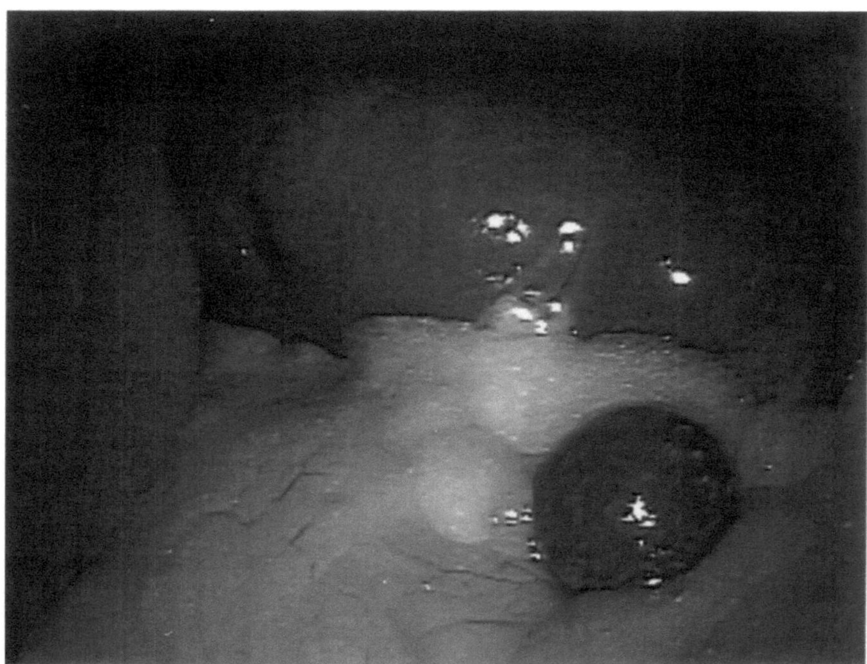

Fig. 3. Accessory spleen in gastrocolic ligament

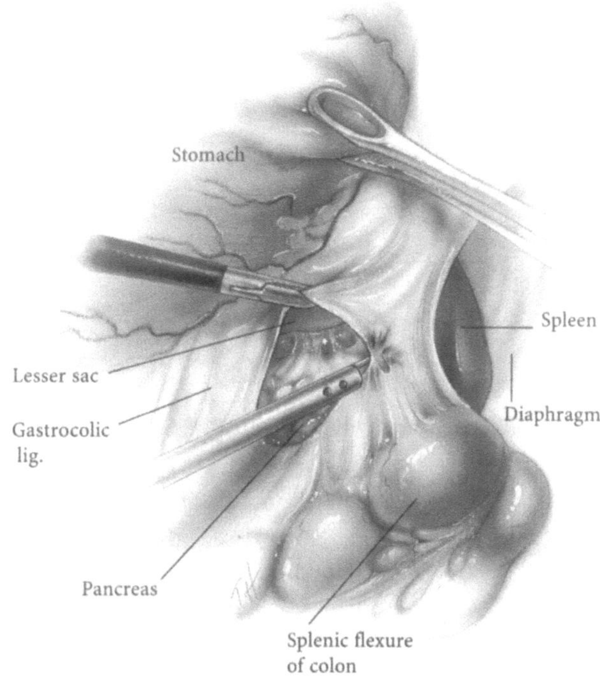

Fig. 4. Elevation of the stomach and view into the lesser sac

complicated splenectomy, it represents the safest course, as hemorrhage during hilar dissection can occur in any situation. Access to the lesser sac is gained by elevating the stomach, using a grasper from the most lateral trocar, and placing inferior traction on the transverse colon with a grasper inserted via the left paramedian 12-mm trocar. The surgeon's left hand (subxiphoid trocar) stabilizes the gastrocolic omentum, and the right hand (midline trocar) pierces, dissects, and coagulates the gastrocolic window using bipolar electrocautery or the harmonic scalpel (Ultracision, Ethicon Endosurgery, Cincinnati, OH; Fig. 4). The lesser sac is entered, and the pancreas is identified and retracted posteriorly and slightly inferiorly with an atraumatic fan retractor inserted through the paramedian 12-mm trocar. The splenic artery or its pulsation should be visible just superior to the pancreas (Fig. 5). Its tortuosity, location, and direction identify it as the splenic artery. The visceral peritoneum is opened with scissors. The artery is dissected free and occluded with a clip, but not divided (Fig. 6).

Splenic Mobilization

The spleen is approached by rotating the table to the right, so that the patient's left side is elevated into the lateral position. An element of head-up positioning may be needed, depending upon the body habitus, to facilitate the division of the splenocolic ligament. This ligament is quite variable: it

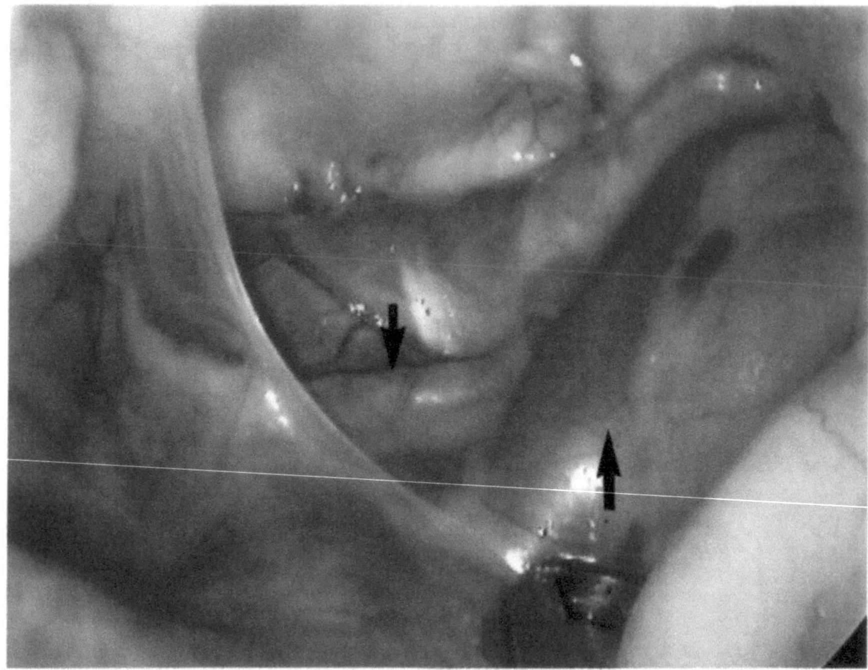

Fig. 5. Splenic artery (*small arrow*) and vein (*large arrow*) in lesser sac

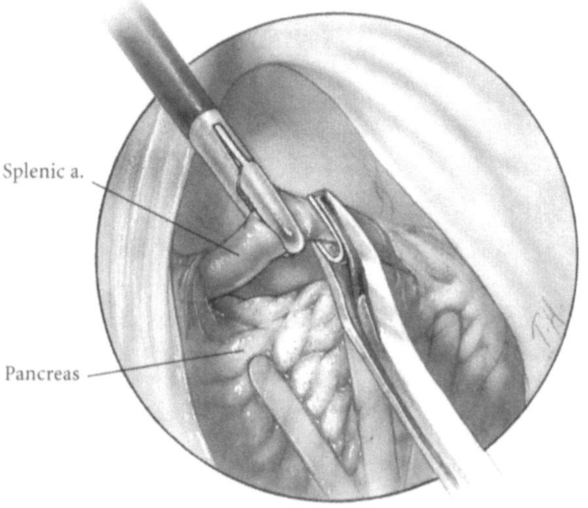

Fig. 6. The splenic artery is clipped

may be thin and avascular, covered by dense omentum, or obscured by the colon, which may even be adherent to the splenic capsule. Exposure is gained in part passively, as gravity causes the viscera to fall away from the spleen, and in part actively. The spleen is lifted gently, either with the surgeon's left-hand grasper (using it as a wand) or with a ring forcep or spleen grasper placed by the assistant through the most lateral trocar. The colon can be put on tension by the assistant's grasper placed through the paramedian trocar, freeing the surgeon's hands. The splenocolic ligament may be divided using scissors, a harmonic scalpel, or an electrocautery hook, taking care to avoid direct or remote electrocautery injury to the colon. The ligament must be divided so that the inferior pole of the spleen is completely visible. The next step is to divide the communicating inferior pole vessels when present. These are small tributaries of the left gastroepiploic vein. The hilum, now more accessible, is once again inspected for accessory spleens.

At this point, the surgeon must choose whether to mobilize the splenorenal ligament, allowing further elevation of the spleen, or to dissect and divide the hilar vessels. In normal-sized or moderately enlarged spleens, we prefer to mobilize the splenic ligaments first, as this facilitates the hilar dissection and vessel ligation. If bleeding is encountered during hilar dissection, it is much easier to control if the spleen has been mobilized. In addition, the endocutter can be inserted rapidly to divide the hilar vessels. In cases of splenomegaly, however, the splenic volume makes it more difficult, if not impossible, to mobilize the splenorenal ligament first. In these cases, the hilar vessels are divided first.

To dissect the splenorenal ligament, the spleen can be grasped with atraumatic lung forceps or a ring clamp or elevated with a fan retractor. Specialized instruments for this purpose are currently being developed. Dissection proceeds from the inferior pole cephalad, progressing as high as possible. An electrocautery hook with suction and irrigation greatly facilitates this part of the procedure. The peritoneal attachment is divided, and a combination of electrocautery and blunt dissection with the hook cautery device is used (Fig. 7). Often, limited exposure makes it necessary to divide some of the vessels to the inferior pole of the spleen before the splenophrenic ligament is reached; with this accomplished, the dissection can be restarted (Fig. 8). In cases of splenomegaly, it is necessary to alternate dissection and ligation several times. The key is that splenic elevation greatly facilitates division of the superior pole vessels and the short gastric vessels by putting them on stretch (Fig. 9). While some surgeons prefer to keep the spleen attached to the diaphragm to enable bag capture, we have not found that to be advantageous.

Hilar Dissection

Anatomy of the splenic artery and its branches supplying the spleen (see chap. by Morgenstern and Skandalakis, this volume) is of particular importance. Michel [16] described two principal patterns in 1942. The distributed

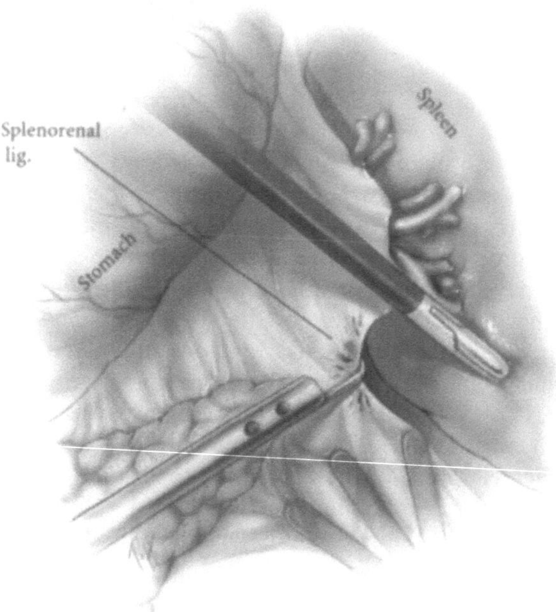

Fig. 7. Dissection of splenorenal ligament

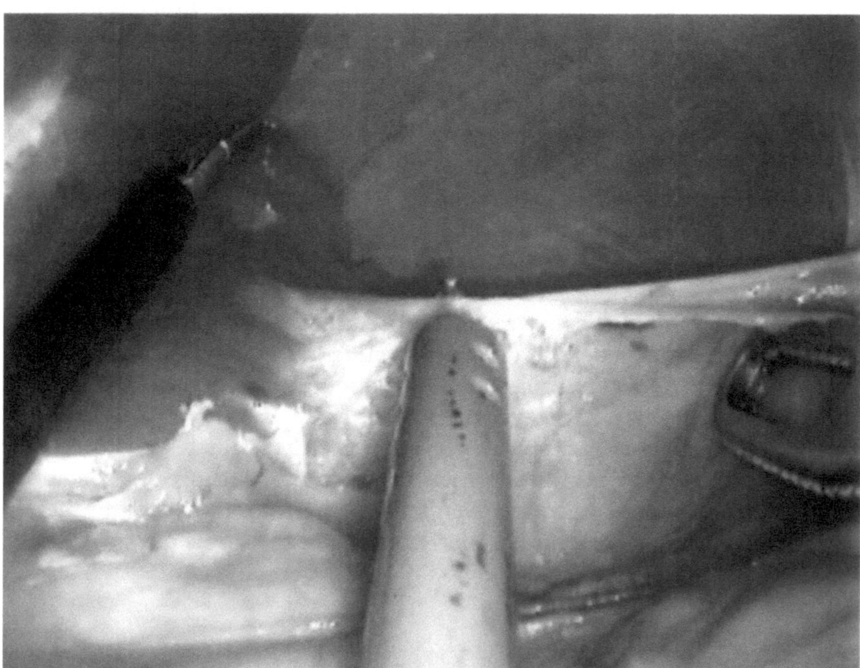

Fig. 8. Division of splenorenal ligament near diaphragm using electrocautery hook suction device. Spleen is reflected medially with grasper, and kidney is reflected posteriorly with ring forceps

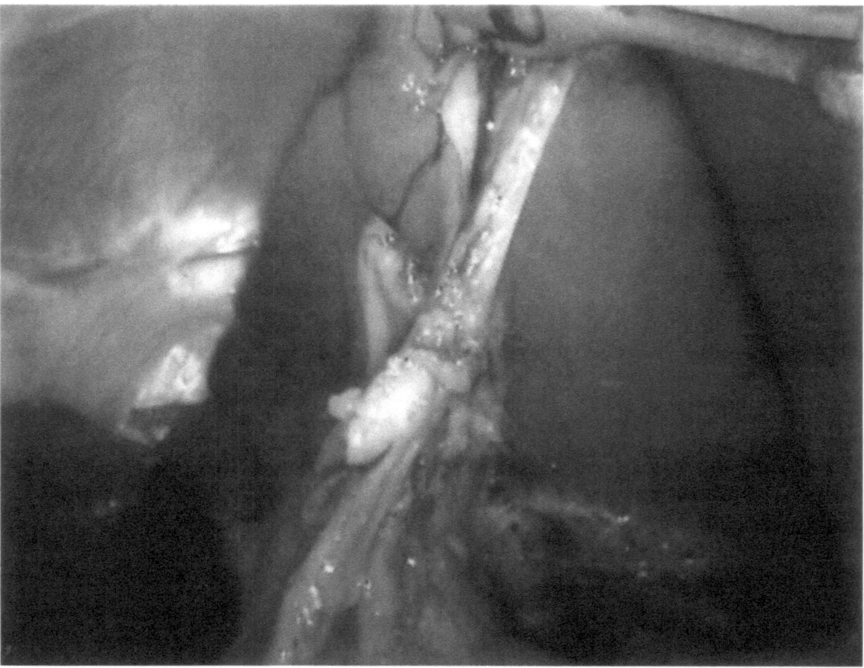

Fig. 9. Spleen elevated with ring forceps after division of splenocolic and splenorenal ligaments

type, present in 70% of the population, is characterized by a short splenic trunk with numerous long branches that enter 75% of the medial surface of the organ. The magistral type, present in 30%, is characterized by a long main splenic artery with short terminal branches that enter only 33% of the medial surface of the spleen. These patterns have important implications in dissection during splenectomy, with the distributed type offering an easier dissection [22]. There are as many as seven principal branches, including the superior terminal, inferior terminal, medial terminal, superior polar, inferior polar, left gastroepiploic, and short gastric arteries. The veins typically run posterior to the arteries [22].

The hilar vessels are dissected with right-angled instruments and divided between clips and/or ligatures. The harmonic scalpel can be used for the short gastric vessels. We have found ligation and division of the vessels with the endocutters to be more secure and far quicker (Fig. 10). The cost of the endocutter (an issue of increasing importance in surgical decisions) is offset by the time savings. On several occasions, conversion to an open procedure has been avoided by using the endocutter to control hemorrhage. Clips can be used, but may become dislodged if handled during the dissection. A further disadvantage of clips is that they prevent complete closure of the endocutter and therefore limit its effectiveness in an emergency.

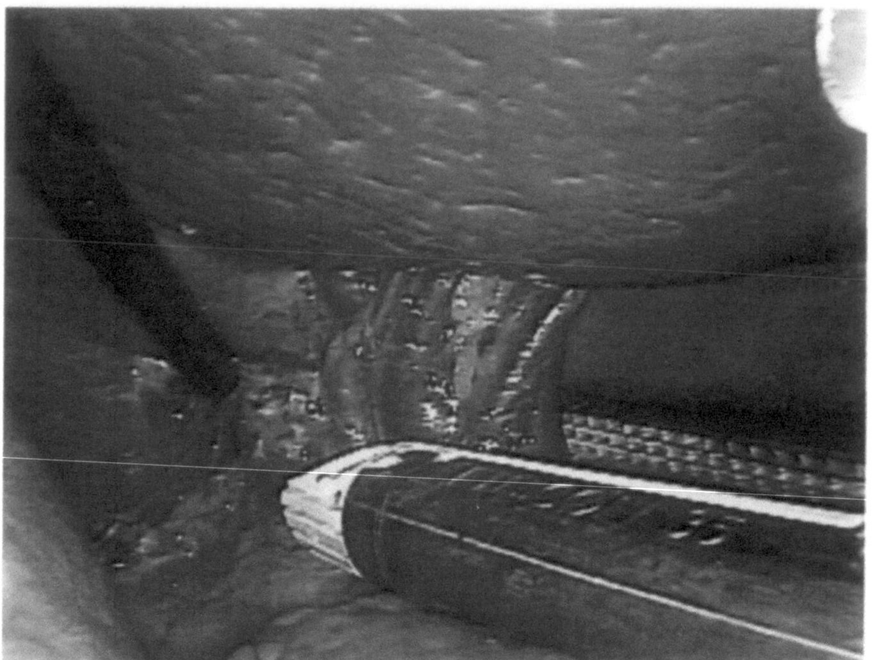

Fig. 10. Division of hilar vessels with endovascular cutter

Once the spleen is detached, it is placed into a sturdy specimen bag (Cook Urologic, New Brunswick, New Jersey). This maneuver can be challenging and is accomplished by rolling the bag, grasping it with a Kelley clamp, and placing it into the abdomen through the 12-mm paramedian trocar site, after the trocar has been removed. The bag is placed into the peritoneal cavity and unfurled in the splenic fossa. The opening is triangulated with three graspers placed through the two upper midline trocars and the left lateral trocar. The spleen is grasped at its lower pole by the ring forceps placed through the paramedian trocar and then inserted into the bag (Fig. 11).

The specimen is extracted piecemeal by morcellation or intact via a small incision. In patients such as those with ITP, where careful pathological analysis is not required, the specimen is morcellated in the bag using ring forceps or a tissue morcellator. It is most important to avoid spilling any fragments in the peritoneal cavity, which could result in splenosis and recurrent disease. To do this safely, the bag is pulled up into the abdominal wall defect at the 12-mm trocar site and is held up tightly against the abdominal wall while the specimen is morcellated manually (Fig. 12).

After morcellation, the 12-mm trocar is reinserted, and the splenic bed is inspected for hemostasis by placing the laparoscope in the 12-mm paramedian port. In patients such as those with Hodgkin's disease, where an intact specimen is important for pathologic analysis, one can extend the umbilical

Fig. 11. Placement
of specimen into bag

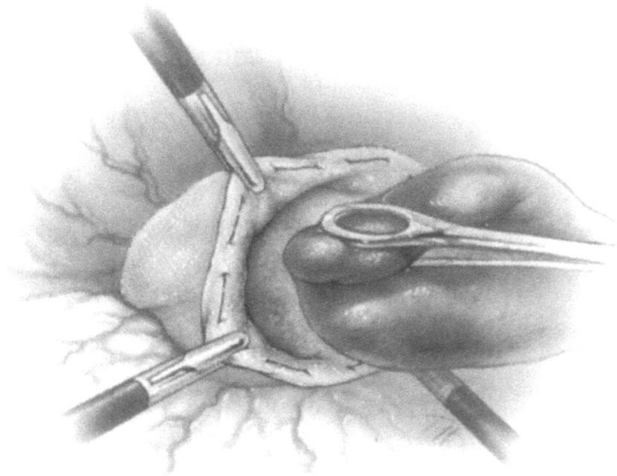

Fig. 12. Exteriorization
of the bag and morcellation
of the specimen

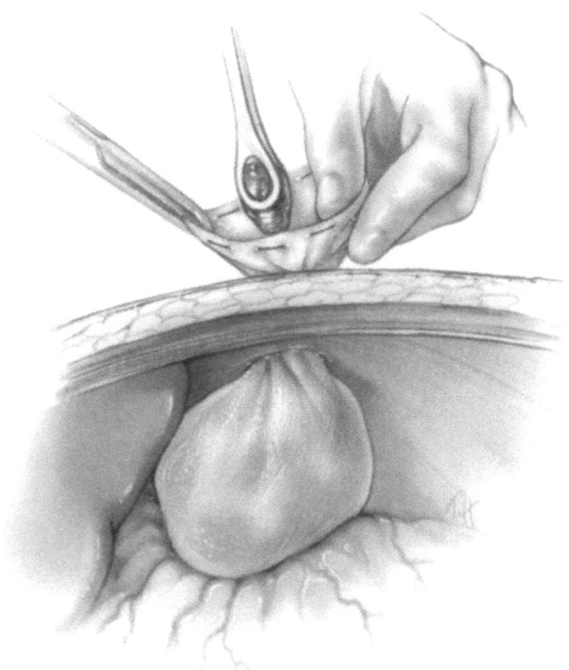

port into a lower midline incision or make a Pfannenstiel incision for extraction. The fascia of all trocar sites of 10 mm or greater is closed with 0-polyglycolic acid suture.

Postoperative Care

The orogastric tube is removed prior to leaving the operating room. Oral feedings are begun the next day. Activity is unrestricted, and ambulation is encouraged. Parenteral analgesia is usually required the first night after surgery, while oral narcotic analgesics are adequate the next day. Platelets and hemoglobin are monitored as determined by the underlying disease and the clinical course.

Collected Experience

Approximately 600 laparoscopic splenectomies have been reported. The largest series are compared in Table 1. The majority were performed for ITP (Table 2); other indications included hereditary spherocytosis, staging of Hodgkin's disease, autoimmune hemolytic anemia, thrombocytopenic thrombotic purpura, abscess, and infarction (see "Indications" above). Overall success rates for the procedures are approximately 90%, with bleeding and splenomegaly the usual reasons for conversion. Comparing LS with OS, authors have reported significantly shorter postoperative hospital stay, no difference in blood loss, earlier recovery of bowel function, but significantly greater operative times [10, 19, 23, 28].

Table 1. Results of laparoscopic splenectomy[a]

Surgeon	Attempted (n)	Successful		Complication		Death (n)
		(n)	(%)	(n)	(%)	
Phillips	60	56	93	7	13	0
Lefor/Flowers	43	35	81	5	14	2
Poulin	40	35	88	4	11	0
Cuschieri	35	34	97	2	6	0
Andrews/Robles	31	29	94	2	7	0
Hashizume	28	28	100	0	0	0
Park	25	23	92	2	9	0
Mulvihill	25	21	84	0	0	0
Schlinkert	14	13	93	2	15	0
Arregui	13	10	5	50	0	

[a] Data provided in personal communications.

Table 2. Laparoscopic splenectomy for idiopathic thrombocytopenic purpura [9]

Author	Attempted	Completed	Success (%)
Cadieri	11	10	91
Emmerman	20	16	80
Gigot	8	7	88
Lee	15	15	100
Phillips	28	27	96
Stanton	18	16	89
Yee	16	14	88

Table 3. Results of laparoscopic splenectomy (LS) for idiopathic thrombocytopenic purpura (LSI) versus LS for other diseases (LSO)

	Operative time (min)	Blood loss (cc)	Splenic weight (g)	Major compli- cation (n)	Hospital days	Days to liquids	Total cost ($)	OR cost ($)
LSI (n=31)	113±50	177±160	156±148	1	2.7±1.3	1.2±0.5	10300 ±500	2700±400
LSO (n=23)	185±88	314±619	715±1089	1	7.4±9.0	1.8±0.7	18500 ±14000	3300±100
p value	<0.05	NS	<0.05	NS	<0.05	<0.05	=0.05	NS

NS, not significant; OR, operating room.

Table 4. Results of laparoscopic splenectomy (LS) versus open splenectomy (OS) for idiopathic thrombocytopenic purpura [9]

	Operative time (min)	Blood loss (cc)	Splenic weight (g)	Major compli- cation (n)	Hospital days	Days to liquids	Direct cost ($)	OR cost ($)
LS (n=2 9)	122±54	203±155	184±156	1	2.9±1.3	1.2±0.5	5509± 3636	2762±418
OS (n=1 8)	103±45	285±196	167±98	0	6.9±3.0	3.2±0.7	9031± 12752	1859±380
p value	NS	NS	NS	NS	<0.001	<0.001	N	NS

NS, not significant; OR, operating room.

However, it is inaccurate to compare the results of LS to OS in a heterogeneous population. Most LS series contain patients with ITP primarily, while OS series include patients with trauma, splenectomy performed in conjunction with other procedures, and a greater number of patients with diseases other than ITP. To emphasize these issues, we first compared LS in ITP patients with LS in patients with other diseases and found that patients with ITP did indeed fare significantly better (Table 3). Those with ITP had significantly decreased operative times (113 vs. 185 min), time to oral intake (1.2 vs. 1.8 days), hospital stay (2.7 vs. 7.4 days), and total cost ($10 300 vs. $18 500).

Next, for an objective comparison, we analyzed the results of LS and OS in patients with ITP only. Table 4 summarizes data from 47 splenectomies for ITP, 29 LS and 18 OS [9]. The size of the spleens did not differ significantly between the two groups. The mean operative time was 122 min for LS and 103 min for OS; the last ten LS cases were performed in 94 min. Estimated blood loss was less in the laparoscopy group, and no transfusions were required, while three patients in the open group required transfusion. Recovery of bowel function, measured as days to tolerance of oral liquids, was significantly earlier after LS. Hospital stay was also shorter, resulting in lower total costs ($5509 vs. $9031), despite the fact that operating room costs were greater in the laparoscopic group ($2762 vs. $1859). Accessory spleens were identified and removed in 20% of LS patients. Platelet response to LS was 93%, and none of the failures in this group was found to have residual splenic tissue on follow-up nuclear scan. Historically, platelet response to splenectomy has been approximately 80% [18], and the response rate after OS in the authors' series was 83%.

Complications

Splenic surgery, open or laparoscopic, can be associated with significant morbidity and mortality. Deaths and complications are the consequences of underlying diseases and their treatments as well as errors in technique and judgment. Expert training and proctoring, proper patient selection, precise anatomical dissection, and diligence in hemostasis will avoid most of the technical problems.

Published series of OS [1, 7, 12, 15, 18] report morbidity rates that range from 15% to as high as 61%. Series of LS [9, 10, 14, 19, 26, 28] report morbidity rates of 0%–14% (Table 2). The mortality rates reported for OS range from 6% to13% and for LS from 0% to 5%. However, most series of OS include splenectomies performed for trauma or iatrogenic operative injury, for which morbidity and mortality rates may be higher (36% and 16%, respectively) [7]. Factors predisposing to complications include the underlying indication for the splenectomy, the patient's age, and associated diseases. For example, patients fared better if the splenectomy was performed for diagnostic purposes or primary hypersplenism (morbidity, 6.4%; mortality, 1%) [7].

Complications specific to LS will be discussed in this chapter; complications of OS are considered in the preceding chapter.

Operative Complications

Cardiovascular Effects of Pneumoperitoneum

Cardiovascular effects of pneumoperitoneum are minimal and rarely result in hypotension or arrhythmia [11]. Hemodynamic problems, usually during insufflation, occur in approximately 0.2% of patients and are associated with vasovagal reflex or decreased venous return. Most often, the problems are minor and can be corrected with administration of fluids or atropine. When significant rhythm disturbances occur, the pneumoperitoneum must be released immediately, and the specific arrhythmia must be treated. Cardiac disease and/or pacemakers are not contraindications.

Bowel Injury

Injury to the bowel is rare and usually occurs during creation of the pneumoperitoneum. Reported frequency, in the gynecology literature, is 0.16%–0.27% [21]. Pneumoperitoneum may be administered by closed technique, using the Veress needle, or by open technique, using a blunt-tipped trocar (Hasson). Use of the open technique does not eliminate the risk of bowel injury, but it does facilitate immediate identification and repair. Patients who have had prior abdominal surgery are at increased risk of accidental enterotomy, regardless of the technique used. Prior abdominal surgery is a relative contraindication to LS.

Veress needle injury to the bowel rarely requires further intervention; such injuries can be managed with close observation. In contrast, intestinal trocar injuries require operative repair. The trocar should be left within the injured bowel so that the injury can be readily identified when the abdomen is opened. While extensive injury to the left colon occasionally requires a diverting colostomy, most bowel injuries are treated by primary repair, either laparoscopic or open.

Vascular Injury

Injury to blood vessels may occur during Veress needle or trocar insertion. Use of the open technique eliminates the risk of injury to major intra-abdominal vessels, as a blunt-tipped trocar is inserted. While Veress needle injury to blood vessels rarely causes significant hemorrhage, trocar injuries to major blood vessels have been the cause of fatal bleeding. Major hemorrhage occurs with injury to the distal aorta or common iliac vessels, and mortality is as high as 15%. Major vascular injuries requiring further intervention occur in 0.64% of laparoscopic procedures [21]. Minor bleeding causing abdominal wall hematomas may occasionally occur from trocar injuries to abdominal wall vessels. These should be identified by careful inspection of the trocar sites prior to the conclusion of the operation; simple ligation of the vessels usually contains the hemorrhage.

Hemorrhage

The most common intraoperative complication of splenectomy is hemorrhage, which occurs in roughly 5% of cases. In our series of LS, it occurred in 6%. Hemorrhage was responsible for 75% of conversions to an open procedure. Defects of clotting factors and platelets cause bleeding from raw surfaces of the splenic bed, diaphragm, retroperitoneum, and less frequently from the pancreatic surface. Occasionally, topical hemostatic agents are necessary. The argon beam coagulator can be extremely useful when diffuse oozing complicates the mobilization of an adherent spleen. Bleeding from a single vessel due to a dislodged or missing ligature may occur and can lead to reoperation. This problem can be avoided by meticulous hemostasis and accurate dissection.

Hemorrhage may occur when the splenic vessels are being encircled [3, 4, 6, 14, 22]. Either the vessel being dissected or a posterior branch can be torn or punctured with a dissector. This risk is lessened by gentle dissection on both sides of the vessel, with a change in position of the laparoscopic viewing angle to visualize the sides and back of the vessel. If bleeding occurs, a grasper is used to apply pressure to the injured vessel until the field has been suctioned, and the operative team has made a plan for ligation of the vessel. Additional trocars may be inserted for better exposure and control. Bleeding from a capsular tear of the spleen is best managed with hemostatic agents or with the argon beam coagulator. Minor bleeding from the splenic bed or ligated hilum can be controlled with pretied loop ligatures, electrocautery, or argon beam coagulation. The use of a cell saver autotransfusion device can minimize the need for transfusion of banked blood. While routine use is costly and unnecessary, the cell saver can be advantageous in patients with conditions that increase the risk for intraoperative hemorrhage such as splenic abscess, AIDS, lymphoma, or coagulopathy.

Injury to Adjacent Organs

Injuries to structures adjacent to the spleen, reported in 1%-3% of OS, have been rare during LS. The magnification of the laparoscopic technique seems to afford a better view of the organs and will probably decrease iatrogenic injuries.

Pancreas. Pancreatic injuries occur in 1%-3% of OS [7] and in as many as 7% of patients with hemolytic malignancies [12]. Signs of pancreatic injury include abdominal tenderness, atelectasis, pleural effusion, and elevated serum amylase and lipase. Pancreatic injuries are avoided by adequate mobilization and elevation of the spleen in a bloodless field before dissection of the splenic pedicle and by ligation of the vessels close to the splenic parenchyma. If a pancreatic injury is suspected, a closed suction drain should be placed.

Stomach, Diaphragm. Gastric injuries occur in less than 1% of splenectomies [7]. These are often due to direct trauma, but occasionally result from devascularization and may occur when dense adhesions, incomplete hemostasis, or splenomegaly hinder precise dissection. Excessive use of cautery or failure to identify the plane between the spleen and the stomach can lead to thermal or ischemic injuries. We injured the left hemidiaphragm while dissecting with scissors through dense adhesions caused by prior splenic infarcts. This type of injury may be more likely in the laparoscopic operation, as manual blunt dissection cannot be used (except in a laparoscopically facilitated technique). Atelectasis, pneumonia, or a subphrenic infection may indicate that one of these injuries exists.

Postoperative Complications

Respiratory

Respiratory complications affect 10%–48% of patients after OS (atelectasis, 16%; pleural effusion, 11%; pneumonia, 7%–13%) [7]. To avoid diaphragmatic irritation from blood and irrigant, the subphrenic space should be aspirated dry at the conclusion of the operation. These complications have been less frequent using the laparoscopic technique, which avoids a subcostal incision. In collected series of LS, atelectasis and pleural effusions occurred in fewer than 4% of cases, and there were no instances of pneumonia. However, ITP patients comprise the majority of cases in most series of LS, and these patients are at lower risk for respiratory complications than are patients in the open series.

Subphrenic Abscess

Subphrenic abscesses are reported to occur in 4%–8% of OS [12, 15], but to date have not been reported in the laparoscopic literature. No laparoscopic cases were performed for trauma, where associated bowel injuries increase the risk of subphrenic infection.

Wound Problems

Wound complications such as hematoma, seroma, and infection occur because of impaired wound healing, coagulation abnormalities, steroid use, and immune defects. Wound infections occur in 3% of OS performed for diagnostic indications, 6% performed for therapeutic indications, and 11% of patients who require perioperative steroids [13, 18]. Infections occasionally lead to incisional hernias and rarely to dehiscence. In our laparoscopic experience, wound complications were seen in only 2% of cases and all were trivial [19]. However, trocar site hernias may occur, and bowel obstruction from incarceration has been reported following other laparoscopic procedures.

Ileus and Small-Bowel Obstruction

Postoperative ileus and small-bowel obstruction have been reported in 1%–10% of OS for Hodgkin's disease, with a reoperation rate of 2%–7% [13]. In the laparoscopic series, there is only one report of a prolonged postoperative ileus [23].

Fever

Postoperative fever unrelated to any of the common postoperative causes has been reported in the open splenectomy literature. It is believed to be secondary to circulating leukoagglutinizing antibodies and is self-limited [7]. This complication has not been reported in the laparoscopic literature.

Thromboembolism

Thromboembolism complicates 2%–11% of OS [7, 15] and is more common in patients who have hypersplenism or myeloproliferative disorders. The presumed causes include eradication of splenic sequestration, removal of regulatory humoral factors produced by the spleen, altered platelet function, thrombocytosis, and thrombus extending from the splenic vein remnant secondary to intimal injury and stasis. Treatment with antiplatelet medication may be of some use if platelets exceed 500 000 per mm^3, but no prospective studies have been performed. In addition, thrombolytic agents and anticoagulants may prove to be lifesaving. One of our patients developed a transient postoperative embolic stroke following LS.

Splenosis

Splenosis is defined as the autotransplantation of splenic tissue in an ectopic position and is usually seen following traumatic splenic rupture in children; the reported incidence is 48%–66% [17]. This is worrisome to the laparoscopic surgeon, because the ideal grasper for the spleen has not been developed, and fracture of the spleen may occur. Splenosis may also result from inadvertent spillage of fragments during morcellation of ITP patients' spleens. Nevertheless, there have been no reports of splenosis following LS.

Overwhelming Postsplenectomy Infection

Overwhelming postsplenectomy infection (OPSI) follows 4% of splenectomies, with a mortality rate of 1.7%. More than 66% of these cases and 80% of deaths occur within the first 2 years of splenectomy. This problem is discussed in detail in the chaps. by Stiehm and Trunkey (this volume). The incidence of this complication following LS should be the same as after OS, but no cases have been reported in the literature to date.

Summary

LS is a procedure in evolution. It is postulated that avoiding an upper abdominal incision and minimizing the operative trauma will decrease the incidence of pulmonary, thromboembolic, and wound complications associated with OS, and early reports seem to support this. As experience is gained with LS, operative times can be reduced to near those of the open procedure. Overall costs are lower with shorter hospital stays, and the patients benefit by having a shorter recovery period with an earlier return to normal activities.

Most LS are now being performed for ITP, because the normal-sized spleen is ideal for the laparoscopic procedure. Longer follow-up of these patients is necessary to determine whether accessory spleens will be missed more frequently and lead to increased rates of recurrence for the disease. Finally, perfection of instrumentation and operative techniques should make the laparoscopic procedure available for enlarged spleens and a wider range of indications.

References

1. Aksnes J, Abdelnoor M, Mathisen O (1995) Risk factors associated with mortality and morbidity after elective splenectomy. Eur J Surg 161:253–258
2. Carroll BJ, Phillips EH, Semel CJ et al (1992) Laparoscopic splenectomy. Surg Endosc 6:183–185
3. Cadiere GB, Verroken R, Himpens J, Bruyns J, Efira M, De Witt S (1994) Operative strategy in laparoscopic splenectomy. J Am Coll Surg 179:668–672
4. Cuschieri A, Shimi S, Banting S,Vander Velpen G (1992) Technical aspects of laparoscopic splenectomy: hilar segmental devascularization and instrumentation. J R Coll Surg Edin 37:414–416
5. Delaitre B (1995) Laparoscopic splenectomy, the hanged spleen technique. Surg Endosc 9:528–529
6. Delaitre B, Maignien B (1992) Laparoscopic splenectomy: technical aspects. Surg Endosc 6:305–308
7. Ellison EC, Fabri PJ (1983) Complications of splenectomy: etiology, prevention and management. Surg Clin N Am 63 (6):1313–1330
8. Emmerman A, Zornig C, Peiper M et al (1995) Laparoscopic splenectomy. Surg Endosc 9:924–927
9. Friedman RL, Fallas MJ, Carroll BJ, Hiatt JR, Phillips EH (1996) Laparoscopic splenectomy for ITP: the gold standard. Surg Endosc 10:991–995
10. Gigot JF, Healy ML, Ferrant A, Michaux JL, Njinou B, Kestens PJ (1994) Laparoscopic splenectomy for idiopathic thrombocytopenic purpura. Br J Surg 81:1171–1172
11. Hanley ES (1992) Anesthesia for laparoscopic surgery. Surg Clin N Am 72:1013–1019
12. Horowitz J, Smith JL, Weber TK, Rodriguez-Bigas MA, Petrelli NJ (1996) Postoperative complications after splenectomy for hematologic malignancies. Ann Surg 223:290–296
13. Jockovich M, Mendenhall NP, Sombeck MD, Talbert JL, Copeland III EM, Bland KI (1994) Long term complications of laparotomy in Hodgkin's disease. Ann Surg 219:615–624
14. Lefor AT, Melvin WS, Bailey RW, Flowers JL (1993) Laparoscopic splenectomy in the management of immune thrombocytopenia purpura. Surgery 114:613–618

15. MacRae HM, Yakimets WW, Reynolds T (1992) Perioperative complications of splenectomy for hematologic disease. Can J Surg 35:432–436
16. Michel NA (1942) The variational anatomy of the spleen and splenic artery. Am J Anat 70:21–72
17. Mintz SJ, Petersen SR, Cheson B, Cordell LJ, Richards RC (1981) Splenectomy for immune thrombocytopenic purpura. Arch Surg 116:645–650
18. Musser G, Lazar G, Hocking W, Busuttil RW (1984) Splenectomy for hematologic disease: the UCLA experience with 306 patients. Ann Surg 200 (1):40–45
19. Phillips EH, Carroll BJ, Fallas MJ (1994) Laparoscopic splenectomy. Surg Endosc 8:931–933
20. Phillips EH, Carroll BJ, Rosenthal RJ (1995) Laparoscopic splenectomy. In: Cameron JL (ed) Current surgical therapy, 5th edn. Mosby, St. Louis, pp 1069–1072
21. Phillips JM (1977) Laparoscopy. Williams and Wilkins, Baltimore, pp 220–246
22. Poulin EC, Thibault C (1993) The anatomical basis for laparoscopic splenectomy. Can J Surg 36:484–488
23. Poulin EC, Thibault C, Mamazza J (1995) Laparoscopic splenectomy. Surg Endosc 9:172–177
24. Rattner DW, Ellman L, Warshaw AL (1993) Portal vein thrombosis after elective splenectomy. An under-appreciated, potentially lethal syndrome. Arch Surg 128:565–569, 569–570
25. Ravikumar TS, Allen JD, Bothe A, Steele G (1989) Splenectomy: the treatment of choice for human immunodeficiency virus-related immune thrombocytopenia? Arch Surg 124:625–628
26. Rhodes M, Rudd M, O'Rourke N, Nathanson L, Fielding G (1995) Laparoscopic splenectomy and lymph node biopsy for hematologic disorders. Ann Surg 222:43–46
27. Sheldon GF, Croom RD, Meyer AA (1991) The spleen. In: Sabiston DC (ed) Textbook of surgery: the biological basis of modern surgical practice. Saunders, Philadelphia, pp 1108–1133
28. Yee LF, Carvajal SH, Lorimier A, Mulvihill SJ (1995) Laparoscopic splenectomy: an initial experience at University of California, San Francisco. Arch Surg 130:874–878

Splenic Trauma

D. D. Trunkey, Frieda Hulka, and R. J. Mullins

"When the milt or spleen is wounded, blacke and grosse blood cometh out at the wound, the patient will be very thirsty, with paine on the left side, and the blood breakes forth into the belly, and there putrifying causeth most maligne and greevous accidents and often times causes death to follow."
Ambrose Pare, Sixteenth Century
"Injuries of the spleen demand excision of the gland."
Theodor Kocher, 1911

"Splenectomy is considered by most authorities to be mandatory for rupture of the spleen following blunt abdominal trauma. Recently some interest has been shown in the possibility of conservative management of this injury... selected cases of splenic trauma in children can be successfully treated without surgery."
C.J. Douglas and *J.S. Simpson*, 1971

The spleen is the abdominal organ most commonly injured in blunt trauma [1]. Patients may be asymptomatic or present with life-threatening shock. The diagnosis and management of splenic injury have been topics of controversy for the past century, with more than 1250 published articles on the subject in the last 30 years. This chapter will consider the major current controversies in splenic trauma, including splenic preservation, splenic repair, nonoperative treatment, radiologic evaluation, and postsplenectomy management.

Splenic Preservation

Historical Perspective

Aristotle was the first to suggest that the spleen had no purpose [2]. Kocher in 1911 stated that all injuries should be treated by excision, as there were no ill effects of splenectomy, and the risk of bleeding was eliminated [3]. This dogma was questioned in 1919 by Morris and Bullock, who showed an increased susceptibility to infection in splenectomized rats challenged with bacillus [4]. That observation and the authors' speculation of its relevance to humans was largely ignored by surgeons; splenectomy was preferred even for minor splenic injury as well as a variety of hematologic disorders until 1952.

The concept of splenectomy as an innocuous procedure was dispelled by King and Schumacher with their description of five children who developed septic complications after splenectomy for congenital hemolytic anemia [5]. Smith et al. reported the first case of sepsis following splenectomy for trauma in 1957 [6]. Accumulating evidence of the infectious risks of splenectomy was the stimulus for development of methods for splenic preservation.

Effect of Splenectomy on Immune Function

The spleen is a major source of immunoglobulin M (IgM) and opsonin (tuftsin and properdin) production. The spleen also acts as a filter for antigens and abnormal blood cells [7] and affects immune cell populations in other lymphoid tissue, primarily T cells [7, 8]. Splenic immunology is discussed in the chapter by Stiehm, this volume.

After splenectomy, alterations in cellular function and splenic filtration affect the ability of the immune system to recognize and eliminate bacteria. A transient increase in T suppressor cells blunts the cellular response to antigen [8, 9], while decreased IgM production diminishes the antibody response to antigens not previously encountered [7, 10–15]. Levels of properdin and tuftsin decrease, impairing opsonization and phagocytosis [16–18]. Impaired antigen clearance of blood-borne particles occurs with the absence splenic filtration [13, 19]. The net effect of these changes in the reticuloendothelial system is an increased risk of infection in postsplenectomy patients.

Infection After Splenectomy

Overwhelming Postsplenectomy Infection

Description. Due to decreased opsonization and impaired clearance of antigens, the asplenic patient is at increased risk of overwhelming bacteremia from encapsulated organisms, both in the early postoperative period as well as many years later. The syndrome of overwhelming postsplenectomy infection (OPSI) is unlike most fulminating bacteremias and septicemias in patients with normal splenic function [20]. Symptoms begin with a sore throat, fever, or malaise and progress quickly to headache, vomiting, and hyperexia; hypotension, coma, and death can follow within 12–18 h. Disseminated intravascular coagulation (DIC) has also been associated with OPSI [21]. The overall mortality is 50%–80% [22–24].

The most common causative organism is *Streptococcus pneumoniae*, accounting for at least 50% of cases [22, 25, 26]. Other organisms include *Neisseria meningitidis, Escherichia coli, Haemophilus influenzae, Staphylococcus,* and *Streptococcus.* Half of OPSI cases occur within 12 months of splenectomy [22, 27]. However, OPSI has been reported as late as 42 years after splenectomy [28].

Incidence. The first evaluation of OPSI risk in asplenic patients was made by Eraklis and Filler [29]. Of 1413 pediatric patients who underwent splenectomy for hematologic disorders or trauma, there were 34 deaths due to infection (2.5%). In the subset of trauma patients, three of 342 died of sepsis (0.87%).

Singer's 1973 review of 2795 splenectomized patients demonstrated a 4.25% incidence of OPSI, with a subsequent mortality of 2.5% [22]. In trauma patients, however, the incidence of OPSI was 1.45%, with a mortality rate of 0.58%. Given that the community mortality from sepsis is 0.01%, the determined risk of death from OPSI after splenectomy for trauma was 58–87 times the expected rate in the general population. However, the true incidence of OPSI and the definition of sepsis used by the authors have formed the basis of a challenge to this extrapolation [27, 30, 31].

Other studies attempting to identify the risk to asplenic patients have shown similar incidence of OPSI in the trauma population. O'Neal and McDonald reviewed 187 splenectomized trauma patients and found a 2.2% incidence of OPSI with no deaths [32]. Sekikawa and Shatney evaluated 619 trauma patients who underwent splenectomy [33]; long-term follow-up in 242 of them demonstrated a 2.5% incidence of sepsis, with no deaths. Chaikof and McCabe showed that 3.7% of pediatric patients and 0.34% of adults developed OPSI [34].

In 1987, Luna and Dellinger published a literature review which included 2531 trauma patients who underwent splenectomy [35]. OPSI was the cause of death in 11 patients, reflecting a mortality rate of 0.4% from OPSI. Most of these series predated the availability of pneumococcal vaccination. Recognizing this, the authors calculated a lifetime mortality rate from OPSI of 0.026% for adults and 0.052% for children. The true risk of OPSI continues to be debated, since the estimated risks have been based upon retrospective studies of selected populations.

Other Postsplenectomy Infections

Asplenic patients also develop other postoperative infections (wound, urinary tract, subphrenic abscess) more frequently than immunocompetent patients. The immune defect responsible for this propensity is probably the transitory increase in suppressor T cells [8], which persists for approximately 10 days after splenectomy [9].

Earlier studies noted a postoperative infection rate in asplenic patients of 8%–13% [36–38]. In 1975, Steele and Lim found a 27% infection rate in patients with splenectomy secondary to trauma [39]. Systemic sepsis developed in 23% of patients postoperatively in series published by Sekikawa and Shatney [33], and Goins et al. showed an increased risk of intra-abdominal abscesses in splenectomized trauma patients [40].

Comparing splenorrhaphy to splenectomy, Feliciano et al. found an increased number of intra-abdominal abscesses in splenectomized patients (6%

vs. 2%) [41]. Although asplenic patients had more associated injuries, more hollow viscus injuries occurred in the splenorrhaphy group. Duke et al. [42] and Shackford et al. [53] in separate studies also demonstrated increased infectious complications in splenectomized patients [42, 53]. These observations concerning infectious complications of splenectomy show that, while the risk of OPSI is low, the risk of other infections is increased, and attempts to save the spleen are justified.

Splenic Repair

Historical Perspective

Despite the widespread use of splenectomy to treat splenic injuries, there are early reports of splenic repair. The first splenorrhaphy was probably performed in 1895 by Zikoff, a Russian surgeon [43]. Few case reports of splenorrhaphy were published until 1930, when Dretzka reported three patients whose splenic injuries were successfully treated with suture repair [44]. Campos Cristo reported a successful splenic salvage by partial splenectomy in 1962 [43]. Morgenstern was the first to describe the use of a hemostatic agent, microfibrillar collagen (Avitene), in treating splenic injuries [45]. The first pediatric splenorrhaphy was reported by Mishalany in 1974 [46].

Splenorrhaphy Versus Splenectomy

Since 1978, more than 40 studies have compared splenorrhaphy with splenectomy [41, 47–87] including 4565 patients with traumatic splenic injury (Table 1). There were 2736 initial splenectomies and 1829 successful splenorrhaphies, with an average salvage rate of 39% (8%–99%). An overall failure rate of 3% resulted in 48 additional splenectomies.

Despite the extensive literature regarding splenorrhaphy, it is difficult to compare studies, because selection criteria and injury grading have been inconsistent. Of the 42 studies cited, only 23 provide the decision criteria used for splenorrhaphy. The two main indications for splenectomy were hemodynamic instability and an "irreparable" injury. After excluding hilar injuries or hemodynamic instability, only 50% of patients were successfully repaired [41, 49–51, 53, 55, 58–60, 62, 65, 68, 69, 72, 76–79, 82, 85, 86].

It has been proposed that operating times are longer for splenorrhaphy than splenectomy, leading to an increase in blood loss [47]. Because of this observation, splenorrhaphy has been discouraged by some in the face of serious associated injuries [41, 64, 66]. However, neither Shackford et al. [53] nor Traub and Perry [56] found a difference in operative times for the two modalities. Further, the success of splenorrhaphy improves as the surgeon's experience increases [62]. The current recommendation is that splenic repair

Table 1. Splenectomy versus splenorrhaphy

Date	Reference	Initial splenec-tomies (n)	Attempted splenor-rhaphies (n)	Repairs successful (n)	Salvage rate (%)	Repair failures (n)	Decision criteria
1978	[47]	0	6	6	–	0	Case reports
1979	[48]	62	22	22	26	0	No comment
1979	[49]	12	18	18	60	0	Reparable, no associated injuries
1981	[50]	33	23	20	36	3	27 serial attempts
1981	[51]	4	20	19	79	1	All patients attempted
1981	[52]	59	33	33	36	0	No comment
1981	[53]	42	43	43	51	0	Grade I–IV No associated injuries
1981[a]	[54]	22	16	15	39[b]	1	Last 3 years, all patients
1982	[55]	85	49	48	36[c]	1	Reparable, stable
1982	[56]	231	41	40	15	1	Surgeon's discretion
1982	[57]	107	33	33	24[b]	0	No comment
1982	[58]	18	39	34	60	5	All patients attempted
1982[a]	[59]	4	3	3	43[b]	0	Reparable
1983	[60]	16	20	18	50	2	Reparable, no associated injuries
1983	[61]	25	13	13	34[b]	0	No comment
1984	[62]	93	85	82	48[c]	3	Reparable, stable patients
1984	[63]	55	12	12	18[b]	0	No comment
1984	[64]	114	10	10	8[b]	0	No comment
1985	[41]	169	136	136	45	0	Reparable, stable patients
1985	[65]	18	9	8	30[b]	1	Stable patients
1986	[66]	170	60	60	26	0	No comment
1986	[67]	107	42	32	28[b]	10	No comment
1986[a]	[68]	2	23	23	92	0	All patients attempted
1986	[69]	25	17	16	38	1	Stable patients
1987	[70]	43	42	41	49	1	No comment
1987	[71]	53	31	30	36[b]	1	No comment
1988	[72]	0	119	118	99	14	Grade II–IV injuries
1988	[73]	20	18	18	47[b]	0	No comment
1988	[74]	12	18	18	60[b]	0	No comment
1988	[75]	33	21	21	39[b]	0	No comment
1989	[76]	63	107	105	61[c]	3	Stable patients
1989	[77]	69	27	27	28[b]	0	Stable patients
1990	[78]	313	240	236	43	4	Grade I–IV, stable patients
1990	[79]	56	111	109	65[b]	2	Minor to moderate injuries, stable patients

Table 1. (Continued)

Date	Reference	Initial splenectomies (*n*)	Attempted splenorrhaphies (*n*)	Repairs successful (*n*)	Salvage rate (%)	Repair failures (*n*)	Decision criteria
1990	[80]	69	43	42	38[b]	1	No comment
1990[a]	[81]	30	13	13	30[b]	0	No comment
1990	[82]	59	32	31	35[b]	1	Reparable, stable patients
1990	[83]	246	164	160	37[b]	4	No comment
1991	[84]	59	5	5	8[b]	0	No comment
1992	[85]	2	9	8	73[b]	1	Nonoperative treatment failure
1992	[86]	49	17	16	26[b]	1	Reparable
1993	[87]	87	39	39	31[b]	0	No comment
Total		2736	1829	1781	39[b]	62	

[a] Pediatric cases only.
[b] Does not include patients not operated on.
[c] Does not include autotransplantation.

should be considered in most instances, but if the surgeon determines that associated injuries are life-threatening, the most expeditious procedure should be performed [67]. Attempts to save the spleen should not be made at the expense of increased operative time or blood loss.

Associated visceral perforation is a relative contraindication to splenorrhaphy [56]. In the collected series, other intra-abdominal injuries occurred in 29%–74% of patients [41, 50, 53, 55–57, 62, 66, 67, 70, 76, 80, 82]. However, the incidence of postoperative infection is lower with splenorrhaphy, even with the presence of hollow viscus injury. In the series published by Traub and Perry, 15% of both splenectomy and splenorrhaphy groups had hollow visceral injuries, yet sepsis was twice as frequent in the splenectomy group [56]. Feliciano et al. found a decrease in intra-abdominal abscesses after splenorrhaphy, despite a larger number of hollow viscus injuries in the same patients [41]. These observations demonstrate that a functioning spleen is more important in prevention of infection than the presence of a perforated viscus with contamination.

Current contraindications to splenorrhaphy include hemodynamic instability, associated injuries which require immediate attention, such as aortic or retrocaval trauma, coagulopathy, and irreparable splenic injury. When these are present, splenectomy should be performed.

Splenic Injury Grading

In 1987, the American Association for the Surgery of Trauma developed an Organ Injury Scaling committee. The widely accepted Organ Injury Scale was

Table 2. Spleen injury scale (1994 revision)

Grade	Injury	
I	Hematoma:	subcapsular, <10 surface area
	Laceration:	capsular tear, <1 cm parenchymal depth
II	Hematoma:	subcapsular, 10–50% surface area; intraparenchymal, <5 cm in diameter
	Laceration:	1–3 cm parenchymal depth which does not involve a trabecular vessel
III	Hematoma:	subcapsular, >50% surface area or expanding; ruptured subcapsular or parenchymal hematoma; intraparenchymal hematoma >5 cm or expanding
	Laceration:	>3 cm parenchymal depth or involving trabecular vessels
IV	Laceration:	involving segmental or hilar vessels producing major devascularization (>25% of the spleen)
V	Laceration:	completely shattered spleen
	Vascular:	hilar vascular injury with devascularized spleen

published in 1989 [89] and has recently been revised [90] (Table 2). It should be noted that there has been no correlation between the injury scale and successful splenic salvage. However, the use of standardized descriptions of injury has clarified reporting in the literature, which was a problem with earlier studies.

Methods of Splenic Repair

Operative Principles

A midline incision allows for full exposure of the spleen and other viscera. For larger splenorrhaphies, the spleen must be mobilized completely to inspect the injury. Control of the hilar vessels with direct pressure or a vascular clamp can minimize blood loss. For small serosal lacerations, the spleen may be left in place, as mobilization may aggravate the injury. The extent of injury determines the manner of repair. Techniques for splenic mobilization and splenectomy are described in the chapter by Hiatt (this volume) and techniques of partial splenectomy and splenic repair are considered further in the chapter by Morgenstern (this volume).

Hemostatic Agents and Coagulation Methods

Hemostatic agents are used for minor splenic injuries and raw surfaces. Various agents include Gelfoam (absorbable gelatin sponge), Surgicel, oxidized

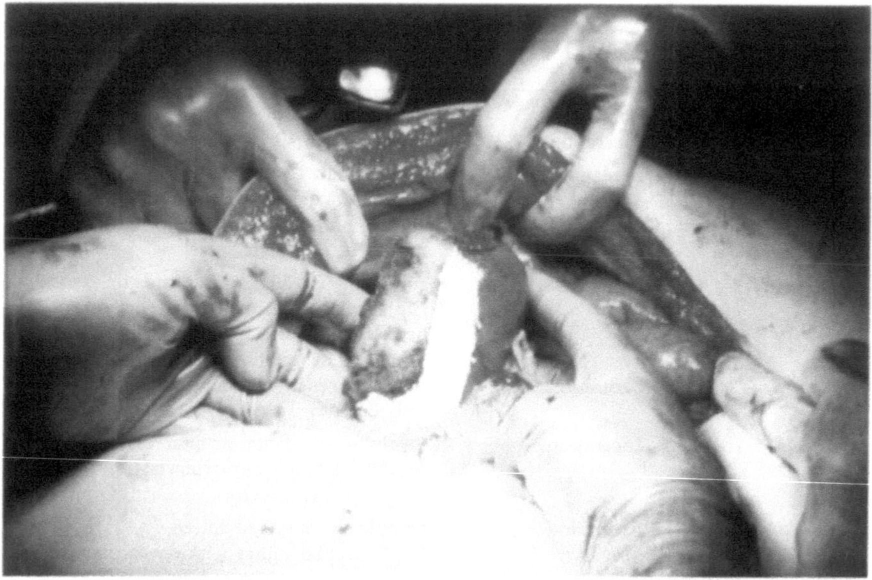

Fig. 1. Splenic repair with Gelfoam (absorbable gelatin sponge) and electrocautery

cellulose, microfibrillar collagen, and fibrin tissue adhesive (Fig. 1), used alone or in conjunction with suture [41, 47, 55, 58, 60, 62, 78, 91–93]. Standard electrocoagulation is the modality used most commonly for hemostasis. In addition, argon beam coagulation and infrared diathermy have also been advocated [94].

Suture Repair

Suture repair is utilized for more severe splenic injuries. Because the splenic parenchyma is fragile and the capsule is thin and lacking in tensile strength, care must be taken when suturing to avoid tearing the capsule and extending the laceration. Absorbable sutures are preferred, and many techniques have been described. Most authors recommend mattress or figure-of-eight sutures [41, 55, 60, 62, 70, 78, 88, 92, 95, 96]. Teflon (polytetrafluoroethylene) pledgets may be used to minimize tearing through the capsule. The omentum can also be included in the repair for hemostasis.

Mesh Repair

For more disruptive injuries, with multiple lacerations or a fractured spleen, suture repair is ineffective. Delany et al. were the first to wrap the spleen with absorbable mesh as an adjunct to splenorrhaphy in 1982 [97]. The spleen is fully mobilized by division of the posterior ligaments and short gastric vessels. The mesh is wrapped around the spleen, with a fenestration for the hilar vessels, and then sutured tightly in a sequential fashion around the periphery (Fig. 2). A tight wrap tamponades venous and parenchymal bleeding. The use of mesh in severe splenic injuries has been shown to increase rates of splenic preservation [98, 99].

Splenic Artery Ligation

Splenic artery ligation has been advocated as an adjunct to splenorrhaphy, especially in the treatment of hilar injuries [100–102]. Because of collateral circulation from the short gastric vessels, splenic artery ligation as a sole treatment for splenic injury is rarely adequate [101], and splenic infarction is a potential problem.

Partial Splenectomy

In the event of a polar injury, partial splenectomy has been used to remove the damaged end (Figs. 3, 4). After amputation of the injured area, hemostasis of the open edge is secured with mattress sutures or a stapling device [41, 43, 47, 60, 78, 96, 98, 103]. This method of repair has the advantage of removing the macerated tissue and allowing visualization of the parenchyma and hilum; direct vessel ligation can then be performed. The residual volume of splenic tissue is important, as it is correlated with resistance to infection [13, 104, 105]. Most studies show that at least one third of the spleen must be salvaged [104]. Partial splenectomy is discussed further by Morgenstern (this volume).

Nonoperative Management

Historical Perspective

Billroth (cited in [43]) suggested that the spleen could heal without intervention: a patient with a concomitant head injury died 5 days after injury, and a splenic injury with a small amount of hemorrhage was found at autopsy. However, prior to this century, mortality for nonoperative management of splenic injuries was 90%–100% [106, 107]. By the 1930s, splenectomy had a mortality rate of 27% [106], and the reported incidence of delayed splenic rupture was 10%–15% [107]. Therefore, operative therapy was advised for all cases of splenic injury [108].

With increasing appreciation of the infectious risks of asplenia, nonoperative management was reconsidered. In 1968, Upadhyaya and Simpson [109] successfully treated 12 pediatric patients with suspected splenic injuries non-

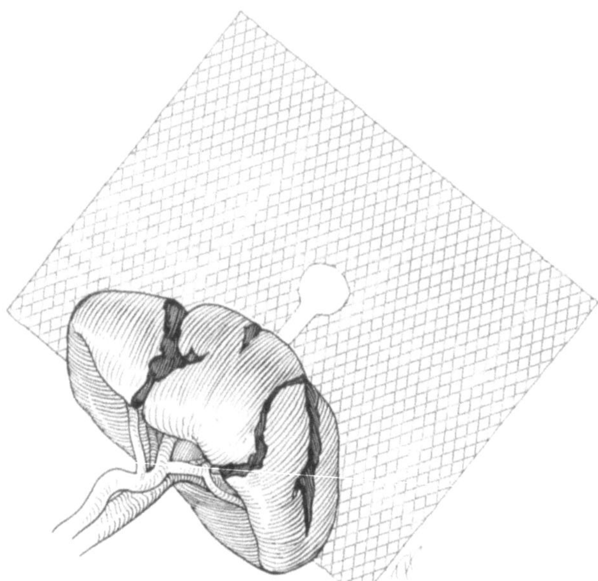

Fig. 2a,b. Splenic repair with polyglycolic mesh. a Preparation of the mesh, with fenestration for hilar vessels. b Splenic wrap; mesh is secured to itself using a running absorbable suture

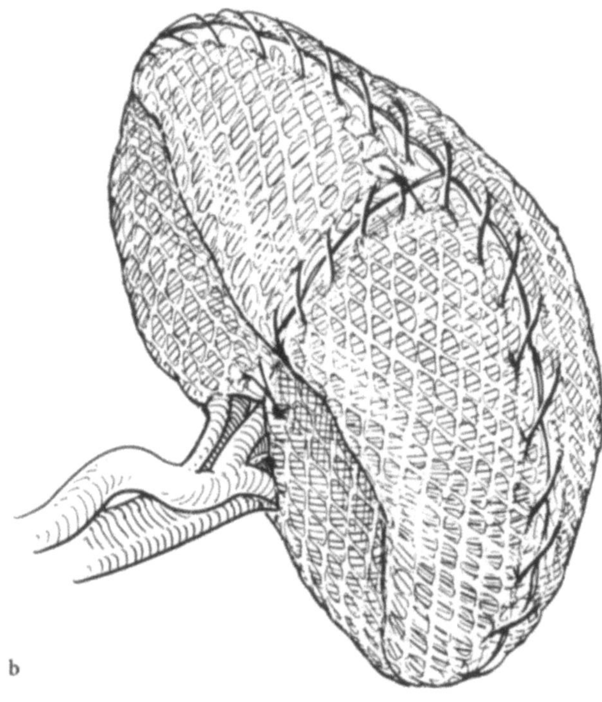

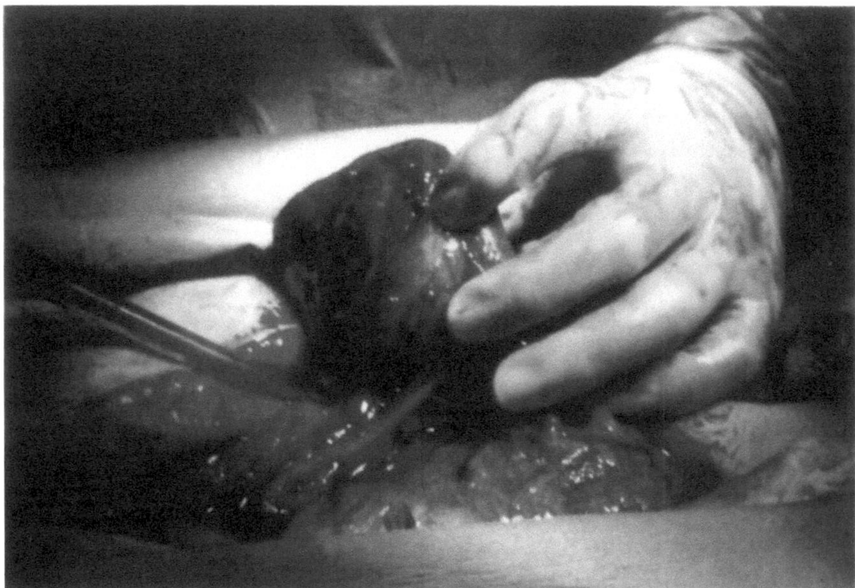

Fig. 3. Splenic injury to the inferior pole

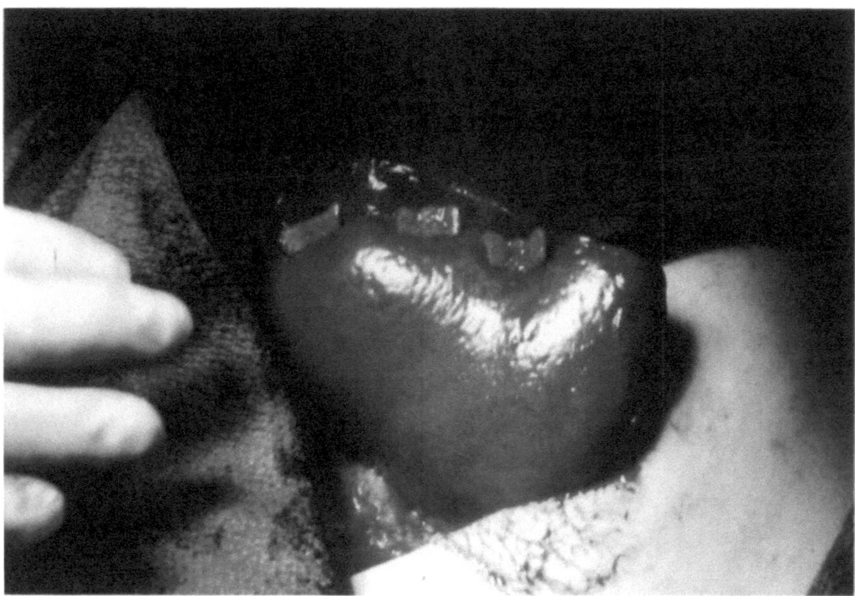

Fig. 4. Partial splenectomy with mattress sutures

operatively. Experience from the Toronto Hospital for Sick Children was reported by Douglas and Simpson [110] in 1971 and included 25 patients with clinical symptoms of splenic rupture, all of whom were successfully treated without operation. Radiographic documentation of splenic injury combined with nonoperative treatment was subsequently used with success in 28 children [111].

Use of nonoperative treatment in nine adult patients was first reported by Solheim in 1979 [112]. The use of abdominal computed tomography (CT) for trauma was introduced in 1980, improving the accuracy of diagnosis and augmenting the success of nonoperative treatment [161].

Children and Adults

Pediatric Series

More than 20 articles regarding nonoperative treatment of pediatric patients have been published [54, 59, 68, 81, 109, 110, 113–127] (Table 3). Of 1228 patients with splenic injury, 785 (64%) were hemodynamically stable and eligi-

Table 3. Nonoperative treatment (pediatric series)

Date	Reference	Total population (n)	Attempted nonoperative treatment (n)	Eligible patients (%)	Failures (n)	Patients receiving blood (n)
1968	[109]	52	12	23	0	N/A
1971	[110]	32	25	78	0	9
1977	[113]	–	6	–	0	4
1977	[114]	39	24	62	1	10
1978	[115]	56	35	63	0	14
1981	[54]	68	30	44	0	N/A
1981	[116]	63	44	70	0	16
1982	[59]	28	28	100	7	9
1984	[117]	128	91	70	0	30
1986	[68]	25	4	16	0	N/A
1987	[118]	87	6	7	0	N/A
1987	[119]	24	18	75	0	N/A
1989	[120]	75	65	87	0	15
1990	[81]	111	68	61	24	30
1990	[121]	23	23	100	0	14
1993	[122]	91	53	58	0	5
1994	[123]	28	25	89	0	N/A
1994	[124]	120	112	93	2	N/A
1994	[125]	59	50	85	0	N/A
1994	[126]	36	11	31	0	2
1995	[127]	83	55	66	5	13
Total		1228	785	64	39	171

N/A, not available.

ble for nonoperative treatment. There were 39 failures (4%). Within the series addressing transfusion requirements, an average of 32% of patients received blood products [59, 81, 110, 113–117, 120–122, 126, 127].

Adult Series

Over 40 articles have been published on nonoperative management of adult splenic trauma [57, 61, 63–65, 67, 71, 73–75, 77, 79, 80, 82–87, 112, 128–147] (Table 4). Of the 5051 patients with splenic injury, 1232 (24%) met criteria for nonoperative treatment. The cumulative failure rate was 14%. In the series describing transfusion requirements, 31% of patients received blood products [61, 65, 67, 71, 73, 77, 79, 80, 84–85, 87, 112, 129, 132, 133, 135–137, 140, 142–144, 147].

Differences

The noted differences between adult and strictly pediatric series were the numbers of patients who satisfied the criteria for nonoperative treatment and the failure rates. Besides the obvious differences in size between children and adults, there are important differences in mechanisms of injury and splenic anatomy which explain the variations.

Gross showed that splenic weight increases tenfold by age 6, but the size of the splenic capsule only increases fivefold [148]. This decrease in the capsule to parenchyma ratio with age leads in turn to a diminished tamponade effect. Disruptive splenic injuries from rib fractures occur with differing frequencies in the age-groups. Mazel reported that children's ribs are elastic and rarely prone to fractures [149]. As the skeleton matures, however, elasticity decreases, and traumatic rib fractures become more common. Bony injuries produce more parenchymal damage, which does not lend itself as well to nonoperative treatment. These differences offer possible explanations for the increased failure rate in the adult population.

Two series further elucidate the effects of age on the success of nonoperative treatment. In a multicenter experience reported by Cogbill [137], 112 patients were treated nonoperatively with 13 failures, 30% of whom were over age 50. In Smith's [86] series of 46 patients treated nonoperatively, all three failures were in patients older than 55 years. This suggests that, as age increases, nonoperative treatment is more likely to fail.

Patient Selection

Hemodynamic stability is the principal criterion for consideration of nonoperative management. If the patient is hypotensive, ongoing hemorrhage is the most likely cause, and prompt exploration is needed. Among the re-

Table 4. Nonoperative treatment (adult series)

Date	Reference	Total population (n)	Attempted nonoperative treatment (n)	Eligible patients (%)	Failures (n)	Patients receiving blood (n)
1979	[112]	15	9	60	0	1
1982	[57]	172	32[a]	19	1	N/A
1983	[61]	55	17	31	0	5
1984	[63]	77	10	13	7	N/A
1984	[64]	154	30	19	21	N/A
1984	[128]	267	11[a]	4	0	N/A
1984	[129]	68	24[a]	35	1	9
1985	[65]	80	55[a]	69	2	N/A
1985	[130]	76	11	14	8	N/A
1985	[131]	53	19	36	2	N/A
1986	[132]	52	13	25	0	6
1986	[133]	60	11	17	3	4
1986	[67]	235	66[a]	28	19	28
1987	[71]	147	63[a]	43	0	4
1987	[134]	70	22[a]	31	5	N/A
1987	[135]	30	7	23	2	3
1987	[136]	–	10	–	3	1
1988	[73]	48	10	21	7	2
1988	[74]	46	16[a]	35	0	N/A
1988	[75]	87	43[a]	49	10	N/A
1989	[77]	143	47	33	6	13
1989	[137]	832	112[a]	13	13	38
1989	[138]	46	36[a]	78	5	N/A
1989	[139]	252	60	24	5	N/A
1990	[79]	193	26	13	1	13
1990	[80]	169	11	11	3	6
1990	[82]	106	15	14	7	N/A
1990	[83]	428	18	4	2	N/A
1990	[140]	45	15	33	0	0
1990	[141]	37	25[a]	68	5	N/A
1990	[142]	51	34	66	1	14
1991	[84]	91	23[a]	25	2	6
1991	[143]	182	23	13	3	7
1991	[144]	56	44[a]	79	5	15
1992	[85]	20	9	20	0	5
1992	[86]	114	46[a]	40	3	N/A
1992	[145]	75	22	29	4	N/A
1993	[87]	185	85	46	8	20
1994	[146]	137	70[a]	51	7	N/A
1996	[147]	97	32	33	0	17
Total		5051	1232	24	171	217

N/A, not available.

[a] Adult and pediatric series.

ported series of splenic injury patients, only 24% of adults and 64% of children satisfied criteria for nonoperative treatment.

Associated intra-abdominal injuries have also been cited as exclusion criteria for nonoperative treatment. These occur with a frequency of 15% (range, 5%–47%) in patients treated nonoperatively [61, 73, 77, 82, 84, 87, 124, 131–133, 135–137, 139–142, 144]. However, the average incidence of associated intra-abdominal injuries in the population who underwent splenectomy or splenic repair was 55% (range, 17%–72%) [41, 49, 50, 53, 55, 56, 62, 66, 70, 150], suggesting that hemodynamically stable patients with splenic injury are less likely to have other intra-abdominal injuries. An explanation for this finding is that the mechanism of injury is less severe, causing less injury to the spleen and fewer intra-abdominal injuries. Unless the associated injury clearly requires operative repair, its presence alone should not preclude nonoperative management. It is obviously essential to identify all associated injuries.

Bleeding Risks

More than 30% of patients treated nonoperatively received blood. When compared to patients undergoing splenectomy or splenorrhaphy, the amount of blood received is often less [63, 67, 71, 126, 127, 129, 138], because the severity of injury for patients requiring operation is usually greater. Prompt exploration with immediate splenectomy has the advantage of achieving timely control of hemorrhage. Some investigators have expressed concern that the risks of blood transfusion with nonoperative treatment will outweigh the risk of infectious complications following splenectomy [35, 80, 84–87, 121, 137].

The risks of blood transfusion include both transfusion reactions and disease transmission. The probability of death from an acute fatal transfusion reaction is 0.00001 per patient [151]. Per unit of blood, the estimated risk of exposure is 0.0003 for hepatitis and 0.000035 for human immunodeficiency virus (HIV) [151, 152]. There are geographic variations, depending on the number of carriers in the area evaluated. Although the potential exposure to these viral infections is small, the question that remains is whether the risk of exposure outweighs the risk from postsplenectomy immunologic deficiencies.

To address the issue, Luna and Dellinger [35] compared the risks of death, transfusion, and treatment failure for nonoperative treatment with the risk of OPSI for operative treatment, including splenectomy and splenorrhaphy. They determined that the risk of death from nonoperative treatment in adults was 0.26%, compared to 0.06% for initial operative treatment. In children, the risk of death for nonoperative treatment was 0.17%, compared to 0.06% for initial operative treatment. The authors concluded that early laparotomy produced lower mortality rates than nonoperative treatment. However, these calculations were based on a nonoperative treatment success rate of 60% and a splenic salvage rate of 63% in adults. In addition, transfusion risks were based upon estimates that 40% of children and 20% of adults treated nonoperatively required blood products.

Success rates for nonoperative management have improved over time. Cogbill [137] recalculated the risk of death using Luna and Dellinger's model but with more favorable success rates for nonoperative treatment. Their calculations demonstrated that the risk of death from nonoperative management was 0.07% in adults and 0.036% in children. The risk of death from nonoperative management based on a multicenter experience compares favorably with the 0.06% risk of death from operative treatment.

Decision analysis represents another method to evaluate the risks of operative versus nonoperative treatment [153, 154]. The analyses defined incidences of selected variables based upon published series. When the model by Feliciano et al. was extrapolated to a population of 100 000 patients, the authors found an increase in transfusion-related deaths, but no difference in OPSI deaths between the two management strategies [153]. A greater number of transfusions was required in patients treated nonoperatively. Therefore, the number of transfusion-related deaths remained higher regardless of the success of nonoperative treatment. Velanovich and Tapper used quality-adjusted life expectancy (QALE) to analyze the treatment modalities [154]. In children, nonoperative treatment and splenorrhaphy had similar QALE despite the transfusion rate in the latter; nonoperative management and splenorrhaphy had longer QALE than splenectomy. Further evaluation of the effects of transfusion on QALE demonstrated that even if 100% of observed patients and none of the splenectomized patients received blood transfusions, the QALE would still be shorter for splenectomy. Therefore, splenic preservation increases life expectancy; however, the risk of blood transfusion may still outweigh the benefit of splenectomy.

The threshold criteria for transfusion have varied in the published series. Earlier studies used a hemoglobin of 10 g or a hematocrit of 30% to prompt transfusion, despite stable vital signs [113, 115, 119, 138, 139]. In more recent studies, an hematocrit of 25% is considered acceptable in stable patients [87, 121, 122, 126, 155]. Many investigators have limited transfusion to fewer than 4 U [61, 67, 77, 79, 84, 116, 117, 129, 133, 139, 144]. The current recommendation is that transfusions required beyond 4 U are an indication for immediate operation. This approach minimizes the patient's exposure to transfusion risks and does not delay the probable need for surgery. Other authors have advocated early operation if blood replacement is even considered [85].

Risk of Missed Injuries

The frequency of intra-abdominal injuries in patients who meet the criteria for nonoperative management is lower than those who require operative treatment (15% vs. 55%). Missed injuries, a theoretical risk of nonoperative management, have occurred in only four of more than 2000 patients included in both adult and pediatric series [121, 133, 137, 144]. Morse and

Garcia considered this problem specifically and concluded that nonoperative management did not increase the risk of missed abdominal injuries in children [124]. Flaherty and Jurkovich reviewed 182 blunt splenic injuries, 33 of which met the observation criteria retrospectively [143]. All patients were explored for hemoperitoneum, and one had an unsuspected bowel injury. While the risk of a missed injury does not preclude the use of nonoperative approaches, the surgeon must observe the patient closely for signs of other injuries which may not be evident at the outset of management.

Delayed Splenic Rupture

Splenic rupture has been defined as delayed if it occurs 48 h or more after injury [157]. The risk of delayed splenic rupture is a potential complication of nonoperative management [114], although some have argued that this is simply a missed diagnosis [156]. MacIndoe reviewed 46 cases of delayed splenic rupture and found a mortality rate of 27% [106]. Zabinski and Harkins reported a 14% incidence of delayed rupture [107]. During the 1960s, the use of diagnostic peritoneal lavage enabled earlier recognition of hemoperitoneum [96, 157], and the incidence of delayed splenic rupture fell to less than 1%.

In series of nonoperative treatment, 56 cases of delayed splenic rupture have been reported, representing less than 1% of patients treated nonoperatively [63, 67, 71, 73, 129–131, 134–138, 142, 144–146]. This incidence compares favorably with published findings in the era preceding nonoperative management and suggests that an increase in delayed splenic rupture has not been seen with application of nonoperative approaches to splenic injury.

Activity Restrictions

In the early experience with nonoperative management of splenic injury, at least 2 weeks of complete bedrest were recommended [110, 113]. Ein et al. were the first to define activity restrictions, including a 2- to 3-week hospital stay and limited activities for at least another month [115]. More recent studies have recommended 48–72 h of intensive care unit (ICU) monitoring, 7–14 days of inpatient care, and 2–3 months of limited activity [84, 86, 87, 124, 125, 129, 135, 136, 138–140, 154].

These recommendations evolved from clinical experience and have not been based on scientific evidence. The review by Lynch et al. of 53 patients treated nonoperatively demonstrated an average hospitalization of 7 days and a stable hematocrit within 2 days [122]. The authors concluded that ICU monitoring was of no benefit and that most patients could have been discharged after 3 days. Activity restrictions were continued after discharge until healing was demonstrated by CT or ultrasonography.

Pranikoff et al. evaluated the use of CT in postinjury management [125]. CT scans performed at 6 weeks after injury showed healing of the majority of fractures and reperfusion of previously nonperfused areas. Follow-up CT scans decreased the length of activity restriction in minor injuries, but did not alter management for more severe injuries. We recommend that postinjury care should include early monitoring for 48–72 h, with serial hematocrits and abdominal examinations. Activity should increase while patients are still in hospital, and healing of the injury by CT should dictate when activity limitations are to be lifted.

Radiologic Evaluation

Historical Perspective

Nonoperative therapy depends upon accurate radiologic evaluation of the abdomen. O'Marra et al. were the first to use radionuclide scintigraphy to evaluate the spleen for injury [158]. Spleen scanning was also recommended as a tool to monitor splenic healing after injury [111, 159, 160]. CT was introduced as another modality to evaluate splenic injury in 1980 [161] (Fig. 5). Subsequent reports demonstrated an accuracy rate greater than 90% in identification of splenic injuries [162–164]. In addition, CT offers information about other intra-abdominal structures and quantitates the volume of hemoperitoneum (Figs. 6, 7). Because of these advantages, CT has become the standard for abdominal evaluation in the stable patient in most centers. Splenic imaging is discussed by Komaiko (this volume).

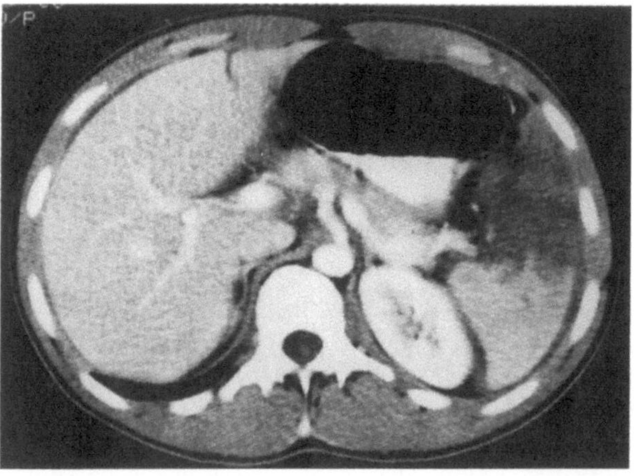

Fig. 5. Abdominal computed tomography (CT) scan demonstrating a splenic injury

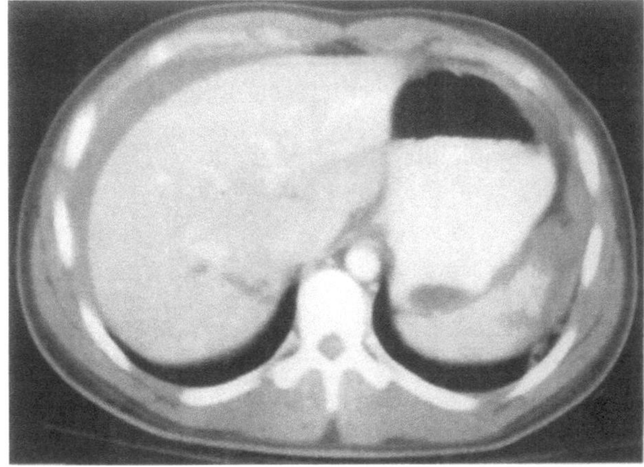

Fig. 6. Abdominal computed tomography (CT) scan demonstrating a splenic injury and hepatic laceration

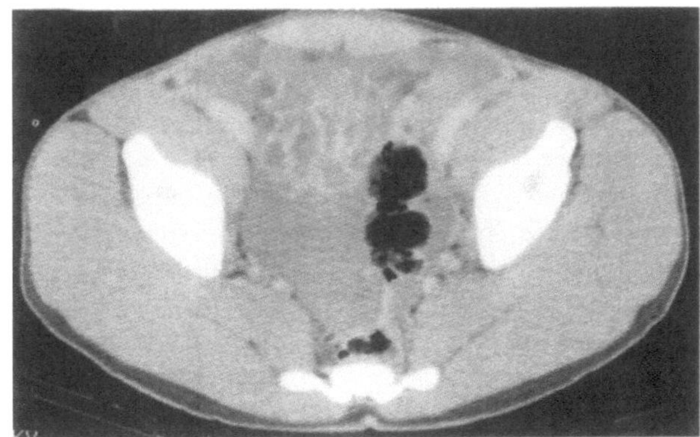

Fig. 7. Abdominal computed tomography (CT) scan with hemoperitoneum extending into the pelvis

Grading Systems

With the emphasis on nonoperative management and the application of CT, scoring systems were developed to grade splenic injuries. These grading systems provide criteria to compare outcomes and guide treatment as well as a means to compare reports by different investigators.

Although CT is highly accurate in identifying the presence of splenic injury, the determination of injury severity has been less accurate. Buntain demonstrated an accuracy of 97% in CT diagnosis of splenic injury, but only 75% in injury grading [74]. Other investigators have found CT grading to underestimate or misgrade splenic injury in 20%–50% of patients [141, 165, 166].

Moreover, CT grading of splenic injuries has not correlated well with successful nonoperative treatment. Resciniti et al. [75] used both splenic injury and presence of hemoperitoneum as elements of a CT scoring system and found that these criteria increased the predictive value of CT evaluation and successful nonoperative management. However, other studies have found poor correlation between splenic injury grading and successful nonoperative management [146, 165, 166]. These observations underscore the very fundamental principle that the ultimate decision to operate must be determined by the patient's condition and not by the degree of injury on CT.

Postsplenectomy Management

Splenosis

Persistence of functioning spleen tissue after splenectomy is a well-known phenomenon. In 1910, Von Kuttner found diffuse functioning nodules at autopsy in a patient who had splenic injury from an abdominal gunshot wound (cited in [167]), as have other authors [168, 169].

The true incidence of splenosis after trauma was evaluated by Pearson et al. [170], who concluded that it was common: more than half of 22 children undergoing splenectomy had absence of Howell-Jolly bodies on peripheral blood smear, which represents hematologic evidence of splenic function, and five demonstrated radionuclide uptake consistent with splenic nodules. Traub et al. reported similar findings, with eight of 19 patients demonstrating splenosis when evaluated 2 years after splenectomy [171]. Case reports of OPSI in patients with documented splenosis or accessory spleens [21, 23, 172] emphasize that the presence of ectopic splenic tissue does not diminish the advisability of splenic preservation, as the presence of functioning splenic tissue does not guarantee intact immunologic function.

Splenic Autotransplantation

Given that residual splenic tissue is common and has some level of function, splenic autotransplantation after splenectomy has been studied. Animal investigations have demonstrated that, while autografts provide improved immunologic protection over splenectomy, subjects with splenic tissue left in situ exhibited the highest level of protection against bacterial challenge [13, 105, 173–176]. The question arises as to how much vascularized splenic tissue is necessary. As was emphasized in the prior discussion of repair techniques, Van Wyck et al. found a correlation between splenic mass and the lethal dose of pneumococcus; a critical mass of at least one third was necessary to restore host resistance [104].

Autotransplantation in humans was first reported in 1981 by Patel et al. [177]. Four patients underwent splenectomy and subsequent autotransplantation; 4 weeks later, there was hematologic evidence of splenic function. Moore reported 43 patients who had splenectomy and autotransplantation [62]. The implants were viable by technetium scanning at 6 months, although one patient died of overwhelming pneumococcal pneumonia. Autotransplantation does not appear to restore all splenic function, particularly immunologic function, and we cannot recommend it as a treatment modality.

Vaccination

A vaccine incorporating 14 pneumococcal capsular polysaccharide antigens became available in the United States in 1977 [178]. Ammann et al. concluded that immunization of asplenic patients could protect them from pneumococcal infection [179], although Broome et al. demonstrated that vaccinated patients could still develop pneumococcal infection with serotypes included in the vaccine [180]. This raised the question of clinical efficacy as distinct from antibody response to vaccination. Butler et al. [178] showed an overall vaccine efficacy of 57% and an efficacy of 77% in asplenic patients in a review that included patients who had received both the original 14 valent vaccine and the newer 23 valent vaccine.

Timing of pneumococcal vaccination also has been debated. Dawes et al. demonstrated adequate antibody responses after immunization in an animal model, with or without the presence of a spleen [181]. Antibody responses of postoperative splenectomy patients were similar to those of normal controls, despite receiving the vaccine within 72 h of operation [182].

Long-term efficacy and the need for revaccination have not been well defined. Butler et al. showed that the efficacy of the vaccine did not decline over time, with 80% efficacy at 9 years or more [178]. However, because there is the potential for a variable response to the vaccine, revaccination has been recommended as early as 2 years [183]. Rutherford et al. demonstrated a doubling of antibody titers in 48% of patients revaccinated 2 years after splenectomy [184]. Current recommendations are revaccination at 6 years for adults and 3–5 years for children [185]. All patients undergoing splenectomy should receive pneumococcal vaccination prior to discharge, and revaccination should be recommended.

Pneumococcus is responsible for 50% of overwhelming infection [22, 25, 26]. Vaccination against other encapsulated organisms, such as *Haemophilus influenzae* and *Neisseria meningitidis*, is a matter of current debate, but may decrease the risk of infection from these organisms. These issues are also discussed by Stiehm (this volume).

Antibiotic Prophylaxis

While antibiotic prophylaxis to prevent OPSI has been recommended by some authors [24, 186], patient compliance with prophylactic regimens is known to be poor [187], and development of resistant bacterial strains is a risk. The efficacy of prophylaxis in prevention of OPSI has not determined.

Summary

The evolution of management of splenic trauma has been discussed. Once regarded as completely dispensable, the injured spleen is now preserved wherever possible in order to avoid the infectious risks of the asplenic state. Prompt exploration and splenectomy are reserved for patients with hemodynamic instability and severe injuries. Splenic preservation includes a range of options, including techniques of splenic repair, partial resection, and nonoperative management of demonstrated injuries. Future investigations will define new operative approaches and improvements in postinjury management, including prophylaxis and treatment of infectious complications.

References

1. Sabiston DC (ed) (1991) Textbook of surgery. Saunders, Philadelphia
2. Peck AL (1955) Aristotle parts of animals 3.12. Harvard University Press, Cambridge MA
3. Kocher ET (ed) (1911) Textbook of operative surgery. Black, London
4. Morris DH, Bullock FD (1919) The importance of the spleen in resistance to infection. Ann Surg 70:513–521
5. King H, Schumacher HB (1952) Splenic studies. I. Susceptibility to infection after splenectomy performed in infancy. Ann Surg 136:239–242
6. Smith CH, Erlandson M, Schulman I, Stern G (1957) Hazard of severe infections in splenectomized infants and children. Am J Med 22:390–404
7. Lockwood CM (1983) Immunological functions of the spleen. Clin Haematol 12:449–465
8. Baker CC, Miller CL, Trunkey DD, Lim RC (1979) Identity of mononuclear cells which compromise the resistance of trauma patients. J Surg Res 26:478–487
9. Tung G, Miller C, Lim RC, Fisher E (1977) Effect of splenectomy on patients' immunocompetent leukocytes. Surg Forum 28:337–339
10. Claret I, Morales L, Montaner A (1975) Immunologic studies in the postsplenectomy syndrome. J Ped Surg 10:59–64
11. Schumacher MJ (1970) Serum immunoglobulin and transferrin levels after childhood splenectomy. Arch Dis Child 45:114–117
12. Downey EC, Shackford SR, Fridlund PH, Ninnemann JL (1987) Long-term depressed immune function in patients splenectomized for trauma. J Trauma 27:661–663
13. Cooney DR, Dearth JC, Swanson SE, Dewanjee MK, Telander RL (1979) Relative merits of partial splenectomy, splenic reimplantation, and immunization in preventing post splenectomy infection. Surg 86:561–569
14. Chaimoff C, Douer D, Pick IA, Pinkhas J (1978) Serum immunoglobulin changes after accidental splenectomy in adults. Am J Surg 136:332–333
15. Andersen V, Cohn J, Sorensen SF (1976) Immunological studies in children before and after splenectomy. Acta Paediatr Scand 65:409–415
16. Constantopoulos A, Najjar VA, Wish JB, Necheles TH, Stolbach LL (1973) Defective phagocytosis due to tuftsin deficiency in splenectomized subjects. Am J Dis Child 125:663–665
17. Spirer Z, Zakuth V, Diamant S, Mondorf W, Stefanescu T, Stabinsky Y, Fridkin M (1977) Decreased tuftsin concentrations in patients who have undergone splenectomy. Br Med J 2:1574–1576
18. Carlisle HN, Saslaw S (1959) Properdin levels in splenectomized persons. Proc Soc Exp Biol Med 102:150–154

19. Hosea SW, Brown EJ, Hamburger MI, Frank MM (1981) Opsonic requirements for intravascular clearance after splenectomy. New Engl J Med 304:245–250
20. Diamond LK (1969) Splenectomy in childhood and the hazard of overwhelming infection. Pediatrics 43:886–889
21. Bisno AL, Freeman JC (1970) The syndrome of asplenia, pneumococcal sepsis and disseminated intravascular coagulation. Ann Intern Med 72:389–393
22. Singer DB (1973) Postsplenectomy sepsis. Persp Pediatr Pathol 1:285–311
23. Gopal V, Bisno AL (1977) Fulminant pneumococcal infections in "normal" asplenic hosts. Arch Intern Med 137:1526–1530
24. Krivit W (1977) Overwhelming postsplenectomy infection. Am J Hematol 2:193–201
25. Dickerman JD (1979) Splenectomy and sepsis: a warning. Pediatrics 63:938–941
26. Francke EL, Neu HC (1981) Postsplenectomy infection. Surg Clin N Am 61:135–155
27. Schwartz PE, Sterioff S, Mucha P, Melton LJ, Offord KP (1982) Postsplenectomy sepsis and mortality in adults. JAMA 248:2279–2283
28. Sass W, Bergholz, Kehl A (1983) Overwhelming infection after splenectomy in spite of some spleen remaining. Klin Wochenschr 61:1075
29. Eraklis AJ, Filler RM (1972) Splenectomy in childhood: a review of 1,413 cases. J Pediatr Surg 7:382–388
30. Condon RE (1982) Post-splenectomy sepsis in traumatized adults. J Trauma 22:169–70
31. Sherman RT (1982) Panel: "splenic injuries". J Trauma 22:507–510
32. O'Neal BJ, McDonald JC (1981) The risk of sepsis in the asplenic adult. Ann Surg 194:775–778
33. Sekikawa J, Shatney CH (1983) Septic sequelae after splenectomy for trauma in adults. Am J Surg 145:667–673
34. Chaikof EL, McCabe CJ (1985) Fatal overwhelming post splenectomy infection. Am J Surg 149:534–539
35. Luna GK, Dellinger EP (1987) Nonoperative observation therapy for splenic injuries: a safe therapeutic option? Am J Surg 153:462–468
36. Horan M, Colebatch JH (1962) Relation between splenectomy and subsequent infection: a clinical study. Arch Dis Child 37:398–414
37. Slater H (1973) Complications of splenectomy. Am Surg 39:221–223
38. McKinnon WM, Sanders HS, Zamora LF, Marion L (1973) Splenectomy: indications, results and complications in 406 patients. Am Surg 39:72–74
39. Steele M, Lim RC (1975) Advances in management of splenic injuries. Am J Surg 130:159–165
40. Goins WA, Rodriguez A, Joshi M, Jacobs D (1990) Intra-abdominal abscess after blunt abdominal trauma. Ann Surg 212:60–65
41. Feliciano DV, Bitondo CG, Mattox KL, Rumisek JD, Burch JM, Jordan GL (1985) A four-year experience with splenectomy versus splenorrhaphy. Ann Surg 201:568–575
42. Duke BJ, Modin GW, Schecter WP, Horn JK (1993) Transfusion significantly increases the risk for infection after splenic injury. Arch Surg 128:1125–1132
43. Sherman R (1980) Perspectives in management of trauma to the spleen: 1979 Presidential address, American Association for the Surgery of Trauma. J Trauma 20:1–13
44. Dretzka L (1930) Rupture of the spleen: a report of 27 cases. Surg Gynecol Obstet 51:258–261
45. Morgenstern L (1965) Experimental partial splenectomy: application of cyanoacrylate monomer tissue adhesive for hemostasis. Am Surg 31:709–712
46. Mishalany H (1974) Repair of the ruptured spleen. J Pediatr Surg 9:175–178
47. Sherman NJ, Asch MJ (1978) Conservative surgery for splenic injuries. Pediatrics 61:267–271
48. Slim MS, Najjar NE, Mishalany HG (1979) Preservation of the injured spleen. Br J Surg 66:671–672
49. Weinstein ME, Govin GG, Rice CL, Virgilio RW (1979) Splenorrhaphy for splenic trauma. J Trauma 19:692–697
50. Pachter HL, Hofstetter SR, Spencer FC (1981) Evolving concepts in splenic surgery. Ann Surg 194:262–269

51. Oakes DD, Charters AC (1981) Changing concepts in the management of splenic trauma. Surg Gynecol Obstet 153:181–185
52. Giuliano AE, Lim RC (1981) Is splenic salvage safe in the traumatized patient? Arch Surg 116:651–656
53. Shackford SR, Sise MJ, Virgilio RW, Peters RM (1981) Evaluation of splenorrhaphy: a grading system for splenic trauma. J Trauma 21:538–542
54. King DR, Lobe TE, Haase GM, Boles ET (1981) Selective management of injured spleen. Surgery 90:677–682
55. Millikan JS, Moore EE, Moore GE, Stevens RE (1982) Alternatives to splenectomy in adults after trauma. Am J Surg 144:711–716
56. Traub AC, Perry JF (1982) Splenic preservation following splenic trauma. J Trauma 22:496–501
57. Hebeler RF, Ward RE, Miller PW, Ben-Menachem Y (1982) The management of splenic injury. J Trauma 22:492–495
58. Scheele J, Gentsch HH, Matteson E (1982) Splenic repair by fibrin tissue adhesive and collagen fleece. Surgery 95:6–12
59. Kakkasseril JS, Stewart D, Cox JA, Gelfand M (1982) Changing treatment of pediatric splenic trauma. Arch Surg 117:758–759
60. Barrett J, Sheaff C, Abuabara S, Jonasson O (1983) Splenic preservation in adults after blunt and penetrating trauma. Am J Surg 145:313–317
61. Morgenstern L, Uyeda RY (1983) Nonoperative management of injuries of the spleen in adults. Surg Gynecol Obstet 157:513–518
62. Moore FA, Moore EE, Moore GE, Millikan JS (1984) Risk of splenic salvage after trauma. Am J Surg 148:800–805
63. Malangoni MA, Levine AW, Droege EA, Aprahamian C, Condon RE (1984) Management of injury to the spleen in adults. Ann Surg 200:702–705
64. Bitseff EL, Adkins RB (1984) Splenic trauma: a trial of selective management. South Med J 77:1286–1290
65. Solheim K, Hoivik B (1985) Changing trends in the diagnosis and management of rupture of the spleen. Injury 16:221–226
66. Flancbaum L, Dauterive A, Cox EF (1986) Splenic conservation after multiple trauma in adults. Surg Gynecol Obstet 162:469–473
67. Mucha P, Daly RC, Farnell MB (1986) Selective management of blunt splenic trauma. J Trauma 26:970–979
68. Gourevitch D, Hadley GP (1986) Splenic conservation after trauma in children. Surg Gynecol Obstet 163:536–538
69. Norby II, Max MH (1986) Splenorrhaphy in patients with abdominal trauma. South Med J 79:1503–1505
70. Kreis DJ, Montero N, Saltz M, Saltz R, Echenique M, Plasencia G et al (1987) The role of splenorrhaphy in splenic trauma. Am Surg 53:307–309
71. Splenic Injury Study Group (1987) Splenic injury: a prospective multi-centre study on non-operative and operative treatment. Br J Surg 74:310–313
72. Beal SL, Spisso JM (1988) The risk of splenorrhaphy. Arch Surg 123:1158–1163
73. Nallathambi MN, Ivatury RR, Wapnir I, Rohman M, Stahl WM (1988) Nonoperative management versus early operation for blunt splenic trauma in adults. Surg Gynecol Obstet 166:252–258
74. Buntain WL, Gould HR, Maull KI (1988) Predictability of splenic salvage by computed tomography. J Trauma 28:24–34
75. Resciniti A, Fink MP, Raptopoulos V, Davidoff A, Silva WE (1988) Nonoperative treatment of adult splenic trauma: development of a computed tomographic scoring system that detects appropriate candidates for expectant management. J Trauma 28:828–831
76. Pickhardt B, Moore EE, Moore FA, McCroskey BL, Moore GE (1989) Operative splenic salvage in adults: a decade perspective. J Trauma 29:1386–1391
77. Elmore JR, Clark DE, Isler RJ, Horner WR (1989) Selective nonoperative management of blunt splenic trauma in adults. Arch Surg 124:581–586

78. Feliciano DV, Spjut-Patrinely V, Burch JM, Mattox KL, Bitondo CG, Cruse-Martocci PC et al (1990) Splenorrhaphy. Ann Surg 211:569–582
79. Pachter HL, Spencer FC, Hofstetter SR, Liang HG, Hoballah J, Coppa GF (1990) Experience with selective operative and nonoperative treatment of splenic injuries in 193 patients. Ann Surg 211:583–591
80. Williams MD, Young DH, Schiller WR (1990) Trend toward nonoperative management of splenic injuries. Am J Surg 160:588–593
81. Lally KP, Rosario V, Malhour GH, Woolley MM (1990) Evolution in the management of splenic injury in children. Surg Gynecol Obstet 170:245–248
82. Rappaport W, McIntyre KE, Carmona R (1990) The management of splenic trauma in the adult patient with blunt multiple injuries. Surg Gynecol Obstet 170:204–208
83. Molin MR, Shackford SR (1990) The management of splenic trauma in a trauma system. Arch Surg 125:840–843
84. Koury HI, Peschiera JL, Welling RE (1991) Non-operative management of blunt splenic trauma: a 10 year experience. Injury 22:349–352
85. Witte CL, Esser MJ, Rappaport WD (1992) Updating the management of salvageable splenic injury. Ann Surg 215:261–265
86. Smith JS, Wengrovitz MA, DeLong BS (1992) Prospective validation of criteria, including age, for safe, non surgical management of the ruptured spleen. J Trauma 33:363–369
87. Jalovec LM, Boe BS, Wyffels PL (1993) The advantages of early operation with splenorrhaphy versus nonoperative management for blunt splenic trauma patient. Am Surg 59:698–705
88. Sherman R (1984) Management of trauma to the spleen. Adv Surg 17:37–71
89. Moore EE, Shackford SR, Pachter HR, McAninch JW, Browner BD, Champion HR et al (1989) Organ injury scaling: spleen, liver and kidney. J Trauma 29:1664–1666
90. Moore EE, Cogbill TH, Jurkovich GJ, Shackford SR, Malangoni MA, Champion HR (1995) Organ injury scaling: spleen and liver (1994 revision). J Trauma 38:323–324
91. Buntain WL, Lynn HB (1979) Splenorrhaphy: changing concepts for the traumatized spleen. Surgery 86:748–760
92. Morgenstern L, Shapiro SJ (1979) Techniques of splenic conservation. Arch Surg 114:449–454
93. O'Connor GS, Geelhoed GW (1986) Splenic trauma and salvage. Am Surg 52:456–462
94. Dunham CM, Cornwell EE, Militello P (1991) The role of the argon beam coagulator in splenic salvage. Surg Gynecol Obstet 173:179–182
95. Sherman R (1981) Rationale for and methods of splenic preservation following trauma. Surg Clin N Am 61:127–134
96. Lucas CE (1991) Splenic trauma: choice of management. Ann Surg 213:98–112
97. Delany HM, Porreca F, Mitsudo S, Solanski B, Rudavsky A (1982) Splenic capping: an experimental study of a new technique for splenorrhaphy using woven polyglycolic acid mesh. Ann Surg 196:187–193
98. Lange DA, Zaret P, Merlotti GJ, Robin AP, Sheaff C, Barrett JA (1988) The use of absorbable mesh in splenic trauma. J Trauma 28:269–275
99. Rogers FB, Baumgartner NE, Robin AP, Barrett JA (1991) Absorbable mesh splenorrhaphy for severe splenic injuries: functional studies in an animal model and an additional patient series. J Trauma 31:200–204
100. Hadley GP (1984) Splenic artery ligation – an adjunct to splenorrhaphy in children. S Afr Med J 66:578–579
101. Keramidas DC (1979) The ligation of the splenic artery in the treatment of traumatic rupture of the spleen. Surgery 85:530–533
102. Conti S (1980) Splenic artery ligation for trauma. Am J Surg 140:444–446
103. Ravo B, Ger R (1988) Splenic preservation with the use of a stapling instrument: a preliminary communication. J Trauma 28:115–117
104. Van Wyck DB, Witte MH, Witte CL, Thies AC (1980) Critical splenic mass for survival from experimental pneumococcemia. J Surg Res 28:14–17

105. Pringle KC, Rowley D, Burrington JD (1980) Immunologic response in splenectomized and partially splenectomized rats. J Pediatr Surg 15:531–536
106. McIndoe AH (1932) Delayed hemorrhage following traumatic rupture of the spleen. Br J Surg 20:249–268
107. Zabinski EJ, Harkins HN (1943) Delayed splenic rupture: a clinical syndrome following trauma. Arch Surg 46:186–213
108. Bailey H (1927) Traumatic rupture of the normal spleen. Br J Surg 15:40–46
109. Upadhyaya P, Simpson JS (1968) Splenic trauma in children. Surg Gynecol Obstet 126:781–790
110. Douglas GJ, Simpson JS (1971) The conservative management of splenic trauma. J Pediatr Surg 6:565–570
111. Howman-Giles R, Gilday DL, Venugopal S, Shandling B, Ash JM (1978) Splenic trauma – nonoperative management and long-term followup by scintiscan. J Pediatr Surg 13:121–126
112. Solheim K (1979) Non operative management of splenic rupture. Acta Chir Scand 145:55–58
113. Aronson DZ, Scherz AW, Einhorn AH, Becker JM, Schneider KM (1977) Nonoperative management of splenic trauma in children: a report of six consecutive cases. Pediatrics 60:482–485
114. Joseph TP, Wyllie GG, Savage JP (1977) The non-operative management of splenic trauma. Aust NZ J Surg 47:179–182
115. Ein SH, Shandling B, Simpson JS, Stephens CA (1978) Nonoperative management of traumatized spleen in children: how and why? J Pediatr Surg 13:117–119
116. Wesson DE, Filler RM, Ein SH, Shandling B, Simpson JS, Stephens CA (1981) Ruptured spleen – when to operate? J Pediatr Surg 16:324–326
117. Filler RM (1984) Experience with the management of splenic injuries. Aust NZ J Surg 54:443–445
118. Buyukunal C, Danismend N, Yeker D (1987) Spleen-saving procedures in paediatric spleen trauma. Br J Surg 74:350–352
119. Muehrcke DD, Kim SH, McCabe CJ (1987) Pediatric spleen trauma: predicting the success of nonoperative therapy. Am J Emerg Med 5:109–112
120. Pearl RH, Wesson DH, Spence CJ, Filler RM, Ein SH, Shandling B et al (1989) Splenic injury: a 5-year update with improved results and changing criteria for conservative management. J Pediatr Surg 24:428–431
121. Consentino CM, Luck SR, Barthel MJ, Reynolds M, Raffensperger JG (1990) Transfusion requirements in conservative nonoperative management of blunt splenic and hepatic injuries during childhood. J Pediatr Surg 25:950–954
122. Lynch JM, Ford H, Gardner MJ, Weiner ES (1993) Is early discharge following isolated splenic injury in the hemodynamically stable child possible? J Pediatr Surg 28:1403–1407
123. Haller JA, Pape P, Drugas G, Colombani P (1994) Nonoperative management of solid organ injuries in children. Is it safe? Ann Surg 219:625–631
124. Morse MA, Garcia VF (1994) Selective nonoperative management of pediatric blunt splenic trauma: risk for missed associated injuries. J Pediatr Surg 29:23–27
125. Pranikoff T, Hirschl RB, Schlesinger AE, Polley TZ, Coran AG (1994) Resolution of splenic injury after nonoperative management. J Pediatr Surg 29:1366–1369
126. Schwartz MZ, Kangah R (1994) Splenic injury in children after blunt trauma: blood transfusion requirements and length of hospitalization for laparotomy versus observation. J Pediatr Surg 29:596–598
127. Coburn MC, Pfeifer J, DeLuca FG (1995) Nonoperative management of splenic and hepatic trauma in the multiply injured pediatric and adolescent patient. Arch Surg 130:332–338
128. Hunter RA, Kiroff GK, Jamieson GG (1984) The injured spleen: should consideration be given to conservative management? Aust NZ J Surg 54:129–135
129. Zucker K, Browns K, Rossman D, Hemingway D, Saik R (1984) Nonoperative management of splenic trauma. Arch Surg 119:400–404

130. Mahon PA, Sutton JE (1985) Nonoperative management of adult splenic injury due to blunt trauma: a warning. Am J Surg 149:716–721

131. Tom WW, Howells GA, Bree RL, Schwab R, Lucas RJ (1985) A nonoperative approach to the adult rupture spleen sustained from blunt trauma. Am Surg 51:367–371

132. Andersson R, Alwmark A, Gullstrand P, Offenbartl K, Bengmark S (1986) Nonoperative treatment of blunt trauma to liver and spleen. Acta Chir Scand 152:739–741

133. Johnson H, Shatney CH (1986) Splenic injuries in adults: selective nonoperative management. South Med J 79:5–8

134. Kidd WT, Liu RCK, Khoo R, Nixon J (1987) The management of blunt splenic trauma. J Trauma 27:977–979

135. Moss JF, Hopkins WM (1987) Nonoperative management of blunt splenic trauma in the adult: a community hospital's experience. J Trauma 27:315–318

136. Wiebke EA, Sarr MG, Fishman EK, Ratych RE (1987) Nonoperative management of splenic injuries in adults: an alternative in selected patients. Am Surg 53:547–552

137. Cogbill TH, Moore EE, Jurkovich GJ, Morris JA, Mucha P, Shackford SR (1989) Nonoperative management of blunt splenic trauma: a multicenter experience. J Trauma 29:1312–1317

138. Delius RE, Frankel W, Coran AG (1989) A comparison between operative and nonoperative management of blunt injuries to the liver and spleen in adult and pediatric patients. Surgery 106:788–793

139. Longo WE, Baker CC, McMillan MA, Modlin IM, Degutis LC, Zucker KA (1989) Nonoperative management of adult blunt splenic trauma. Ann Surg 210:626–629

140. Klin B, Rivkind A, Krausz Y, Rabinovici R, Chisin R, Eyal Z (1990) Nonoperative management of blunt splenic trauma in adults. Int Surg 75:50–53

141. Malangoni MA, Cue JI, Fallat ME, Willing SJ, Richardson JD (1990) Evaluation of splenic injury by computed tomography and its impact on treatment. Ann Surg 211:592–599

142. Villalba MR, Howells GA, Lucas RJ, Glover JL, Bendick PJ, Tran Oanh et al (1990) Nonoperative management of the adult ruptured spleen. Arch Surg 125:836–839

143. Flaherty L, Jurkovich GJ (1991) Minor splenic injuries: associated injuries and transfusion requirements. J Trauma 31:1618–1621

144. Oller B, Armergol M, Camps I, Rodriguez N, Montero A, Inaraja L et al (1991) Nonoperative management of splenic injuries. Am Surg 57:409–413

145. Schweizer W, Bohlen L, Dennison A, Blumgart LH (1992) Prospective study in adults of splenic preservation after traumatic rupture. Br J Surg 79:1330–1333

146. Kohn JS, Clark DE, Isler RJ, Pope CF (1994) Is computed tomographic grading of splenic injury useful in the nonsurgical management of blunt trauma? J Trauma 36:385–389

147. Erzurum VZ, Raimonde AJ (1996) Trends in splenic salvage in a community teaching hospital. Contrib Surg 48:31–34

148. Gross P (1964) Zur kindlichen traumatischen Milzruptur. Beitr Klin Chirurg 208:396–401

149. Mazel MS (1945) Traumatic rupture of the spleen. J Pediatr 26:82–88

150. Livingston CD, Sirinek KR, Levine BA, Aust JB (1982) Traumatic splenic injury. Arch Surg 117:670–674

151. Heymann SJ, Brewer TF (1993) The infectious risks of transfusion in the United States: a decision analytic approach. Am J Infect Control 21:174–82

152. Donahue JG, Munoz A, Ness PM, Brown DE, Yawn DH, McAllister HA et al (1992) The declining rise of post-transfusion hepatitis C virus infection. New Engl J Med 327:369–373

153. Feliciano PD, Mullins RJ, Trunkey DD, Crass RA, Beck JR, Helfand M (1992) A decision analysis of traumatic splenic injuries. J Trauma 33:340–348

154. Velanovich V, Tapper D (1993) Decision analysis in children with blunt splenic trauma: the effects of observation, splenorrhaphy or splenectomy on quality adjusted life expectancy. J Pediatr Surg 28:179–185

155. Shackford SR, Molin M (1990) Management of splenic injuries. Surg Clin N Am 70:595–620
156. Blaisdell FW. Discussion in Olsen WR, Folley TZ (1977) A second look at delayed splenic rupture. Arch Surg 112: 422–425
157. Olsen WR, Polley TZ (1977) A second look at delayed splenic rupture. Arch Surg 112:422–425
158. O'Marra RE, Hall RC, Dombroski DL (1970) Scintiscanography in the diagnosis of rupture of the spleen. Surg Gynecol Obstet 130:1077–1084
159. Lutzker LG, Chun KJ (1981) Radionuclide imaging in the nonsurgical treatment of liver and spleen trauma. J Trauma 21:382–387
160. Mishalany HG, Miller JH, Woolley MM (1982) Radioisotope spleen scan in patients with splenic injury. Arch Surg 117:1147–1150
161. Mall JC, Kaiser JA (1980) CT diagnosis of splenic laceration. Am J Roentgenol 134:265–269
162. Karp MP, Cooney DR, Berger PE, Kuhn JP, Jewett TC (1981) The role of computed tomography in the evaluation of blunt abdominal trauma in children. J Pediatr Surg 16:316–323
163. Berger PE, Kuhn JP (1981) CT of blunt abdominal trauma in childhood. Am J Roentgenol 136:105–110
164. Jeffrey RB, Laing FC, Federle MP, Goodman PC (1981) Computed tomography of splenic trauma. Radiology 141:729–732
165. Mirvis SE, Whitley NO, Gens DR (1989) Blunt splenic trauma in adults: CT-based classification and correlation with prognosis and treatment. Radiology 171:33–39
166. Umlas SL, Cronan JJ (1991) Splenic trauma: can CT grading systems enable predictions of successful non surgical treatment. Radiology 178:481–487
167. Cahill CJ, Wastell C (1990) Splenic conservation. Surg Ann 22:379–404
168. Widmann WD, Laubscher FA (1971) Splenosis: a disease or beneficial condition? Arch Surg 102:152–158
169. Brewster DC (1973) Splenosis: report of two cases and review of the literature. Am J Surg 126:14–19
170. Pearson HA, Johnston D, Smith KA, Touloukian RJ (1978) The born again spleen. New Engl J Med 298:1389–1392
171. Traub A, Giebink GS, Smith C, Kuni CC, Brekke ML, Edlund D et al (1987) Splenic reticuloendothelial function after splenectomy, spleen repair and spleen autotransplantation. New Engl J Med 317:1559–1564
172. Davis C, Alexander RW, DeYoung HD (1963) Splenosis: a sequel to traumatic rupture of the spleen. Arch Surg 86:523–533
173. Goldthorn JF, Schwartz AD, Swift AJ, Winkelstein JA (1978) Protective effect of residual splenic tissue after subtotal splenectomy. J Pediatr Surg 13:587–590
174. Cooney DR, Michalak WA, Michalak DM, Fisher JE (1981) Comparative methods of splenic preservation. J Pediatr Surg 16:327–338
175. Cooney DR, Swanson SE, Dearth JC, Dewanjee MK, Telander RL (1979) Heterotopic splenic autotransplantation in prevention of overwhelming postsplenectomy infection. J Pediatr Surg 14:336–342
176. Schwartz AD, Goldthorn JF, Winkelstein JA, Swift AJ (1978) Lack of protective effect of autotransplanted splenic tissue to pneumococcal challenge. Blood 51:475–478
177. Patel J, Williams JS, Shmigel B, Hinshaw JR (1981) Preservation of splenic function by autotransplantation of traumatized splenic mass. Surgery 90:683–688
178. Butler JC, Breiman RF, Campbell JF, Lipman HB, Broome CV, Facklam RR (1993) Pneumococcal polysaccharide vaccine efficacy. JAMA 270:1826–1831
179. Ammann AJ, Addiego J, Wara DW, Lubin B, Smith WB, Mentzer WC (1977) Polyvalent pneumococcal polysaccharide immunization of patients with sickle-cell anemia and patients with splenectomy. New Engl J Med 297:897–900
180. Broome CV, Facklam RR, Fraser DW (1980) Pneumococcal disease after pneumococcal vaccination. New Engl J Med 303:549–552

181. Dawes LG, Malangoni MA, Spiegel CA, Schiffman G (1985) Response to immunization after partial and total splenectomy. J Surg Res 39:53–58
182. Caplan ES, Boltansky H, Snyder MJ, Rooney J, Hoyt NJ, Schiffman G et al (1983) Response of traumatized splenectomized patients to immediate vaccination with polyvalent pneumococcal vaccine. J Trauma 23:801–805
183. Lawrence EM, Edwards KM, Schiffman G, Thompson JM, Vaughn WK, Wright PF (1983) Pneumococcal vaccine in normal children. Am J Dis Child 137:846–850
184. Rutherford EJ, Livengood J, Higginbotham M, Miles WS, Koestner J, Edwards KM et al (1995) Efficacy and safety of pneumococcal revaccination after splenectomy for trauma. J Trauma 39:448–452
185. Immunization Practices Advisory Committee (1989) Pneumococcal polysaccharide vaccine. MMWR 38:64–76
186. Powell RW, Blaylock WE, Hoff CJ, Chartrand SA (1988) The efficacy of postsplenectomy sepsis prophylactic measures: the role of penicillin. J Trauma 28:1285–1288
187. Brooks RE, Notario G, McCabe RE (1988) Hospital survey of antimicrobial prophylaxis to prevent endocarditis in patients with prosthetic heart valves. Am J Med 84:617–621

Partial Splenectomy

L. Morgenstern

> "Beside your stomach may be seen
> A pulpy organ called the spleen.
> The body seems to jerk without it
> But since its role is still in doubt, it
> Is prudent on the part of man
> To keep it in him if he can."
> Author unknown

Partial splenectomy figures prominently in the early history of splenic surgery. As described in "The History of Splenectomy" (Morgenstern, this volume), it was performed more frequently and more successfully than total splenectomy by a diverse group of ordinary surgical practitioners during the eighteenth and nineteenth centuries. The conditions under which it was performed, however, were unique to earlier times; in all early recorded instances, partial splenectomy was done for portions of spleen which had prolapsed through wounds of the abdomen and had become mortified by prolonged extraperitoneal exposure. Such exploits were reported by Clark in 1676 [1], Ferguson in 1735 [2], O'Brien in 1816 [3], and Markham in 1874 [4], among others. Although notable as unusual and daring undertakings in times gone by, they hardly qualify as partial splenectomies in the present surgical sense.

Fifty years ago, any procedure on the spleen other than the total extirpation for trauma or disease was unthinkable. Although splenorrhaphies for trauma had been performed earlier in the century by Mayo [5] and others [6, 7], partial splenectomy was not a recognized surgical procedure. It was in 1962 that Marcel Campos Christo of Brazil reported the first true partial splenectomies, describing eight partial splenic resections for trauma [8]. Then in 1966 Morgenstern reported a subtotal splenectomy for myeloid metaplasia [9]. Thereafter an increasing number of reports worldwide attested to the feasibility and safety of partial resection [10–15]. As convincing evidence of the immunologic importance of the spleen accumulated, splenic salvage procedures, including partial splenectomy, have become commonplace in many major surgical centers throughout the world.

Indications

General Principles

Partial splenectomy is a much more difficult procedure than total splenectomy. It requires greater technical expertise, more operative time and usually entails greater blood loss. The decision, therefore, to undertake partial splenectomy must be tempered by good surgical judgment, with a careful weighing of the risks versus benefits of partial resection as compared with total splenectomy.

In general, partial splenectomy should be considered primarily in younger age groups, particularly children. This does not imply that if splenic salvage can be performed safely and expeditiously in any age group that it should not be done. In older age groups, however, the risks of overwhelming post-splenectomy sepsis after total splenectomy are so small that unusual measures for surgical preservation requiring inordinate operative time or increased transfusion requirements are not warranted. Clinical judgment should dictate which procedure is of greatest benefit to the patient.

Partial Splenectomy for Trauma

Trauma remains the principal indication for partial splenectomy. In grade IV injuries to the spleen, when portions of the spleen are obviously completely devitalized by separation from their blood supply, resection of devitalized segments is indicated. When the principal site of injury involves the main hilar vessels, 50% or more of the spleen may be devitalized and should be resected. The technique for such a procedure will be described below.

Inclusion of frankly devitalized segments within an all-inclusive mesh envelope is not advised. Subsequent necrosis and abscess formation are likely sequelae when major portions of devitalized spleen are wrapped *en masse* with viable segments.

Splenic Cysts

Nonparasitic splenic cysts, which may be discovered at any age, do not require total splenectomy. They may be removed in their entirety [16] with a remnant of adjoining spleen (partial splenectomy) or removed subtotally, leaving a minor remnant of the cyst still affixed to the spleen (cystectomy or "splenic decapsulation") [17]. Although the latter procedure is one of lesser complexity, long-term follow-up studies are still not available as to ultimate outcome. Partial splenectomy, on the other hand, encompassing the entire cyst is curative.

Partial splenectomy has also been reported for hydatid (echinococcal) cysts [18]. This approach is still being evaluated. The risk of leaving residual daughter cysts or other developing cysts in the salvaged remnant is still unknown. It is not as clear an indication for partial splenectomy as the nonparasitic splenic cyst.

Questionable Indications

Hodgkin's Disease

Staging laparotomy for Hodgkin's disease is less frequently performed now than previously, since most patients are now treated with radiotherapy and chemotherapy. When staging is performed, particularly in children, partial splenectomy has been proposed as an alternative to total splenectomy to obviate the risks of subsequent sepsis. Such an approach has been reported in studies by Hoekstra [19]. However, the number of missed lesions varies from 1% [20] to 12% [21].

At present, partial splenectomy is not an accepted technique for the staging of Hodgkin's disease because of the uncertainty of residual lesions in the splenic remnant. Further outcome studies, weighing the risks of possible induced immunodeficiency against the benefits of accurate staging, will determine the feasibility of partial splenectomy for this disease.

Gaucher's Disease

Subtotal splenectomy for the massive splenomegaly associated with type I (nonneuronapathic) Gaucher's disease has been reported by Rubin et al. [22], Bar-Maor et al. [23], Morgenstern et al. [24], Fleshner et al. [25] and Guzzetta et al. [26]. The indications for the procedure were splenomegaly and pancytopenia. The rationale for subtotal splenectomy, particularly in children, was postulated as the preservation of splenic immunologic function, some protection against massive hepatic and osseous deposition of glucocerebroside and relief from incapacitating splenomegaly. Follow-up studies by Cohen et al. [27] and Morgenstern et al. [28] have described moderate regrowth of the splenic remnant, but with some relief from bone crises and possibly some protection against sepsis. The availability of enzyme therapy with glucocerebrosidase since 1990 has radically altered the indications for total or partial splenectomy for type I Gaucher's disease. Enzyme replacement therapy obviates the need for splenectomy in most cases [29]. However, the cost may be prohibitive, ranging from $100000 to $400000 annually. As a temporizing measure, therefore, for children and adults in whom replacement therapy is not an option, subtotal splenectomy should still be considered when massive splenomegaly and pancytopenia mandate some form of intervention.

Hematologic Diseases

Partial or subtotal splenectomy has been reported for myeloid metaplasia [9] but has not received acceptance as a valid indication. Partial splenectomy has also been performed in homozygous beta thalassemia [30, 31] to reduce blood requirements and obviate the risk of postsplenectomy sepsis. Outcome studies to validate this approach are still pending. Selective splenic embolization to achieve results comparable to surgical partial splenectomy has been favorably reported [32]. Disadvantages of this method are the pain consequent to splenic infarction and the danger of postnecrotic abscess formation. In idiopathic thrombocytopenic purpura, although some reports have advocated partial splenectomy in children [33, 34], no such approach has been generally accepted at this time.

Other hematological conditions in which partial splenectomy has been performed include hereditary spherocytosis [35], sickle cell beta thalassemia [36] and the prevention of azothioprine-induced neutropenia in young patients awaiting renal transplantation. The use of cyclosporine has obviated the lattermost indication.

Miscellaneous conditions for which partial splenectomies have been performed include solitary splenic abscess [37], spleen-related portal hypertension [38, 39], splenic hamartoma [40], and splenic schistosomiasis [41]. Although individual clinical reports are encouraging, many more outcome studies will be required to justify the choice of partial splenectomy in these conditions.

Relative Contraindications

In general partial splenectomy should not be undertaken in the presence of multivisceral injury, especially if the peritoneal cavity has been contaminated. Likewise, it is foolhardy to pursue the prize of splenic salvage in the elderly if such a course inordinately prolongs operating time, increases blood loss, or otherwise places the patient at risk.

In hematologic conditions of immunologic etiology, such as idiopathic thrombocytopenic purpura or autoimmune hemolytic anemia, partial splenectomy is an unproven and unwarranted procedure.

Techniques

Partial splenectomy may be performed "open", by laparotomy, or by laparoscopy. At this time the greater experience by far is with the open technique.

Preoperative Measures

Informed Consent

Since partial splenectomy is a relatively recent variant in splenic operations, full preoperative disclosure of the nature of the procedure, its risks, benefits and expected outcomes should be discussed with the patient and documented in the patient record. The benefits, particularly for children, include retention of immunologic function and protection against the rare, but well-documented condition of overwhelming postsplenectomy sepsis. The spleen is the largest reticuloendothelial organ in the body and there may be as yet undiscovered benefits of retaining its function.

Among the risks which should be mentioned is the possibility that partial splenectomy may be technically impossible and total splenectomy might be required. Other risks include hemorrhage, in the operative or postoperative period; the possibility of torsion of the splenic remnant (a rare complication); and for those indications in which insufficient data have been collected, the still unknown long-range outcome if partial splenectomy is done.

Preoperative Immunization

If the partial splenectomy is elective, prophylactic immunization should be given as for total splenectomy. These include immunizations given against *Pneumococcus, Hemophilus influenzae* and *Meningococcus.* These should be administered at least 2 weeks preoperatively.

Preoperative antibiotic prophylaxis should follow the present standard for all major abdominal procedures. One preoperative dose of cephalosporin and one postoperative dose suffice.

Preoperative Autologous Blood

In preparation for elective partial splenectomy, it is advisable to store 1 to 2 units of autologous blood obtained 2–4 weeks before operation. Although with present techniques major blood loss is rare, autologous blood in reserve is insurance against unexpected hemorrhagic complications.

Open Technique

Incision (see Fig. 1 in the chapter by Hiatt, this volume)

In emergency laparotomy for trauma, the vertical midline incision is the preferred standard. Although atraumatic delivery of a small spleen is more difficult with this incision, mandatory exploration for other injuries dictates this choice.

For small or moderate-sized spleens, if elective partial splenectomy is contemplated, the left subcostal incision is best for exposure and mobilization of the spleen. In rare instances, when exposure through this incision is not adequate, the incision may be extended vertically in the midline (left-sided "Kehr" incision). This gives the widest possible exposure. Transthoracic extension of the incision, whether vertical or transverse, should never be necessary, even with massively enlarged spleens.

For massively enlarged spleens the vertical midline incision is satisfactory and even preferred by some surgeons (the author among them). The hilar and gastroepiploic vessels are easily accessible and the spleen, however large, is usually mobilized with little difficulty.

In infants and small children, the left upper quadrant transverse incision is satisfactory for most splenic operations, including partial splenectomy.

Step I: Preliminary Splenic Artery Ligation

Control of splenic arterial inflow should be the first step, when time and circumstances permit, in performance of a partial splenectomy. The splenic artery is easily approached through the gastrocolic omentum, as the vessel courses tortuously on the superior aspect of the pancreas. It is encircled by a vessel-loop which can be tightened once the splenic procedure has begun. To occlude the splenic artery, the vessel-loop is pulled taut and fixed in that position by a large hemoclip. Alternatively, the ends of an encircling 0 silk ligature can be manipulated through a Rummell tourniquet for intermittent occlusion of the artery at the will of the operator.

Step II: Atraumatic Mobilization of Spleen

For partial splenectomy by the open technique, it is imperative that the spleen be completely mobilized to the surface of the incision (Fig. 1), allowing manipulation in all planes and full access to all surfaces. This requires division of the splenic "ligaments", described in the chaps. by Morgenstern and Skandalakis (this volume), which tether the spleen in the left upper quadrant and incision of the retroperitoneum 1–2 cm parallel to the posterior splenic surface. The surgeon, positioned on the patient's right, then carefully manipulates the spleen superomedially with the right hand, maintaining utmost care that the splenic capsule is not torn during the mobilization. Although most of the splenic ligaments and peritoneal attachments can be divided by scissors or electrocautery, visible larger vessels should be clipped before division.

Once fully mobilized, the splenic vasculature is assessed. Although splenic vessels have a segmental distribution (Fig. 2), the nature of this distribution varies markedly. The types of splenic blood supply are described in the chaps. by Morgenstern and Skandalakis (this volume). The splenic arterial

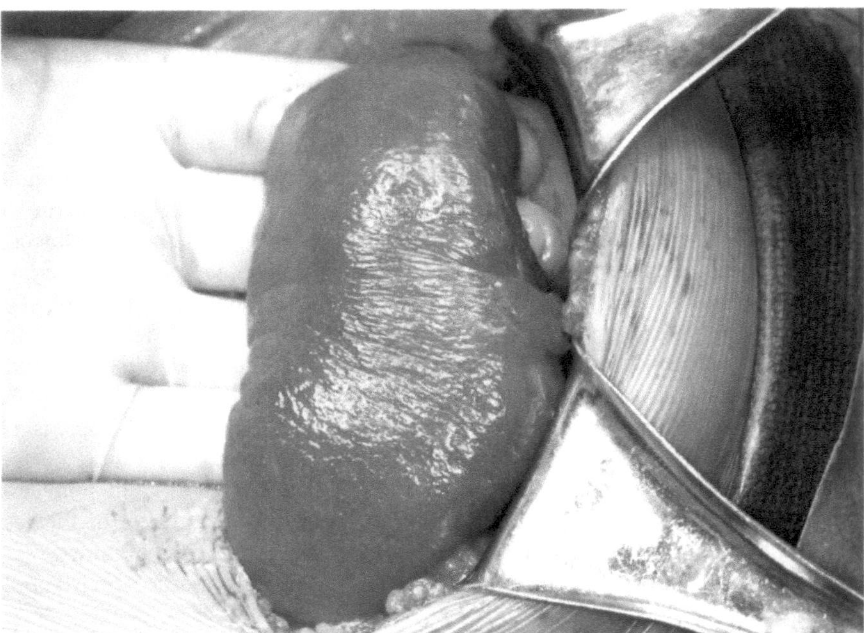

Fig. 1. Extent of mobilization required for partial splenectomy or splenorrhaphy. Spleen should be mobilized to surface of wound allowing access to hilar vessels and all splenic surfaces

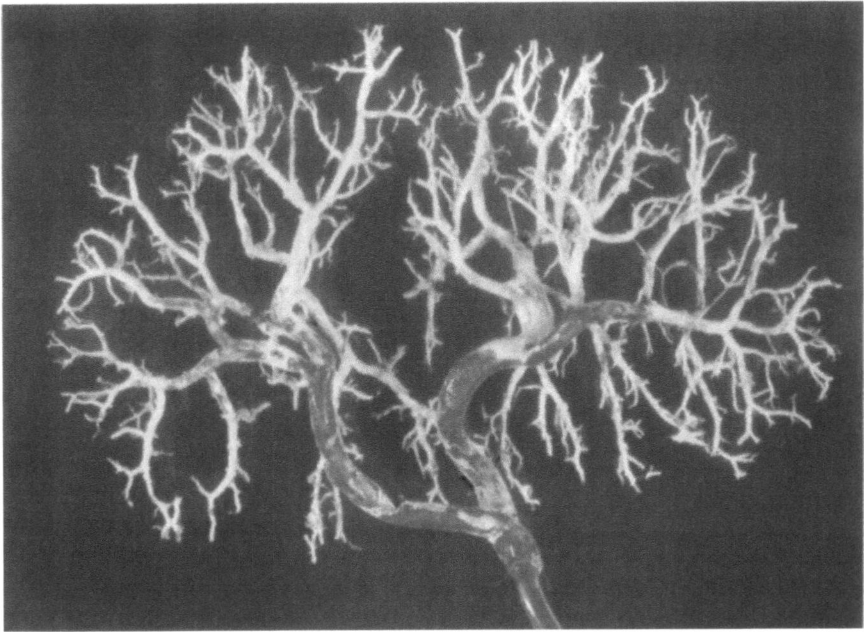

Fig. 2. Vascularization of normal human spleen showing one pattern of segmental distribution. In this spleen, ligation of superior polar artery (first branch) would have devascularized upper half of spleen

branch most accessible for ligation, when indicated, is the superior polar branch. Ligation of this branch usually devascularizes the superior pole of the spleen. In massively enlarged spleens it should not be mistaken for the main splenic artery.

Sites of ligation of the splenic vessels depend on the segment selected for preservation. During ligation of the segmental vessels the vessel-loop encircling the splenic artery is left untightened. As the segmental vasculature is divided, the bluish color of the devascularized splenic parenchyma delineates a clear line of demarcation between viable and nonviable spleen. Vessels are ligated in tandem until the desired size of the remnant is obtained. The choice of the polar segment to be preserved (upper or lower) depends on the operative findings, the nature of the disease, and character of the vasculature. In general, preservation of the upper pole or upper half of the spleen allows less likelihood of postoperative torsion, as the splenic remnant is returned to a more or less natural position in the left upper quadrant.

In traumatic cases, the line of demarcation between viable and nonviable may already have been created by traumatic division or avulsion of the segmental vessels (Fig. 3). In such cases, as hemostasis is being obtained, care must be taken not to ligate any additional segmental vessels which supply the remnant.

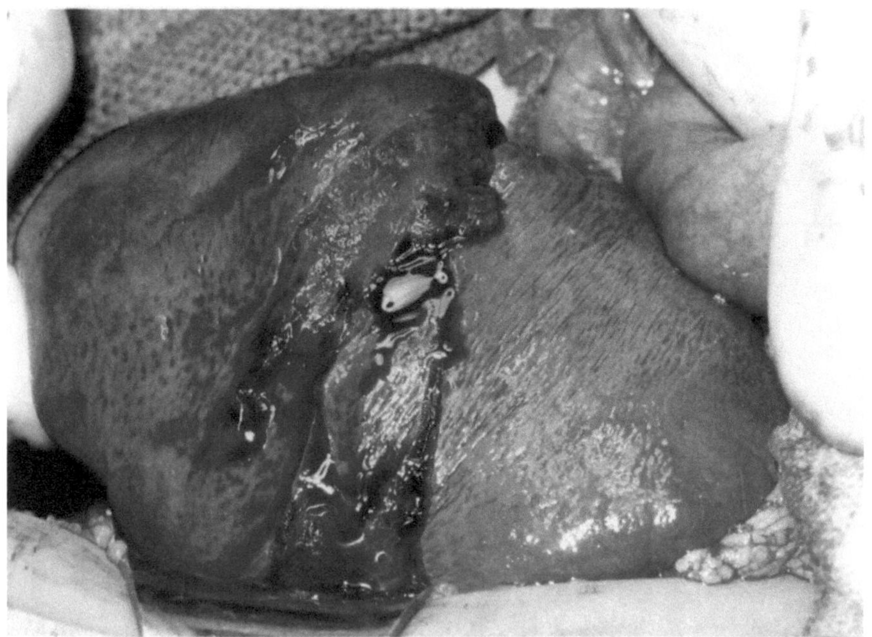

Fig. 3. Traumatic laceration of spleen with avulsion of superior pole vessels. Devascularized upper half (*left*) was resected

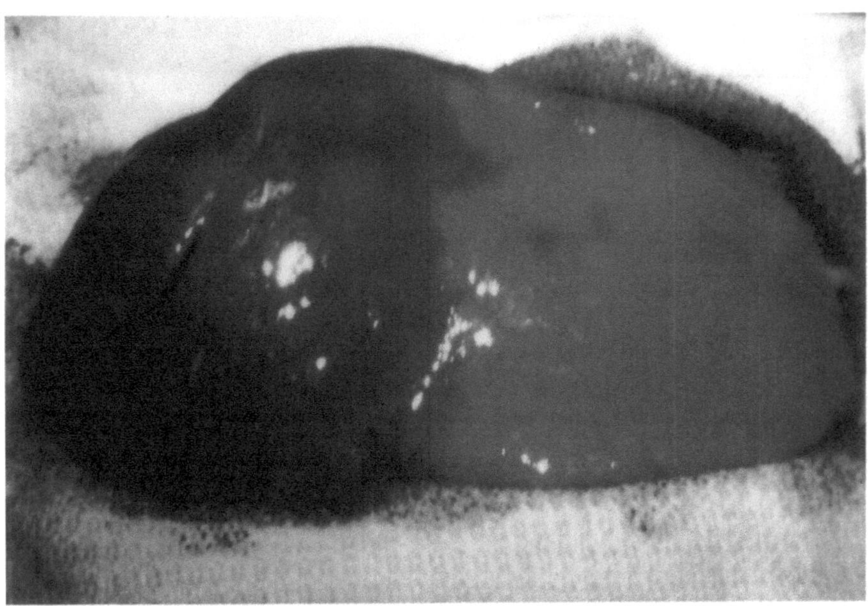

Fig. 4. Clear line of demarcation after ligation of segmental vessels, indicating levels of transection for partial splenectomy

Step III: Transection

Once the line of demarcation is clear (Fig. 4) and the site of transection has been decided upon, the vessel-loop is tightened and fixed in the taut position. Transection of the spleen should commence at least 1 cm on the *cyanotic* side of the line of demarcation.

There are several methods of transection which are applicable.

Method I

The splenic capsule is incised sharply and the line of transection slowly deepened into the parenchyma. Beyond the capsule, transection is best accomplished by finger or with a scalpel handle, clamping or clipping all vessels as they are encountered (Fig. 5). Once the spleen has been completely transected the taut vessel-loop is released, allowing ready identification of all residual bleeding vessels. Arterial bleeders may be grasped with fine forceps and clipped with mini-clips. Transected venules retract toward the parenchymal surface and are best controlled by fine figure-of-8 sutures (Fig. 6). Small residual bleeders may be controlled by electrocautery or argon beam coagulation. Application of a topical hemostatic agent such as surgicel, avitene, or other collagen hemostatic agents is optional. If the splenic parenchyma is absolutely dry, no topical hemostatic agent is necessary.

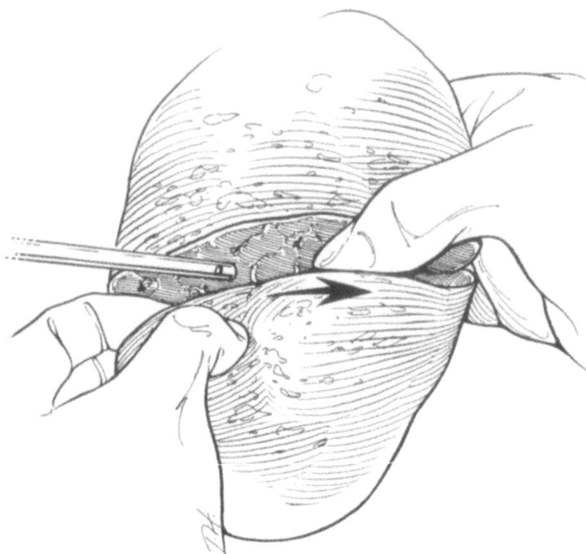

Fig. 5. Incision of spleen at line of demarcation and extension of dissection into splenic parenchyma

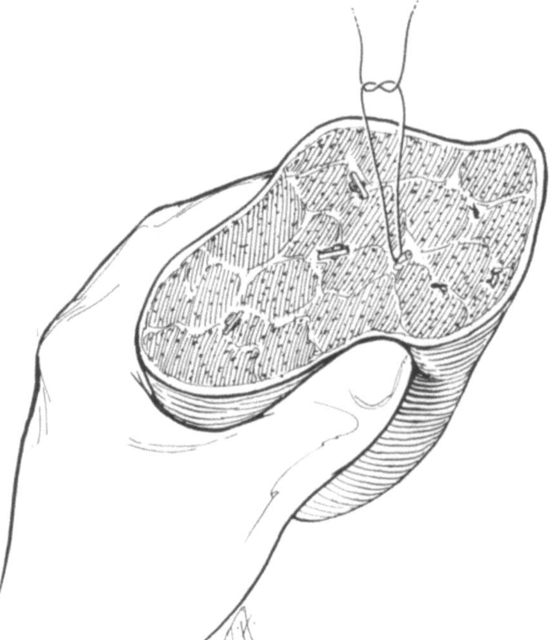

Fig. 6. Securing hemostasis of intraparenchymal vessels or raw splenic surface with hemoclips and fine silk sutures

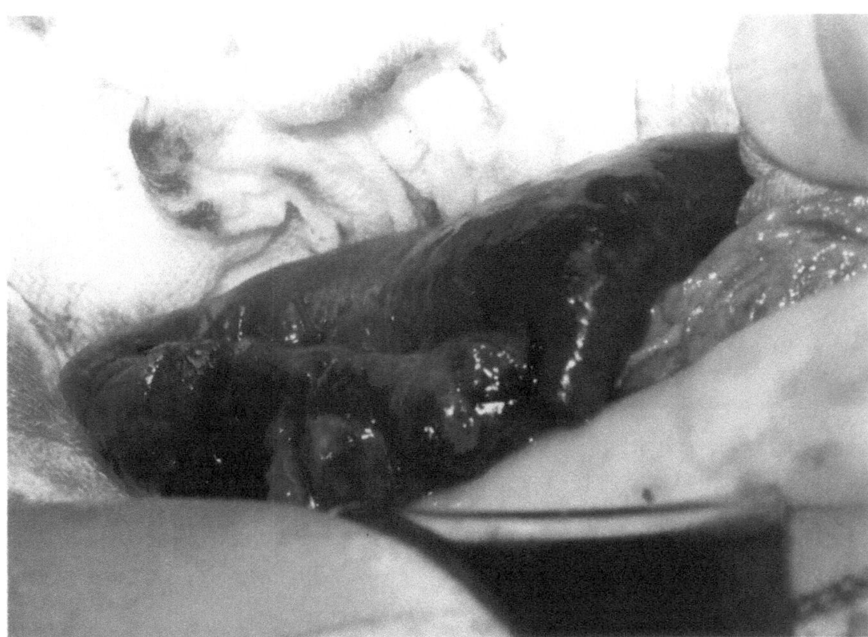

Fig. 7. Row of horizontal mattress sutures of 2-0 chromic catgut placed 1.5 cm from edges of divided parenchyma. Bolsters beneath sutures are preferred by some sutures, though not absolutely necessary

Method II: Horizontal Mattress Suture

Hemostasis on the raw surface of the splenic remnant can also be achieved by a row of mattress sutures placed parallel to the resected edge (Fig. 7). These sutures, of 2-0 chromic catgut, are placed at least 1 cm from the edge of the divided parenchyma, encompassing 1.5 cm of tissue with each suture for the entire width of the remnant. These mattress sutures may be interlocking, or be placed in close enough proximity to one another to preclude bleeding from intervening tissue.

The use of pledgets of gelfoam, surgicel or teflon on the knotted side to allow tightening of the suture without tearing of the delicate capsule or cutting through the parenchyma has been recommended for routine use with mattress suture by some surgeons. This is a matter of individual preference. If the parenchyma is gradually and carefully tightened, pledgets or bolsters should not be necessary. If the parenchyma is fragile and capsular breaches occur when the suture is tightened, pledgets or bolsters below the knots are indicated.

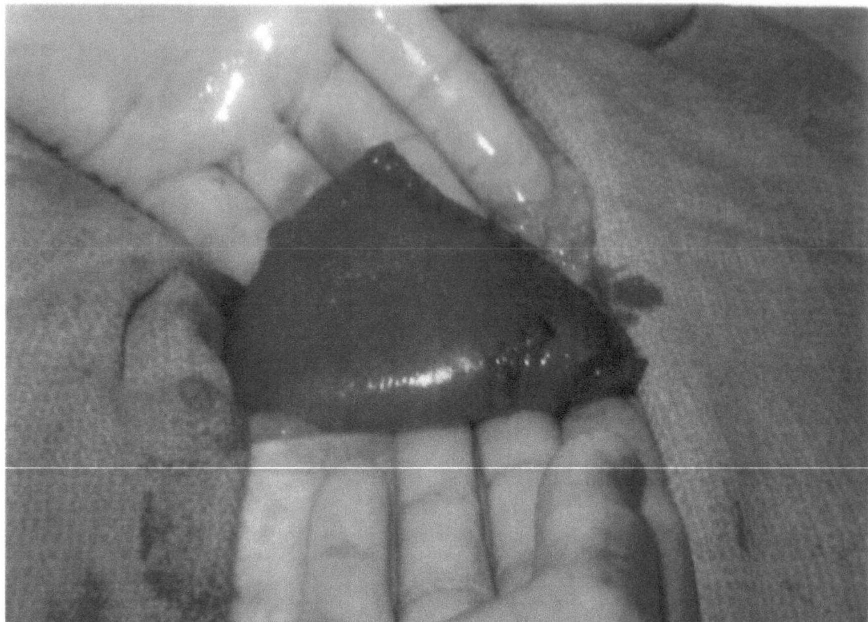

Fig. 8. Alternative closure of transected spleen with continuous locking suture of 2-0 chromic catgut

Method III: Continuous Suture

In an occasional splenic remnant, especially in cases of trauma, the configuration of the spleen at the site of transection is such that the edge may be approximated as with a splenorrhaphy. A 2-0 continuous, interlocking suture of 2-0 chromic catgut can achieve satisfactory hemostasis. This method can only be used when the width of the transected parenchyma is more than 1.5 cm (Fig. 8). The running suture should commence and continue in a line at least 1.0 cm from the transected edge. Care must be taken not to exert undue tension on the continuous suture during placement lest it tear through the capsule and parenchyma. This technique has been used successfully on several occasions by the author.

Method IV: Surgical Stapling

Stapling techniques for partial splenectomy have been described by Breil et al. [42], Bergholt et al. [43] and Üranus et al. [44], the latter author describing its use in 15 partial resections. Although at first glance the stapling technique seems applicable to spleens which are "thin" enough to accept the stapler, Üranus has adopted a technique of compressing the splenic parenchyma at the proposed transection site between thumb and forefinger until it becomes "thin" enough to accept the stapler. The TA-55 stapler was used in all but one of the stapled resections and the TA-90 in the remaining case. There were no postoperative complications. Üranus has employed this technique for traumatic rupture, splenic cysts, diagnostic resection, and iatrogenic injury. The method, when applicable, is rapid and hemostatically effective.

Method V: Argon Beam

Experimental hemisplenectomy in rabbits using the argon beam coagulator for effective hemostasis on the transected surface was reported by Stylianos et al. and Dunhametas in 1991 [45, 46]. This method has since been used clinically by Hayes-Jordan and Organ (1996, personal communication) in partial splenectomies for trauma. Further experience with this technique will be necessary before its adoption in standard surgical practice. This does not apply to the use of the argon beam coagulator as an adjunctive device for surface hemostasis, in combination with the hemostatic techniques described above. Its effective use for surface hemostasis, especially for coagulation of smaller vessels, has been well demonstrated.

A caveat must be kept in mind for any method which is dependent upon induced tissue coagulation, be it electrocoagulation, heat-induced coagulation, or argon beam coagulation. The coagulum has the potential of separating from normal splenic parenchyma, sometimes within 1 week of the postoperative period. In the author's opinion, no system of surface hemostasis is as yet known to be as safe for secure control of larger vessels as the methods employing sutures or staples as described above.

Other Methods, Other Adjunctive Hemostatic Agents

The use of the ultrasonic surgical aspirator (Cavitron, Valley Lab, Boulder, CO) has also been described for splenic transection [47], its principal use having previously been in major hepatic resections. Advantages of such a technique in partial splenectomy are said to include more accurate identification and control of individual vessels during division of the parenchyma and hence less operative blood loss. In the hands of individuals accustomed to its use, it may afford some advantage over finger or scalpel-handle transection.

There is a vast array of topical hemostatic agents available to the surgeon for adjunctive use on oozing surfaces. These include well known agents such as surgicel, microfibrillar collagen (Avitene), topical thrombin and a host of collagen products. Some surgeons prefer to wrap the surgical remnant in dexon mesh for further compression of the parenchyma and insurance against postoperative hemorrhage. If satisfactory hemostasis has been achieved, as previously described, the dexon mesh wrap or envelope is unnecessary. It does provide one advantage which may be of use in selected cases, namely, the ability to anchor the remnant to the diaphragm or retroperitoneum and thus preclude the possibility of torsion. It may be of use, therefore, in instances where the remnant and its pedicle appear exceptionally prone to torsion.

Use of autologous splenic capsule to cover the raw splenic surface has been described by Brown and Mukherjee [48]. The autologous capsule is obtained from the amputated splenic tissue. It is doubtful that this has any distinct advantage over omentum, which quickly becomes adherent to the surface of the reposited splenic remnant.

Drains

Unless there is a compelling reason for the use of a drain for reasons other than the splenic procedure, there is no need to drain the left upper quadrant following partial splenectomy. Drains are notoriously deceptive in signaling postoperative hemorrhage and their presence may encourage rather than prevent infection. Only when the possibility of pancreatic injury exists, either prior to or during the splenic operation, should a drain be employed for diagnostic and therapeutic purposes.

Should a drain be necessary, the drainage should be collected in a sterile collecting bag affixed to the skin. In cases of suspected or known pancreatic injury, the drainage fluid should be studied for amylase content.

Laparoscopic Partial Splenectomy

Laparoscopic partial splenectomy has been described in experimental animals by Üranus et al. [49] and clinically by Poulin et al. [50]. The technique and instrumentation are of course very different than those of the open technique. There is no reason to suppose that partial splenectomy will not be among the operations successfully performed with endoscopic techniques. Laparoscopic splenectomy is discussed in the chapter by Phillips (this volume).

Follow-up Studies

In the immediate postoperative period, the operation of partial splenectomy alone is insufficient reason for admission to an intensive care unit. Routine floor care, with daily observation of vital signs, symptoms and hemograms are sufficient. In the absence of other reasons for prolonging hospitalization, discharge should be possible by the fifth day. Unless there is a suspicion of nonviability of the remnant, imaging studies during this period are not needed.

Following discharge, function of the splenic remnant should be discernible on blood smears, with special attention to red cell morphology. With a functioning remnant of sufficient size there should be no nucleated or pitted red blood cells nor Howell-Jolly bodies. Elevation of the platelet count, which occurs after splenic trauma and splenic surgery, whether or not the spleen is removed, returns to normal within weeks. There is no need to treat an elevated platelet count, even if the platelet count has risen as high as $10^6/mm^3$ or higher.

If there is a question of viability or diminished function, imaging studies with technetium-99 are helpful in assessing splenic function. Ultrasound and computed tomography are useful only in elucidating complications, such as fluid or abscess. They cannot assess function. Serial imaging studies to determine spleen size and function are of academic interest. They have no specific utility unless the remnant is affected by the underlying disease, such as Gaucher's disease.

Postoperative Physical Activity

There is no absolutely reliable indicator of splenic healing which guarantees safety against rupture from any type of mechanical stress or trauma. Empirically, it seems appropriate to advise the patient to refrain from contact sports, or any activity which might reasonably harm the splenic remnant, for a period of 3 months. The latter types of activities might be skiing, jumping, jogging, and similar pastimes. In industrial workers, extraordinarily heavy lifting and straining should be similarly interdicted. After 3 months, no further restrictions need be imposed.

Conclusion

Partial splenectomy is a procedure which has proven safe, feasible and indicated for the preservation of splenic function in carefully selected clinical situations. It has proven its worth in trauma and splenic cysts and is especially applicable in children and younger age groups. In older individuals it must be judiciously employed, with a careful weighing of risks and benefits. Although the major experience with this operation to date has been by laparotomy, there is little question that it will eventually be adapted to laparoscopic techniques. The experience in the last half of this century has taught us that the spleen is no longer surgically inviolable nor is it easily expendable. The salvage of a functional remnant of spleen, as described in this chapter, has been a major contribution in splenic surgery.

References

1. Clark DT (1673–4) De lienis resectione in cane (et homine) vivo. (Observatio 164–165) Misc Curiosa Acad Nat Curios S1 (4–5):198–199
2. Ferguson J (1732–44) An account of the extirpation of a part of the spleen of a man. Philos Trans R Soc Lond 9:149
3. O'Brien E (1816) Case of removal of the human spleen, without injury or derangement of the animal economy. Med Chir J Rev Lond 1:8–9
4. Markham HC (1874) Excision of a portion of the spleen-recovery. Med Rec 97:482–483
5. Mayo WJ (1910) Principles underlying surgery of the spleen. JAMA 54:14–18
6. Von Esmarch F, Kowalzig E (1901) Surgical technic. In: Sena N (ed) A textbook on operative surgery. MacMillan, New York, p 739
7. Da Costa JC (1919) Modern surgery, 8th edn. Saunders, Philadelphia, p 1203
8. Campos Christo M (1962) Segmental resections of the spleen: report on the first eight cases operated on. O Hosp 62:575–590
9. Morgenstern L, Kahn FH, Weinstein IM (1966) Subtotal splenectomy in myelofibrosis. Surgery 60(2):336–339
10. Morgenstern L, Shapiro SJ (1979) Techniques of splenic conservation. Arch Surg 114:449–454
11. Oakes DD, Crane Charters A (1981) Changing concepts in the management of splenic trauma. Surg Gynecol Obstet 153:181–185
12. Feliciano DV, Spjut-Patrinely V, Burch JM, Mattox KL, Bitondo CG, Cruse-Martocci P, Jordan GL (1990) Splenorrhaphy: the alternative. Ann Surg 211(5):569–580
13. Morgenstern L (1990) Technique of partial splenectomy. Probl Gen Surg 7(1):103–12
14. Lucas CE (1991) Splenic trauma: choice of management. Ann Surg 213(2):98–112
15. Witte CL, Esser MJ, Rappaport WD (1992) Updating the management of salvageable splenic injury. Ann Surg 215(3):261–265
16. Morgenstern L, Shapiro SJ (1980) Partial splenectomy for nonparasitic splenic cysts. Am J Surg 139:278–281
17. Touloukian RJ, Seashore JH (1987) Partial splenic decapsulation: a simplified operation for splenic pseudocyst. J Pediatr Surg 22(2):135–137
18. Nangalia R, Al-Salem AH (1993) Splenic salvage in hydatid disease. Ann Saudi Med 13(1):88–90
19. Hoekstra HJ, Kamps WA (1989) Indications for staging laparotomy and partial splenectomy (review). Cancer Treat Res 41:121–127
20. Tubbs RR, Thomas F, Norris D, Firor HV (1987) Is hemisplenectomy a satisfactory option to total splenectomy in abdominal staging of Hodgkin's disease? J Pediatr Surg 22(8):727–729
21. Dearth JC, Gilchrist GS, Telander RL, O'Connell MJ, Weiland LH (1978) Partial splenectomy for staging Hodgkin's disease: risk of false-negative results. N Engl J Med 299(7):345–346
22. Rubin M, Yampolski I, Lambrozo R, Zaizov R, Dintsman M (1986) Partial splenectomy in Gaucher's disease. J Pediatr Surg 21(2):125–128
23. Bar-Maor JA (1993) Partial splenectomy in Gaucher's disease: follow-up report. J Pediatr Surg 28(5):686–688
24. Morgenstern L, Phillips EH, Fermelia D, Weinstein IM (1986) Near-total splenectomy for massive splenomegaly due to Gaucher disease: a new approach. Mt Sinai J Med 53:501–505
25. Fleshner PR, Aufses AH Jr, Grabowski GA, Elias R (1991) A 27-year experience with splenectomy for Gaucher's disease. Am J Surg 161:69–75
26. Guzzetta PC, Ruley EJ, Merrick HFW, Verderese C, Barton N (1990) Elective subtotal splenectomy: indications and results in 33 patients. Ann Surg 211(1):34–42
27. Cohen IJ, Katz K, Freud E, Zer M, Zaizov R (1992) Long-term follow-up of partial splenectomy in Gaucher's disease. Am J Surg 164(4):345–347

28. Morgenstern L, Verham R, Weinstein I, Phillips EH (1993) Subtotal splenectomy for Gaucher's disease: a follow-up study (review). Am Surg 59(12):860–865
29. NIH Technology Assessment Panel on Gaucher's Disease (1996) Gaucher disease: current issues in diagnosis and treatment. JAMA 275(7):548–553
30. Kehila M, Khelif A, Kharrat H, Ennabli S, Abderrahim T (1994) La splenectomie partielle au cours des thalassemies majeures. A propos de 19 cas. J Chir (Paris) 131(2):99–103
31. de Montalembert M, Girot R, Revillon Y, Jan D, Adjrad L, Ardjoun FZ, Belhani M, Najean Y (1990) Partial splenectomy in homozygous beta thalassaemia. Arch Dis Child 65(3):304–307
32. Stanley P, Shen TC (1995) Partial embolization of the spleen in patients with thalassemia. J Vasc Interv Radiol 6(1):137–142
33. Specht U, Mau H, Winter H, Jahn S, Volk H, Cario WR (1988) Partial splenectomy for treatment of chronic idiopathic thrombocytopenia in childhood. Folia Haematol (Internationales Magazin für Klinische und Morphologische Blutforschung) 115(4):509–514
34. Jahn S, Bauer B, Schwab J, Kirchmair F, Neuhaus K, Kiessig ST, Volk HD, Mau H, von Baehr R, Specht U (1993) Immune restoration in children after partial splenectomy. Immunobiology 188(4–5):370–378
35. Tchernia G, Gauthier F, Mielot F, Dommergues JP, Yvart J, Chasis JA, Mohandas N (1993) Initial assessment of the beneficial effect of partial splenectomy in hereditary spherocytosis. Blood 81(8):2014–2020
36. Nouri A, de Montalembert M, Revillon Y, Girot R (1991) Partial splenectomy in sickle cell syndromes. Arch Dis Child 66(9):1070–1072
37. Bhattacharyya N, Ablin DS, Kosloske AM (1989) Stapled partial splenectomy for splenic abscess in a child. J Pediatr Surg 24(3):316–317
38. Louis D, Chazalette JP (1993) Cystic fibrosis and portal hypertension interest of partial splenectomy. Eur J Pediatr Surg 3(1):22–24
39. Petroianu A (1993) Subtotal splenectomy and portal variceal disconnection in the treatment of portal hypertension. Can J Surg 36(3):251–254
40. Havlik RJ, Touloukian RJ, Markowitz RI, Buckley P (1990) Partial splenectomy for symptomatic splenic harmatoma (review). J Pediatr Surg 25(12):1273–1275
41. Kamel R, Dunn MA (1982) Segmental splenectomy in schistosomiasis. Br J Surg 69:311
42. Breil Ph, Bahnini MA, Fékété F (1986) Partial splenectomy using the TAr stapler. Surg Gynecol Obstet 163:575–576
43. Bergholt T, Westphall IT, Standberg C, Bruun E (1992) Partial spleen resection using a stapler. (In Danish. Original title: Partiel miltresektion ved hjaelp af haeftemaskine). Ugeskr Laeger 154(14):938–939
44. Üranus S, Kronberger L, Kraft-Kine J (1994) Partial splenic resection using the TA-stapler (review). Am J Surg 168(1):49–53
45. Stylianos S, Hoffman MA, Jacir NN, Harris BH (1991) Sutureless hemisplenectomy. J Pediatr Surg 26(1):87–89
46. Dunham CM, Cornwell EE III, Militello P (1991) The role of the Argon Beam Coagulator in splenic salvage. Surg Gynecol Obstet 173:179–182
47. Moorman DW, Evans DM, Wright DJ (1988) Segmental splenectomy using the ultrasonic aspirator. Am J Surg 155:266–267
48. Brown DA, Mukherjee D (1988) Partial splenectomy with autologous capsule graft. Surg Gynecol Obstet 166:555–556
49. Üranus S, Pfeifer J, Schauer C, Kronberger L, Rabl H, Ranftl G, Hauser H, Bahadori K (1995) Laparoscopic partial splenic resection. Surg Laparosc Endosc 5(2):133–136
50. Poulin EC, Thibault C, DesCôteaux JG, Côté G (1995) Partial laparoscopic splenectomy for trauma: technique and case report. Surg Laparosc Endosc 5(4):306–310

Subject Index

Abscess splenic   73–75, 85, 144–151, 212
- bacterial   146–147
- - table   147
- figures   74–75, 149
- fungal   147, 156
- incidence   144
- partial splenectomy for   266
- presentation   145–146
- table   145
- treatment   149–151
Abscess, subphrenic   206–207, 229, 235–236
Accessory spleens   22–23, 26, 62, 215
- figures   19, 63, 216
Acquired immunodeficiency syndrome
    (AIDS)   212, 247
Agenesis of spleen   54
Alglucerase, for Gaucher's disease   166
Alpha-interferon   119
Amebic infection   147–148
Amyloidosis   82, 170–171
Anaerobes   146
Anemias, congenital   133
Angiitis, leukoclastic   47
Angiography   61, 186–187
- splenic embolization procedures   85,
    166, 188, 189, 203–205, 211, 213
- figure   204
Angiosarcoma   78
Anomalies of spleen   21–24, see specific
    anomalies
Antibiotics, after trauma   253
Antigen   54
Arteriography see angiography
Arteriovenous fistula, splenic   176, 188–
    189
Aspirin   137
Asplenia   21, 53, 55, 62
Autoimmune hemolytic anemia   10, 22, 26,
    41, 133–134
Autoimmune neutropenia   41
Autotransplantation, splenic   58, 252–253
Avitene   275

Bacillary angiomatosis   96
Banti's disease   11
Bessel-Hagen   10
Beta-glucosidase   163
Billroth, Theodor   9
Biopsy percutaneous   84–85, 93, 107–108
Bone marrow transplantation   119–120, 167
Bryant, Thomas   7
Bullock, FD   233

Calcification, splenic   65, 74
- figure   66
Campos Christo, Marcelo   12, 263
- figure   12
Candida   147
Capsule of spleen   15, 54
Castleman's disease   41
Ceroid histiocytosis   45
Clark, Timothy   5
Complications see splenectomy,
    complications
Computed tomography   61–85, 106, 148,
    182, 186, 250–252, 275
- grading systems   69, 71, 251–252
- percutaneous abscess drainage   151
Consumptive coagulopathy see
    disseminated intravascular coagulation
Cordal macrophages, disorders of   43
Cords of Billroth   43, 54
Coumarin (warfarin)   137
"Criminal fold"   20
Crosby, William   11
Cruger, Daniel   5
Cyclophosphamide   117
Cystic hygroma   94
Cysts of spleen   8, 23–24, 48, 71–73, 99–
    102, 123
- figure   72
- nonparasitic   99–101
- - figure   100, 101
- parasitic   65, 71, 102
- partial splenectomy for   13, 264–265

Dextran 206
Dipyridamole 137, 206
Disseminated intravascular coagulation 93–94
Dorsch 6
Drains, use following splenectomy 203, 207, 276

Echinococcus granulosus 102, 147
Embolization, as cause of splenic rupture 30
Embryology of spleen 21
Endoscopy, upper gastrointestinal 180, 182
Entameba histolytica 147–148
Epstein-Barr virus 151
Essential thrombocythemia 41, 43, 45
– figure 44

Felty's syndrome 138
Ferguson, John 6
– figure 6
Fibroma 78
Fine-needle aspiration see biopsy
Flow cytometry 26
Fludarabine 117
Frozen sections 26
Functions of spleen 27–28, 54–55
– deficiency of 55–58
– – immunologic 56
– – infectious 56–57
– – table 57
– filtration 27, 28, 234
– hematopoietic 27, 54
– immunologic 27, 28
– reservoir 27
– table 28

Galen 3, 25, 53
Gastrointestinal bleeding
– with splenic arteriovenous fistula 188
– with splenic artery aneurysm 185
– with splenic vein thrombosis 178–183
Gaucher's Disease 11, 138–139, 163–167
– diagnosis 164
– enzyme replacement therapy for 165–167
– figure 163
– partial splenectomy for 13, 166, 265
Germinal centers 33–35, 54
Glucocerebrosidase 163
Granulomas of spleen 37–38
– table 38
Hamartoma 23, 48, 97–99, 123
– figure 49, 98
– partial splenectomy for 266
Heinz bodies 54

Hemangioendothelioma 9, 48
Hemangioma 48, 78, 92, 122
– figure 92
Hemangiopericytoma 96
Hemangiosarcoma 48, 123
– figure 49
Hematoma
– figure 85
– intrasplenic 69
– perisplenic 70, 71
– subcapsular 70
Hematopoiesis, extramedullary 84
Hemochromatosis 84
Hemoglobinopathies 66
Hemolytic anemia see autoimmune hemolytic anemia
Hemophilus influenzae 53, 234, 253, 267
Hemostasis, topical 12
Hemosuccus pancreaticus 186
Heparin 137, 206
Hereditary elliptocytosis 41, 131
Hereditary spherocytosis 10, 41, 42, 131–132
– figure 43
Hippocrates 53, 143
Hodgkin's disease 39–40, 112–114, 137
– partial splenectomy for 13, 265
– staging laparotomy for 39, 212–213, 222
Howell-Jolly bodies 28, 54, 208
Hypersplenism 28, 41, 43, 94, 124, 136, 198–199
– table 31
Hyperviscosity syndrome 117
Hyposplenia 22, 55
Hyposplenism 28
– table 28

Immunoglobulins 55, 234
Infarction of spleen 30, 47, 75–77, 212
– figure 76–78
Infectious mononucleosis 35
– figure 36
– spontaneous rupture and 37
Infiltrative disorders 170–171
Intestinal obstruction 208
Irradiation, splenic 115, 120, 122
Idiopathic thrombocytopenic purpura (ITP) 11, 22, 26, 37, 41, 134–135
ITP
– AIDS and 134
– laparoscopic splenectomy for 13, 212, 222, 224–226
– – tables 224–225
– platelets and 134
– surgery for 134, 198
Ivemark syndrome 53, 55

Kasabach-Merritt syndrome   93
Kaznelson, Paul   11, 131
Kuchler   7

Laparoscopic splenectomy *see* splenectomy,
   laparoscopic
Leukemia
- chronic lymphocytic   115
- chronic myelogenous   45, 46, 118
- - figure   119
- hairy cell   41, 45, 116-117, 137
- - figure   46, 47, 117
Ligaments of spleen   18-21, 175, 177, 201-
   203, 219
- figure   201-202
- phrenico-colic   21
- spleno-omental   20
- splenocolic   19, 219
- splenocolic figure   221
- splenogastric   20
- splenopancreatic   21
- splenophrenic   20
- splenorenal   20, 219
- splenorenal figures   20, 220-221
Littoral cell angioma   93
Liver-spleen scan *see* radionuclide
   scintigraphy
Lobulations, splenic
- figure   63
Lymphangioma   78, 93-95, 123
- figure   94
Lymphatics of spleen   21
Lymphocytes, T and B   54-55
Lymphoma   11, 31, 38-39, 79-80, 212
- figures   32, 65, 80, 81, 82
- Hodgkin's *see* Hodgkin's Disease
- immunoblastic   39
- marginal zone cell type   38-39, 111-112
- non-Hodgkin's   108-110
- - figure   109, 110
- primary splenic (PSL)   110-111
Lymphoproliferative disorders   30, 40-41,
   108-117
Lysosomes   161

MAd-CAM-1   54
Magnetic resonance imaging   77, 80, 182
Matthias, Nicolaus   5
Meningococcus *see* Neisseria meningiditis
Metastases to spleen   79, 124
- figure   79
Micheli   10, 131
Morgagni   5
Morgenstern, Leon   12, 20, 263
Morris, DH   234
Moynihan   11

Mycobacterial infection   11, 154
Myelofibrosis   120-122
- figure   121
Myeloid metaplasia, agnogenic   45, 46
- figure   33, 48
Myeloproliferative disorders   26, 33, 45-46,
   118-122, 136-137

Neisseria meningiditis   234, 253, 267
Neutropenia, autoimmune   41
Niemann-Pick diseases   167-169
- figure   168

O'Brien, E.   8
- figure   10
Opsonins   234
Overwhelming post-splenectomy infection
   (OPSI)   12, 53, 207, 230, 234-235
- organisms   53, 234

Pancreas   18, 21, 202
- injury during splenectomy   208, 228
- pancreatic fistula   18
- pancreatic pseudocyst   18, 72
- - figure   73
- pancreatitis   18, 72
- splenic artery aneurysm and   186
- splenic vein thrombosis and   178-179,
   182
Paracelsus   4
Parenchyma of spleen   17
- radiologic appearance of   61
Partial splenectomy   8, 12, 16, 57, 98, 99,
   100, 102, 241, 263-277
- drains, use following   276
- figures   269-274
- follow-up studies   276
- indications   264-266
- techniques   266-276
- - open   268
- - laparoscopic   276
- trauma and   264
Pèan, Jules   8
- figure   9
Peliosis   48, 95
Penicillin prophylaxis   58
Phase contrast microscopy   28
Phillips, Edward   13
Plasma cells   55
Plasmodium   147
Platelets therapy with   139, 199
Pliny   3
Pneumococcus *see* Streptococcus
   pneumoniae and Vaccinations
Pneumocystis carinii   66, 154
Polyarteritis nodosa   47

Polycythemia vera 45
Polysplenia 22, 62
- figure 19, 63
Porphyria erythropoietica 139
Portal hypertension 81, 94, 121, 136–137,
    161, 175–183, 183, 184–185, 188
- figure 83
- sinistral (left-sided) 177
- types 176
Pregnancy splenic artery aneurysm
    and 184–187
Prolapse of spleen 5, 8
Protozoal infection 147
Pseudotumor inflammatory 48, 96–97
Pseudotumor mycobacterial spindle
    cell 97
Pulp see splenic pulp

Quittenbaum, Carl 6
- figure 7

Radionuclide scintigraphy 61, 106, 107,
    148, 277
Red blood cell membrane 28
Red pulp see Splenic pulp
Reed-Sternberg cells 112
Reigneur, O. 8
Repair of spleen 11, 12, 236–241, see also
    partial splenectomy
- contraindications 238
- table 237–238
- techniques 239–241
- - argon beam 275
- - figures 242–243
- - mesh 240–241
- - stapling 274–275
- - suture 240, 273–274
Rupture of spleen 30–33, 37, 39, 94, 124,
    151–152
- delayed 68, 249
- figures 250–251

Sarcoidosis 138
Schistosomiasis 147
- partial splenectomy for 13, 266
Septicemia 30
Sequestration, splenic 84
Shape of spleen 15
Short gastric vessels (veins and ar-
    teries) 17, 219
Sickle cell disease 47, 53, 66, 132–133
- partial splenectomy for 266
Situs inversus 22
- with polysplenia, figure 19
Size of spleen 15
Spherocytes 42

Sphingomyelinase deficiency 168
Splenectomy, blood picture after, table 30
Splenectomy complications of 205–208
- arteriovenous fistula 188
- bleeding 139, 205
- DIC 57
- infection 206–207, 234
- intestinal 208
- respiratory 206
- splenosis 207–208
- subphrenic abscess 206–207, 234
- thrombosis 206
- wound 207, 234
Splenectomy for hypersplenism 29, 198–208
- table 205
Splenectomy incisions for 199–200
- figure 200
Splenectomy, laparoscopic 13, 23, 100,
    114, 211–231
- complications 226–230
- - bowel injury 227
- - fever 230
- - hemorrhage 227–228
- - infection 230
- - intestinal obstruction 229
- - operative 226–228
- - organ injury 228
- - of pneumoperitoneum
- - postoperative 229–230
- - respiratory 229
- - splenosis 230
- - subphrenic abscess 229
- - vascular injury 227
- - wound 229
- - thromboembolism 230
- indications 212
- positioning 211, 213–214
- - figure 214–215
- postoperative care 223–224
- results 224–226
- trocar placement 214–215
- - figure 216
Splenic abscess see abscess, splenic
Splenic artery 16, 219, 221
- aneurysm 176, 183–188
- - liver transplantation and 183, 187–
    188
- - rupture of 185
- branches 16–17
- figure 16, 18
- ligation 200, 215, 217, 270
Splenic index 61, 108, 114
Splenic pulp 54, 109
- tables 34, 36
- red 18, 28, 30
- - disorders of 41

– – table   42
– white   18, 28, 30, 33
– – atrophy of   34
– – diseases of   33–35, 38
– – figure   34
Splenic vein   17, 18
– thrombosis   137, 176–183
– – algorithm   184
– – figure   181
Splenogonadal fusion   22
Splenomegaly   8, 11, 17, 23, 65, 74, 80, 81,
    82, 94, 105–107, 118, 121, 136, 138, 152,
    161, 164, 170, 176, 178, 188
– open splenectomy for   197–208
Splenoportography   61, 179–180
– figure   180
Splenorenal shunt   17
Splenorrhaphy see repair of spleen
Splenosis   26, 58, 207–208, 230, 252
Staging laparotomy   39, 113, 138, 212–213,
    232
Stomach, injury during splenectomy   208,
    228
Storage disorders   161–170
– table   162
Streptococcus pneumoniae   53, 234, 253, 267
Surfaces of spleen   15
Sutton, J. Bland   10
Systemic mast cell disease   139

Tangier disease   169–170
Thalassemia   132
Thalassemia partial splenectomy for   266
Thorotrastosis   83
Thrombocytopenia   121
Thrombocytosis   137
Thrombotic thrombocytopenic purpura
    (TTP)   47, 135–136, 198
Torsion, splenic   64
Trauma   5, 8, 11, 12, 13, 22, 184–185, 188,
    233–254, see also partial splenectomy,
    repair of spleen, rupture of spleen
– blood transfusion and   247–248
– imaging of   67–71, 250–252
– – figure   68, 250

– nonoperative management of   11, 13,
    18, 241–252
– – bleeding risks   247–248
– – missed injuries   248–249
– – patient selection   245–247
– – tables   244, 246
– postsplenectomy management
    252–253
– quality-adjusted life expectancy
    (QALE)   248
– splenic injury grading   238–239, 251–
    252
– – table   239
Tuberculosis   11
Tuftsin   55
Tumors of spleen   30
Two-chlorodeoxyadenosine (2-CDA)   116,
    117

Ultrasonography   61, 71, 74, 99, 106, 148,
    275
– duplex doppler   182, 186

Vaccinations   57, 139, 198, 213, 253, 267
Varices esophageal   179
– gastric   178
Vasculitis   30, 47
Vesalius   4
Vessels of spleen   12, 175, 201 (see also
    specific vessels)
– figures   203, 218, 269
Viard   4
Viral infections   151–152

Waldenstrom's macroglobulinemia   117
Wandering spleen   8, 11, 23, 63, 131
Weight of spleen   15, 26, 54
Wells, Thomas Spencer   7, 8, 131
– figure   8
White pulp see splenic pulp
Wilson   6

Zacarello, Adriano   4, 197
– figure   5
Zambeccari   5

Springer
and the
environment

At Springer we firmly believe that an international science publisher has a special obligation to the environment, and our corporate policies consistently reflect this conviction.

We also expect our business partners – paper mills, printers, packaging manufacturers, etc. – to commit themselves to using materials and production processes that do not harm the environment. The paper in this book is made from low- or no-chlorine pulp and is acid free, in conformance with international standards for paper permanency.

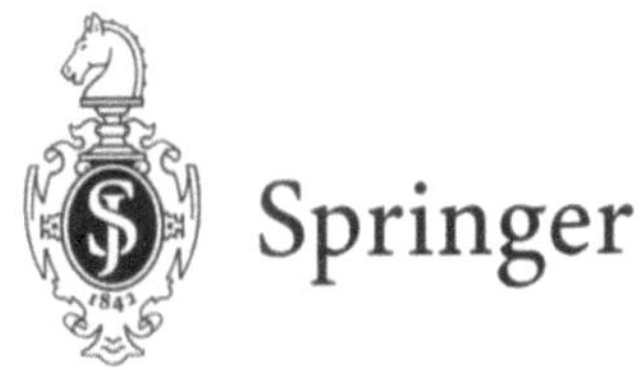

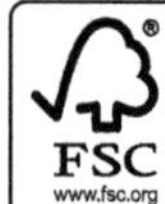